To Audrey,
God bless + keep you in
health + wellness!
Dr. Gayle + Porter

"African American women who are in their prime years have long needed a complete guide of their own on health and wellness. Finally, we can prevent early deaths and major illnesses by managing stress levels and getting rid of unwanted attitudes. Truly, *Prime Time* will empower a woman's life."

—**Audrey B. Chapman**
**Author of *The 7 Attitude Adjustments for Finding a Loving Man***

"Authoritative and informative, *Prime Time* is a valuable guide to midlife health and wellness for African American women. Women of all races would benefit from its recommendations and wisdom. Unique questionnaires in every chapter allow readers to personalize information. Each woman can evaluate her own health risks and behaviors and take important steps to maintain the best possible health. The authors are experts in their fields and in presenting medical and psychological information in an easy-to-read and enjoyable style. *Prime Time* is an ideal gift for relatives and friends who are approaching or established in midlife."

—**Roselyn Payne Epps, M.D., M.P.H., M.A.**
**Past President, American Medical Women's Association**
**Coeditor, *Women's Complete Healthbook***

"The late summer and early fall of life is a wonderful season to work before the rest of winter. It is a time to gather the harvest, it is quality time, our time—Prime Time— " . . . for such a time as this" (Esther 4:14).

"Marilyn and Gayle, my 'Esthers,' have written a book for me, a book that speaks to my intellect, my sensitivity, and my spirituality. As a pediatrician, I know the importance of anticipatory guidance and my Prime Time Sisters not only support me through this new passage of my life, they encourage and celebrate me. The legacy of the 'slave health deficit' must be broken if we are to address the disparities plaguing the African American community. I want to exhibit for my daughter the self-love and self-care that is necessary for us to enjoy the blessings God has intended for us. So often the scientific breakthroughs have little or no application in our lives. These Esthers nurture the nurturer, providing strategies for how we, as middle-aged Black women, can break the generational curses that have cut short the lives of our loved ones.

"Thank you, Gayle and Marilyn. I owe you big time."

—**Lucille C. Norville Perez, M.D.**
**President Elect, National Medical Association**

"Health has been a big issue in our African American community for some time. I am glad this book has been written to extend women's lives in the country and address the persistent disparities. It is a wonderful book and will make a difference in our communities."

—**Stedman Graham**

"Almost six years ago I had an encounter with cancer. In my left lung there was an ugly (as if there is any other kind) tumor. Quick action on the part of my doctors saved my life. I may have helped by being aware that something was wrong.

"*Prime Time* is a great help to all of us; those who pay attention and those who should pay attention. The old saying 'a stitch in time saves nine' is never more accurate than in concerning our health. This is a book everyone needs because everyone has a woman in our lives that we love and want to keep with us: ourselves, our aunts, our mothers, our grandmothers. Marilyn Gaston and Gayle Porter have done a wonderful service for us all."
—**Nikki Giovanni**

"I commend the authors of *Prime Time* for creating a long overdue—and much needed—reference for African American women at midlife.

"African American women have historically given their personal physical and emotional needs low priority. This down-to-earth, comprehensive guide will provide African American women with the tools to achieve and maintain personal wellness. By following *Prime Time*'s practical advice and honestly completing the self-tests and quizzes, women can embark on a personal journey of physical and emotional well-being and explore the joys of successfully transitioning to middle age.

"I wish to thank Dr. Marilyn Gaston and Dr. Gayle Porter for their vision and hard work in creating this invaluable reference on health and wellness."
—**Audrey F. Manley, M.D., M.P.H.**
**President, Spelman College**
**Former Acting Surgeon General and Acting Assistant Secretary for Health**
**Rear Admiral (Retired), United States Public Health Service**

"Powerful and far reaching, *Prime Time* is a perfect mind-body book for all African American women who are facing or thinking about this key time of life transition. With *Prime Time*, you will fully blossom into your own."
—**Marcellus A. Walker, M.D.**
**Author of *Natural Health for African Americans***
**Founder, africanamericanhealth.com**
**Founder, African American Health Foundation**

"I commend Dr. Gaston and Dr. Porter for their informative and inspiring book. It is a rich guide and resource for African American women to help them enjoy longer, healthier, and more fulfilling lives.

"In our national quest for a healthier American and the reduction of disparities in health status, Drs. Gaston and Porter have made a solid contribution."
—**Louis W. Sullivan, M.D.**
**President, Morehouse School of Medicine**
**U.S. Secretary of Health and Human Services, 1989–1993**

"*Prime Time* is a must-read for all women who want to be in charge of their lives and their health destiny."
—**Byllye Y. Avery**
**Founder, National Black Women's Health Project**

# Prime Time

THE AFRICAN AMERICAN WOMAN'S COMPLETE GUIDE TO MIDLIFE HEALTH AND WELLNESS

Marilyn Hughes Gaston, M.D.

and

Gayle K. Porter, Psy.D.

**Edited by Sheryl Hilliard Tucker**

ONE WORLD

THE BALLANTINE PUBLISHING GROUP · NEW YORK

A One World Book
Published by The Ballantine Publishing Group
Copyright © 2001 by Marilyn Hughes Gaston, M.D., and Gayle K. Porter, Psy.D.
Foreword copyright © 2001 by Joycelyn Elders, M.D.

www.randomhouse. com/BB/

Photographs courtesy of Amikaeyla Proudfoot Gaston

Grateful acknowledgment is made to the following for permission to reprint previously published material:

*Impact Publishers, Inc.:* Excerpt from *The Assertive Woman* (3rd Edition) by Stanlee Phelps and Nancy Austin. © 1997 Stanlee Phelps and Nancy Austin. Reproduced for The Ballantine Publishing Group by permission of Impact Publishers, Inc., P.O. Box 6016, Atascadero, CA 93423. Further reproduction prohibited.

*Kate Rushin:* Excerpt from "The Tired Poem: Last Letter from a Typical Unemployed Black Professional Woman" from *The Black Back-Ups*, Firebrand Press. Copyright © 1993 by Kate Rushin. This poem originally appeared in *Conditions: Five, The Black Women's Issue*, 1979, and *Home Girls: A Black Feminist Anthology*, 1983 (JP). Reprinted by permission of the author.

*Handy Brothers Music Co., Inc.:* Excerpt from the lyrics of "One Hour Mama" by Porter Grainger. Reprinted by permission of Handy Brothers Music Co., Inc. International Copyright Secured. Francis, Day & Hunter, Ltd.

*Amy Hill Hearth:* Excerpt from *Having Our Say: The Delany Sisters' First 100 Years* by Sarah and A. Elizabeth Delany with Amy Hill Hearth (Kodansha, 1993). © 1993 by Amy Hill Hearth, Sarah Louise Delany, and Annie Elizabeth Delany. © 2000 by Amy Hill Hearth. Reprinted by permission.

*Random House, Inc.:* Excerpt from "My Man Bovanne" from *Gorilla, My Love* by Toni Cade Bambara. Copyright © 1971 by Toni Cade Bambara.

*Seal Press:* "Poem for Flight" from *Forbidden Poems* by Becky Birtha. © 1991 by Becky Birtha. Reprinted by permission of Seal Press.

*Sandra Y. Lewis, Psy.D.:* "Sisterhood Affirmation" reprinted by permission of Sandra Y. Lewis, Psy.D., Vice President, Program, International Black Women's Congress.

*Cecelia Williams Bryant:* Excerpt from *Kiamsha—A Spiritual Discipline for African-American Women* by Cecelia Williams Bryant. Reprinted by permission of the author.

Library of Congress Cataloging-in-Publication Data

Gaston, Marilyn H.
    Prime time : the African American woman's complete guide to midlife health and wellness / Marilyn Hughes Gaston and Gayle K. Porter.
        p.    cm.
    ISBN 0-345-43215-0
    1. Afro-American women—Health and hygiene.    2. Middle aged women—Health and hygiene.
    I. Porter, Gayle K.    II. Title.

RA778.4.A36 G37 2001
613'.04244'08996073—dc21                                                    00-066803

Manufactured in the United States of America

First Edition: May 2001

10  9  8  7  6  5  4

This book is dedicated to the women who have influenced our lives and role-modeled the belief that dreams can become realities.

—Marilyn and Gayle

It is specifically dedicated to my beloved ancestors and other family members: my mother, Dorothy Mildred Dent Hughes; my father, Myron A. Hughes; my grandmothers, Anna Dent and Lula Vaughn; my godmother, Ruth Showes; my aunt Clarabelle Patterson; my uncle, Bradley Dent; and my brothers and their wives, Mike Hughes and Elaine Hughes, and Myron Clark and Gwen Clark. And to my future generation: my children, Amikaeyla Proudfoot Gaston and Damon Gaston, and my nieces and nephews.

—M.H.G.

For your love, support, and wisdom, I thank: my mother, Willistine Porter; my aunts, Esther Johnson, Mamie Dade, and Cora Pruitt; my cousin, Eldoris Mason; my grandmother, Janie Perry; my great-grandmother, Mamie Oglesby; my mentor, Sister Miriam Wilson; my siblings, Carole, Earl, Lisa, and Antonia; my nieces and nephews; and my Sisterfriend, Marilyn Peals-O'Hara.

—G.K.P.

# Contents

# Acknowledgments

We would like to acknowledge the Prime Time support we received in making our dream a reality. This endeavor would not have been possible without our incredible agent, Victoria Sanders, and our two wonderful editors, Sheryl Hilliard Tucker and Leslie Meredith. We would like to give special thanks to Cheryl Woodruff, who saw the vision for the book and helped us expand the conceptual frame.

Faye Williams and Cassandra Burton, owners of Sisterspace bookstore, encouraged, cajoled, and pushed us to start and finish this project.

The sisters who participated in our focus groups helped us stay grounded in reality. Though different groups of women across the country gave us major input, the following sisters gave us extended blocks of time: Gwendolyn Keita, Joanna Banks, Dorothy West, Clarice Reid, Cheryl Reese, D. Taylor, Laura Thomas, Sylvia Kinard, Vonda Smith-Hill, Anita Marshall, Ricci Morgan, Cheri Waters, Norma Taylor, Diane Graham, and Dorothy Davis.

We were computer illiterates when we started this process and might still be had it not been for the guidance and support of Kemba Maish and Andy Zuckerman.

We would also like to thank our two "Honorary Prime Time Sisters": Peg Cahill, who read and edited the book and said it should be for every woman;

and Joan Zuckerman, who supplied suggestions for the book, fed us multiple meals, and "loaned" us her husband.

We are grateful for the love and support of our sister mentors Naomi Chamberlain and Olivia Hooker, who encouraged us every step of the way.

We also want to thank Denise Jones for her typing support, Audrey Chapman for her advice, and all of the sisters who gave us permission to use their pictures or work.

Finally, we want to thank our families, friends, and colleagues for the support they provided throughout this endeavor.

# Foreword

*Prime Time* is a truthful, sometimes painful, but always uplifting look at the health of African American women as we enter and survive the middle years. It helps us to look back at our past, see the many trials and tribulations that we have overcome, and realize that we can be in control of our destiny. It helps us see that too often we spend so much time just surviving that we don't get around to thriving in life. It also teaches us to celebrate our boldness and joys.

Amazingly, doctors and women don't know much about why the symptoms of menopause occur and how declining levels of estrogen affect the body as we age. We don't know much because menopause hasn't been studied until now. We women haven't discussed it until recently, because it was taboo—and in fact, all information about sex and our female bodies, our powerful reproductive systems, was taboo. Women in general and African American women in particular have not had the same benefits from health studies and research on health risks as men. And African American women have been underserved by health care. This book remedies the lack of information on the potential health risks of midlife African American women.

Health is about much more than the absence of disease. It is about jobs, environment, education, economics, religion, politics, community, family, and social well-being. To improve the health of the black community as a whole, we must improve the health of all black women in particular. We African American women have more chronic disease, live in poorer neighborhoods, enjoy less access to health care, have less education, and suffer from a greater number of life-stressing problems. Women's health care is not limited to pregnancy and childbearing, nor is it separate from general health care. Women's health is about knowing our bodies and our choices and empowering ourselves. We spend half of our life trying not to get pregnant, but reproductive health is important whether a woman chooses to become a mother or not.

Gynecological tests for women should include Pap smears and pelvic exams, screening for cervical cancer and any other abnormalities. Monthly breast self-exams, yearly clinical breast exams, and yearly mammograms for women forty and over are the most effective tools available to detect cancers early, and early detection yields the best hopes for long-term survival. Yet we don't want to just live longer, we want to live better. After age forty, many African American women face the terrible threes: midlife, menopause, and divorce. We need to address these changes and we need to be able to enjoy our lives at this time. We are finally free of menstruation and the fear of pregnancy, but we've taken on a new set of problems, such as:

• How should we address the potential health risk of declining estrogen levels, and how should we control menopause symptoms such as hot flashes?

• What are the advantages and disadvantages of hormone replacement therapy (HRT)?

• How do we handle conflicting information about treatment choices?

• How should we view the menopausal transition?

African American women have had to be beasts of burden for a long time, but we survived slavery, overt segregation, poor schooling, being overworked and underpaid, and having to watch our children grow up without an opportunity to be children. We've had to go on, and we need to keep going on. We know what we've come through, and we must realize exactly where we are in order to find ways to get where we want to be during this millennium. The problems of poverty, obesity, drugs, teenage pregnancy, STDs and AIDS, and ignorance are often lifestyle choices that begin in adolescence and affect health for the rest of our lives.

We have been so busy taking care of our men, our children, our parents, our relatives, and our neighbors that we've forgotten ourselves. We have been so busy downstream pulling out bodies from an apparent accident upstream that we didn't go upstream to fix the bridge that was causing the disaster. Since we have forgotten ourselves, everybody else forgot us, too.

It's time for us to begin to take charge of our lives. We have the know-how, we have the resources, and we have the power to get it done. What we may not have are the strategies and the push to get us out of our rut—and this book gives them to us. *Prime Time* helps us to assess our lives and decide where we are, set goals for where we want to be, and create strategies on how to get there.

We've come a long way, baby, but we've got a long way to go. We pushed, pulled, laughed, cried, and did whatever we had to do for our families, friends, and neighbors. It's time we put the same amount of energy into our own physical, emotional, spiritual, and material well-being and begin to take charge of our lives.

Our average life expectancy has increased from thirty-five years in 1900 to seventy-six years in 1998. Until now we didn't worry about the middle years, because they didn't exist. Now that we are living into our seventies, eighties, nineties, and beyond, however, we must prepare to be more than beasts of burden, bearing children, taking care of other women's children, putting food on the table for our children, taking care of grandchildren, and waiting to go to the nursing home.

The only thing a person has to do to age and grow old is not die, but I believe it is best for us to become sages as we age, to help others along the way. *Prime Time* helps us to do just that. It helps us to help ourselves by learning about the lives of many women—urban and rural, professional and nonprofessional—from across the country. It treats African American women with respect for what we are attempting to do, rather than blaming us for past decisions. It teaches us how to learn from each other, solve problems for ourselves, and think about what we really want for ourselves and our community. But most of all, it teaches us the importance of expanding Sarah's circle, forming a Prime Time Sisterhood as opposed to just climbing Jacob's ladder alone.

*Prime Time* teaches us how to live in a way that prevents crisis, rather than just surviving from one crisis to another. It shows us how to manage stress, how to recognize disease, and how to use the health-care system. Most of all, it teaches us how to take charge, take care of ourselves, and care enough about ourselves and our loved ones to share in the responsibility for our own health.

—Joycelyn Elders, M.D.

# PART I

# Now Is the Time

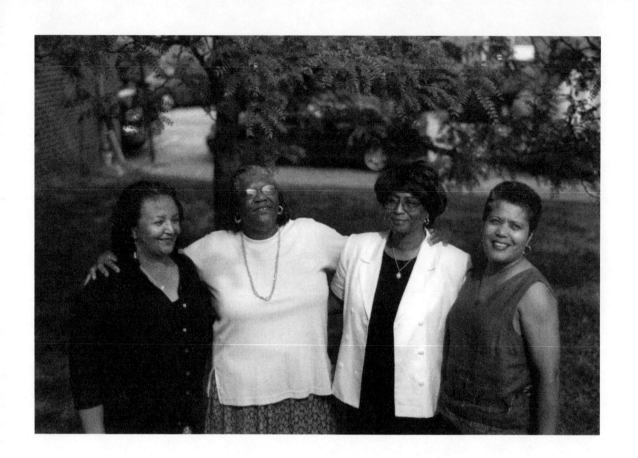

# Chapter 1

# YOUR PRIME TIME JOURNEY

*The real act of discovery consists not in finding new lands but in seeing with new eyes.*

—Unknown

Finally, here is a book about *us!*

It is for and about us—the almost six million African American women who are experiencing the opportunities and challenges of the middle years. Yes, there are millions of us, but there is very little information published about our unique physical and emotional health issues.

African American women have had no *Golden Girls* television program to reflect and celebrate the diversity, the richness, the joy, the pain, the laughter, and the love that are part of the lives of many of us who are over forty. To paraphrase Barbara Smith, Gloria Hull, and Beverly Smith, editors of *But Some of Us Are Brave*: As African American women in the middle years, we are often part of all women, all Blacks, or Black women of all ages, but rarely is there just a space for us.

This book—*Prime Time*—is our space.

## NAVIGATING THE PRIME TIME YEARS

Like you, we, too, are African American women in our middle years. Together we authors have more than sixty years of experience in providing health services to the African American community. Marilyn is a medical doctor with more than thirty-five years of experience in primary health care. She has provided direct health care to African American communities and served as medical director of health programs supervising the care of families. Marilyn has planned and administered health programs for African Americans at the local, state, and national level and has served on the faculties of three medical schools teaching students and residents.

Gayle is a clinical psychologist who has been on the faculty of two medical schools, providing clinical supervision to medical students, psychology interns, and psychiatry residents. With more than twenty-five years as a mental health professional, Gayle has served as a director of two outpatient mental health clinics and been involved in numerous research projects while managing a private practice that includes providing individual and group counseling and psychotherapy to numerous Black women.

We have made changes and midlife corrections in our own lives. Marilyn stopped smoking after twenty-five years: "Yes, even though I am a physician who knew well the negative effects of smoking, I was forty-five when I was finally able to stop."

Gayle started exercising on a regular basis when she turned fifty: "I knew when I was in my thirties that exercise had a positive impact on my emotional and physical well-being, but it wasn't until I reached the middle years that I started to own my responsibility for keeping myself healthy."

Our personal and professional experiences have convinced us that we are now in the prime of our lives. And so are you!

At this age, we're all wiser and more confident than in our younger years. Most of us are healthier and more financially solvent than our mothers or grandmothers. A growing number of us have enjoyed educational and professional opportunities of which our foremothers could only dream. Yet, despite our advances, there remain major disparities between the rates of *morbidity* (disease) and *mortality* (death) for Caucasian and for African American women. We have more chronic emotional and physical health problems, and we die earlier. We also endure the stress of racism, sexism, and ageism, which negatively affect our well-being.


## OUR MISSION TOGETHER

An appearance on a Black Entertainment Television (BET) program, *Our Voices: Prime Time Beauty Inside and Out*, which focused on African American women in midlife, intensified our need to understand these intolerable disparities and to be a catalyst for change.

We had been recommended to the producers of the call-in talk show because of our expertise in African American women's physical and emotional health. Both of us had been speakers and panelists on numerous local, national, and international programs related to this topic.

The panel of four women (all in our middle years) was moderated by Doris McMillon, an award-winning journalist. The other two panelists were Sharon Pratt Kelly, the former mayor of Washington, D.C., and actress Pam Grier. Ms. Grier discussed the difficulties faced by seasoned women film stars. Her comments indicated that most scripts with female characters reflected Hollywood's infatuation with pubescent girls. Ms. Kelly described her experiences as a businesswoman and a politician. These all are demanding careers for anyone, but especially for African American midlife women, who often are expected to juggle their professions and nuclear and extended family responsibilities without complaint.

However, despite the specific concerns expressed by each of us, there were clear declarations about the benefits of this age. Ms. Grier said that she was happier, felt better, and was more aware of herself than she had ever been. Ms. Kelly talked about her decision to take time to make important lifestyle changes—"I'm exercising more, drinking eight glasses of water a day, and just being still." We all felt that we were truly in the prime time of our lives.

Following the show, we were deluged with invitations to present lectures and seminars on this theme. We received numerous calls from African American and Caucasian women and men across the country. The women expressed their delight at seeing a program that illuminated and documented their experiences and asked provocative questions, such as "Am I being selfish because I'm tired of taking care of everyone else?" "I didn't know Black women were dying at a younger age than other women. Why?" "Do Black women get osteoporosis? I thought only white women did."

The men bombarded us with questions about how they could be helpful and supportive of the significant midlife women in their lives. They also asked very directed questions about their relationships with women in midlife, such as "Is she ever going to want sex again?" "Is she mad all the time because she's going through the change, or is it something else?" All of the callers requested more information, specifically, articles, books, or tapes about this topic. But because there are so few articles—and no books—

focusing specifically on the second half of life for African American women, we were frustrated by our inability to help our audience more.

And so we decided to write a book that would help us midlife Black women integrate our minds, bodies, and spirits and save our own lives.

To find out more about the reasons for the untimely deaths and high incidence of illness of our sisters, we authors held focus groups with other midlife African American women between the ages of forty and seventy. What our sisters perceive as their primary stressors and concerns was quite consistent. As a group, we worry about our physical and mental health, our finances, changes in our physical appearance, and our personal relationships or lack of them. Our focus group participants also emphasized their need for strategies to help them confront the challenges and resolve the stress that most of us face in our middle years.

The most significant conclusion of these discussion groups was that racism and sexism are not the primary negative influences in Black women's lives. Their comments confirmed that two other factors are more deleterious to our physical and emotional health: **We don't make ourselves our number one priority, and we live unhealthy lifestyles.** These culprits contribute in major ways to the development of unhealthy bodies and minds and to our overall dis-ease (a state of being either ill or simply not at ease). Most of us spend so much of our time, energy, and money focused on the well-being of others—our spouses or partners, children, parents, relatives, friends, and jobs—that we have very little time, energy, or money left to care appropriately for our own physical and emotional needs.

Armed with this information, and knowing we can change our lives and take responsibility for our own health, we established two primary goals for this book. **First,** we want *Prime Time* to help you make your own physical and emotional needs your main priority. How often do you put your needs second or even last after tending to the needs of your family and friends and your responsibilities at work? We want you to be aware of when you're taking a step backward or off course along your Prime Time journey, so you can adjust your stride and get back to living healthier and living longer.

**Second,** we want this book to help you make "midcourse corrections" in how you're living so you can maximize the Prime Time of your life. Your midcourse corrections can include making positive changes in how you think about yourself, how you view the period of middle age, how you incorporate a philosophy of wellness in your life each and every day, and how you change habits that are negative or self-destructive.

All African American women—and this includes you, no matter what your educational, social, or financial status might be—can live a healthier, longer, happier, and more balanced life. Accentuating the positive and celebrating the opportunities of this time in your life will also help you respond more effectively to its challenges. As we go through the book, we will look at each challenge in more detail, and introduce some midlife women who have successfully confronted these issues.

## ISN'T IT TIME FOR YOUR MIDLIFE CORRECTION?

You took the first step on your Prime Time journey when you bought this book. The next step is to use this book to plan this exciting passage through your middle years. Think of *Prime Time* as a road map designed to help you chart the landscape through which you must travel during this time of your life. The information, self-assessment tools, and advice that you'll find in our book will help you:

1. Assess where you are
2. Identify where you want to go
3. Develop practical, realistic strategies to improve your mind, body, and spirit
4. Reinvent yourself as a healthy, physically active, assertive, and fulfilled woman who is enjoying her Prime Time years

Don't be discouraged if you need to reinvent yourself several times before you are securely on the Prime Time path. Change takes practice—*but you can do it*. Let *Prime Time* be your travel companion.

We authors know from our own experience that traveling the path through midlife can be challenging, especially if you're determined to make substantial changes in the way you live and learn to put your needs first. That's why we encourage you to develop a support system of women—a Prime Time Sister and a Prime Time Circle of Sisterfriends—who can help you use the recommendations in this book to make critically necessary changes in the way you think and the way you live.

## HOW TO GET THE MOST OUT OF PRIME TIME

*Prime Time* is for you and about you. It is yours. We want you to own it. That's why we invite you to write in this book, work in it, and think in it. Use it like a journal; it belongs only to you, no one else. Taking the self-scoring quizzes and filling out the worksheets will give you insights into the current state of your health and help you assess how healthful your lifestyle is. *Prime Time*'s easy-to-use forms will help you document your family's medical history, create your own personal wellness calendar, and record pertinent personal health information and medical test results that you need to share with your doctors and other health-care providers. As you can see, working through the book will also provide testimony to your progress.

We also advise you to start keeping a separate health journal or notebook to capture any of your thoughts and insights that can't fit onto the pages of *Prime Time*. By recording these musings or concerns, you can express and explore your fears in a safe way, sort out new goals and commitments from old habits, weigh your options, and put new ideas in perspective. Use your health journal or notebook to jot down whatever comes to mind. Ask yourself questions, then write what your inner voice tells you.

*Prime Time* is divided into seven parts. Part I, "Now Is the Time," documents the statistics we discovered about the lives and health of African American women in midlife. It establishes why you need to take heed of the unacceptable disparities in health between Black women and women of other racial and ethnic groups so that you can do something about it.

Part II, "Reframing Your Priorities," examines how we Black women think of ourselves and why too many of us view midlife as a negative, powerless time. Our primary objective in the first few chapters is to help you examine your assumptions about being a midlife African American woman and to change any ideas and attitudes that are not serving your health. We want you to develop a new paradigm for seeing your life. We very much believe that you will see how to celebrate the joy as well as embrace the challenges of being who you are *now*, not who you were twenty years ago.

Please be open to rethinking who you are and what you want out of the rest of your life. Keeping an open mind will help you benefit from the hundreds of Prime Time Prescriptions that we offer throughout this book. When you take charge of your mind and beliefs, you take charge of your life and your health. And when you think about it, the only person you can truly be in charge of is yourself. **You—in charge of you—are a force to be reckoned with.**

This section also establishes the underlying principle of *Prime Time*: *Health is not simply freedom from physical disease, but also a positive emotional and spiritual state. To be wholly healthy, you need to acknowledge and nurture all components of your being—physical, emotional, and spiritual—and acknowledge their interdependence.* That's why we offer holistic recommendations—advice for you as a whole person—for getting and staying healthy, as well as for preventing illness from taking root in your body, mind, and spirit.

Finally, Part II explains why it's critical for you to make meaningful lifestyle changes at this time of your life and how these changes can enhance the already tremendous power you have by establishing healthy practices that reduce your chances of developing a disease or getting ill. Preventive practices are the best way to put your own needs first.

Part III, "Putting Self-Care Into Action," underscores the importance of the annual medical visit and exam and provides an explanation of the elements of a thorough exam and critical medical tests. It also addresses risk factors (such as smoking, lack of exercise, or obesity) that increase your chance of developing a chronic illness or disease. This section will help you design your own Personal Prime Time Wellness Plan.

Part IV, "You Can Save Your Own Life," contains chapters that explain the statistics, risk factors, and effective treatments associated with the top four causes of death for African American women: heart disease, cancer, stroke, and diabetes. Throughout the book, we refer to these diseases as the Big Four.

Part V, "Staying Sane in a World that Can Seem Insane," focuses on the paradox inherent in trying to be a strong Black woman. Far too many of us learn from childhood to care for the needs of others at the expense of our own personal well-being. In this section, *Prime Time* provides traditional and nontraditional tactics to avoid, minimize, or overcome stress, depression, and anxiety—serious mental health concerns that plague too many African American sisters in midlife.

Part VI, "Coping With Midlife's Passage," looks at the challenges of menopause and explores the controversial findings about hormone replacement therapy. We also offer advice on how to function as a sexually assertive woman and cope with other common concerns of this period in our lives, such as memory loss, urinary incontinence, loss of vision, and arthritis.

Part VII, "Living in Health and Wellness," will help you become a smarter health-care consumer and a more informed partner with your health-care providers. We cover a broad range of topics, from choosing your doctors and other members of your health team to navigating your medical insurance company's bureaucracy.

Although we wrote this book primarily for African American women in our age group, younger women can benefit from our preventive lifestyle recommendations. We hope you share what you learn from *Prime Time* with all of the important people in your life.

Zora Neale Hurston, the famous writer and anthropologist, described Black women as the "mules of the earth," carrying other people's loads and usually being at the end of the line—never at the beginning. Unfortunately, some of the choices that Black women make and the chances we take often keep us at the wrong end of the line of good physical and emotional health. However, making critical midlife corrections such as the ones we prescribe throughout this book, can and will put you at the front of the line of health and well-being. Then, and only then, you will be a "mule no more."

# Chapter 2

# MIDLIFE IN BLACK

*Just the time to re-program my life; to figure how to*
*make a living doing what I wanna do instead of wasting away in some*
*brain-eroding day gig; to adjust to safe sex and menopause and touches of*
*arthritis; to appreciate less as more.*
—Hattie Gossett, *The Terrifyingly Terrific Teens to the Fiercely 40s and 50s*

Our personal and professional experiences have convinced us that once Black women decide to take charge, we can make profound changes in our own lives and those of our families and communities. Just the fact that we have survived racism and sexism, which to some extent affect the lives of all African American women, proves that we have, as Black feminist theorist bell hooks writes in *Sisters of the Yam: Black Women and Self-Recovery,* "transcended and transformed the people, places and things which could have prevented our growth."

To truly appreciate where we are today, we must first understand and acknowledge the place from which we came. Since we were brought to America as slaves beginning in 1619, our numbers have significantly increased. We are living longer and healthier lives than our mothers and foremothers. In 1790, when the first U.S. census was taken, there were approximately four hundred thousand women of African descent in America. Two hundred years later, in 1990, the Census Bureau recorded more than sixteen million of us. The most dramatic increase in our numbers has occurred among women over forty-five years of age. In fact, as we enter the twenty-first century, there are now almost six million African American women between forty and seventy years of age.

In 1900, life expectancy was forty-nine years for Caucasian women but only thirty-five years for African American women—a disparity of fourteen years. Today, life expectancy for African American women is seventy-five years, and for Caucasian women it is eighty years—a difference of only five years. Major medical advances, lifestyle modifications, better nutrition, and improvement in social status have all contributed to our longevity; however, the disparity still exists.

## DEMANDING SOCIAL, ECONOMIC, AND POLITICAL CHANGE

The most significant cause for celebration, however, is our metamorphosis from slaves to citizens. Just think about the number of African American women political candidates and elected and appointed officials—1972 presidential candidate Shirley Chisholm, U.S. representatives Maxine Waters and Eddie Bernice Johnson, delegate Eleanor Holmes Norton, former U.S. secretary of labor Alexis Herman, former U.S. senator Carol Mosely Braun, and former surgeon general Joycelyn Elders, to name just a few. There's no doubt that Black women have played a catalytic role in demanding change in the social, economic, and political status not just of African Americans but of poor and oppressed people throughout this country and around the world. (If you want to learn more, pick up Paula Giddings' moving history *When and Where I Enter: The Impact of Black Women on Race and Sex in America*.)

African American women have managed to achieve leadership positions in government, business, politics, civil rights, and the nonprofit world despite a corrupted social and legal system that justified overt acts of racism and sexism against our foremothers and many of us as younger women. Oppressive laws often restricted or prevented us from fulfilling our personal and professional goals. Fortunately, many of these laws were changed or eliminated through the social and political activism of middle-aged "she-roes," from Sojourner Truth and Harriet Tubman to Rosa Parks and Fannie Lou Hamer.

The educational achievements of African American women attest to the effectiveness of social activism and changes in law. From 1940 to 1998, the proportion of Black women over twenty-five years old who had finished high school increased from 8 percent to 80 percent. The increase in the college completion rate was also significant. In 1940, only 1 percent of all African American women had completed college. By 1998, the rate had increased to

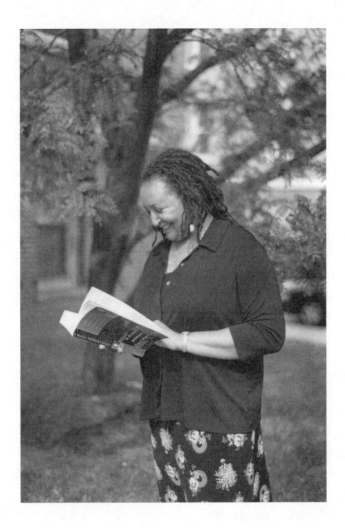

15 percent. Throughout the 1990s, publications such as *Money* magazine have ranked Spelman College in Atlanta—a college that was founded to educate African American young women—one of the best institutions of higher education in the United States.

Education continues to be a key factor in expanding professional and financial options for Black women. Since 1975, the economic status of African American women over forty, especially those with college degrees, has significantly improved. In fact, while researching this point, we discovered some information that truly surprised us. Did you know that the average annual and estimated hourly earnings of African American women over forty years old with a college degree surpasses those of our Caucasian peers? The average annual income for this group has increased during the last twenty-five years from $8,000 to $28,000, whereas the average income of

Caucasian women over forty with college degrees increased from $6,800 to $26,000! The primary explanation for this finding is that, unlike many Caucasian women, college-educated African American women who are now at midlife tended not to stop working when they married or had children. Thus, many of us have seniority over our Caucasian peers who entered or reentered the workforce at a much older age. The other reason is that antidiscrimination laws finally forced companies to hire and promote a few of us into better-paying positions. Unfortunately, the economic picture isn't as bright for the many non-college-educated African American women, who usually earn less than their Caucasian counterparts.

As a result of our improved financial status and increased visibility, we African American women are expanding our sphere of influence. For instance, powerful Black women are taking lead positions in social and political events on a national and international level. Oprah Winfrey, Marion Wright Edelman, Cathy Hughes (owner of the largest Black radio broadcasting company in the United States), and Camille Cosby are just a few African American she-roes who provide much-needed leadership on issues ranging from child abuse to voter registration to gun control. All four of these women are in their middle years.

## OUR STORIES

Now that we (Marilyn and Gayle) are in our Prime Time, our appreciation for the complexity of midlife has deepened. We fully understand why these years are considered a period of discovery, growth, and integration.

We find many reasons for celebrating our midlife. We are more confident, more secure, and happier than ever before. We have been blessed with wonderful people in our lives who surround us with love. We love our jobs and are proud of our professional accomplishments. Both of us have lives full of caring, love, and service to others.

We also hear the satisfaction of our friends and peers sitting around kitchen tables and in beauty shops, churches, book clubs, and our focus groups. We really don't want to be twenty again. Remember Moms Mabley's legendary question: "What good ol' days? I was there, where was they at?"

We can enjoy our Prime Time because, over the years, we have struggled to put ourselves first! Learning to do this without feeling guilty or anxious, however, was initially very difficult for us, because we're both personal and professional helpers and healers. We had to turn to role models, books, friends, and therapy to help us reframe our priorities. And then it took patience, persistence, and practice to put the me-first notion into action. As Prime Time Sisters, we also turned to each other for support as we made these changes.

Now, we can rejoice in our ability to put our needs first. We're more comfortable using our time, energy, and money to promote our own physical, emotional, and spiritual well-being. We celebrate our increased assertiveness. We feel less conflicted whenever we agree or disagree with a request from our sisters, brothers, cousins, parents, friends, or coworkers. (Marilyn is still working on that when it comes to her children.) We enjoy knowing what brings us joy, understanding how to relax, and "feeling free to sweat," as Lydia Alexander wrote in *Wearing Purple*, a delightful book of letters by four midlife African American women—Lydia Alexander, Marilyn Harper, Otis Owens, and Mildred Patterson.

Like most folks, we appreciate positive remarks about our appearance. However, when they're linked to our age ("You don't look like you're in your fifties!"), we find ourselves repeating Gloria Steinem's comment on her fiftieth birthday: "But this is what fifty looks like!"

Midlife brings a variety of concerns, some of which are trivial. We have struggled with gray hair and the to-color-or-not-to-color question. Each of us has made a different decision—Gayle is still coloring, while Marilyn has finally stopped after throwing away the last (number 5,031) bottle of Lady Clairol. Insignificant? Yes. However, we bet many of you also are wrestling with this issue, maybe every morning or at least each time you visit the hair salon.

This new awareness of our needs has convinced us to start wearing clothes and shoes that we find comfortable and attractive. And we're finding more midlife sisters who agree with this excerpt from *Wearing Purple*: "It seems clear to me that now is the time to consider my own specific style of dress. My highest priority is comfort. I refuse to wear restrictive clothes such as control-top panty hose, or walk around on three-inch heels. From now on I intend to stick with flowing lines, big sleeves, and loose tops . . . when I'm not in sweats."

Yet along with the joys of midlife come very real concerns about our own health and mortality. These have been the most profound and difficult issues to address. Injuries and surgeries can take much longer to heal at midlife than when we were younger. Decreasing energy and increasing responsibility for those who once cared for us have taken their toll. We are the "sandwich generation," caught between our aging parents, with their many needs, and our adult children, who are not quite comfortably independent, and we face important decisions on a daily basis.

To help us make these decisions, we draw on our memories of the women who were role models for us during our youth. We were poor and lived in the projects, but these women demonstrated that we could do and be whatever we dreamed. We were surrounded by middle-aged African American women who made major contributions to their families and communities. We witnessed the strength and determination of these women, who often worked two jobs to move us out of the projects into a house in a "good neighborhood"; picketed segregated schools, stores, and swimming pools; initiated new community projects; and played bid whist and bridge on Saturday nights. Arising early on Sunday morning to attend church, where they sang in the choir and chaired church committees, they then came home and cooked dinner for the family and the neighborhood. They seemed to find joy and purpose in all aspects of their lives and were respected by everyone for their wisdom and experience.

These African American sages also broke through racial and gender "glass ceilings," made career changes, obtained General Education Diplomas (GEDs), stopped smoking after forty years, and served as advocates for themselves and other poor families and seniors. And in honor of their hard work and dedication, some, like Esther Johnson (Gayle's aunt), had a building named after them.

Yet these same role models—our mothers, grandmothers, aunts, and their friends—paid the same physical and emotional toll for being strong Black women as many midlife women today. Many of them were ill or dying from diabetes, hypertension, cancer, or heart disease—illnesses that had been untreated or undertreated in part because of poverty, racism, and sexism, but also because they neglected their own health and needs. As we learned more about the links between mind and body that give rise to health or illness, we saw the connection between their obesity and silent depression, their irritability and anxiety over financial difficulties, their fatigue and premature death. Remembering the historic words of Fannie Lou Hamer, "I'm sick and tired of being sick and tired," we understood the dying, diabetic grandmother in the movie *Soul Food* when she turned to her grandson and said, "I'm just so tired."

Each of us has had specific and general personal reasons for rejoicing and grieving during the Prime Time of our lives.

## GAYLE'S STORY

I'll never forget the joy I felt on my fortieth birthday. I had achieved two personal and family milestones. I had acquired a doctorate in clinical psychology, becoming the first person in my known family—for, as African Americans, we're never quite certain about all of our kin—to reach that educational level. I had lived a year longer than my maternal grandmother, who died at thirty-nine years of age. Turning forty was part of the mythology of the women in my family. Even though my mother and my aunts were in their sixties and seventies, experiencing the premature death of their mother, a sister, and numerous female relatives had left them unable to completely exhale until another baby girl had achieved that mystical number—forty!

During my forties, I had several professional positions that allowed me to develop and direct programs that increased the availability of mental health services for poor and minority children and their families. Through my pro bono work and my private practice of psychotherapy, I had an opportunity to focus on issues related to African American women. My personal life was full of love and support both given and received from family and friends. Life was very good!

And then I hit my fifties. Within two years I had had two major surgeries and experienced the deaths of two of my oldest and dearest friends. It was then that I truly understood the bittersweetness that is sometimes associated with the middle years.

Accepting that sadness, like joy, is a part of living, I continued to pursue my career and build a busy, satisfying life. For me, having one job isn't enough—my intellectual curiosity and determination to help others and share what I have learned over the years keeps my schedule packed with a variety of activities: I am a licensed clinical psychologist with a private practice that focuses on working with African Americans, especially women.

I have been on the faculties of the Johns Hopkins College of Medicine and Howard University. Currently, I am a principal research analyst and senior mental health advisor for the American Institutes for Research.

# MARILYN'S STORY

I entered the middle years with a bang. I had never been happier. Professionally, I was fulfilled and making important contributions to sickle cell disease research. Personally, I was married and had two wonderful children. My fifth decade and the first half of the sixth both met many of my expectations and presented some disappointments. My children graduated from college. My husband and I divorced. I left my job as director of the Division of Medicine in the U.S. Public Health Service to pursue my dream job. As the director of the Bureau of Primary Health Care, Health Resources and Services Administration, and an assistant surgeon general of the U.S. Public Health Service, I currently administer a $4 billion national program that helps poor, underserved, and minority people obtain health care across the nation.

When I reached my fifty-fifth birthday, for the first time I didn't want to celebrate; in fact, I felt sad and withdrawn. I was also totally absorbed with thoughts of my mother and my grandmother. I focused on their trials and tribulations in general, and their health problems in particular. My preoccupation lasted through my birthday, January 31, and the first week of February. After experiencing the same reaction on my fifty-sixth and fifty-seventh birthdays, I finally realized the reason. February 6 marks the anniversary of two deaths—that of my grandmother in February 1942 and my mother's in February 1967. As if that weren't enough of a coincidence, they both died at the age of fifty-seven! And the sad thing is, both of their deaths would be preventable today. My grandmother died of rheumatic heart disease that she contracted in childhood before the discovery of penicillin, and my mother died of cancer of the cervix prior to widespread knowledge and use of the Pap smear. Consequently, my own fifty-seventh birthday brought up anxieties and fears about my actual and potential health issues and my mortality. Eventually, my friends, family, and years of experience helped me to gain insight into the causes of my sadness and to work through my issues of aging, so that I was able to once again celebrate my birthdays with joy and gratitude.

## THE PRIME TIME CHALLENGE

Black women in midlife face a myriad of concerns that cross socio-economic lines—they are as relevant to sisters who didn't finish high school as to college-educated African American women. For most of us these center around:

1. Health—physical and emotional
2. Personal finances
3. Being single
4. Personal and professional relationships
5. Physical appearance
6. Caretaking

These concerns are similar to those of Caucasian women, particularly the problems of ageism and sexism. Yet our challenges are further aggravated in a dramatic and negative way by racism and our individual response to each problem.

As a group, we represent one of the poorest segments of the American population. We are more likely to approach our middle years unmarried and without a steady partner. In addition to our caretaking responsibilities for our parents and children, we take on the care of extended family members and friends, further draining our already precious resources of money and time. Many of us don't fully appreciate the true beauty of Black women, and thus we become overly critical of our physical appearance.

All of these factors influence the difference in the health and wellness of African American women compared to other racial and ethnic groups. The disparity between Black women and other women remains a major source of concern. As a group, we have more persistent health problems and we die at an earlier age. This was a fact when we entered the past century a hundred years ago, and the disparity still exists today.

Reports from the Department of Health and Human Services on Black and minority health reveal that African American women have higher death rates from the Big Four causes of death than all other women—Caucasian, Asian/Pacific Islander, Hispanic, and American Indian women. The statistics that follow clearly demonstrate the severity of these diseases, as well as mental health concerns, among Black women.

- African American women are twice as likely to die from strokes as Caucasian women are.
- African American women and men are 30 percent more likely to die from cancer than any other racial or ethnic group. Cancer is the top cause of death for African American women in our middle years.
- One in every four African American women in midlife has diabetes—that is double the rate of White women. Black women are also twice as likely to develop the complications associated with diabetes: heart disease, stroke, kidney failure, blindness, and amputation of the legs or feet.
- Approximately 50 percent of all African American women report depressive symptoms during their lifetime. This is almost twice the rate of depressive symptoms experienced by males and almost 50 percent higher than Caucasian women.
- Anxiety disorders are two to three times more common in African American women than in Black men.

In addition, we are more apt than our peers to have multiple physical and emotional problems. For example, we are more likely to have both heart disease and depression, hypertension and anxiety, hypertension and depression. We also have more risk factors—such as hypertension, obesity, stress, and lack of exercise—that give rise to physical and emotional problems. This demonstrates how important it is for you to pay attention to your mind and body.

## AGNES' STORY

Agnes, sixty, has experienced bouts of depression throughout her adult life. She has never been to a mental health professional because she has not wanted to admit to anyone that she couldn't handle her own problems. When she and her partner of ten years broke up, Agnes regained the thirty pounds that she had spent years trying to keep off, and she became quite depressed. Controlling her hypertension also became a major problem.

While trying to lift a lamp, Agnes realized that she was having pain again in her upper back and some shortness of breath. She had attributed her growing sense of fatigue and difficulty breathing to her weight gain and allergies. However, she was in such distress that a friend insisted they go to the emergency room. There Agnes was diagnosed as having a heart attack.

How many women like Agnes do you know? Agnes demonstrates the connection between depression and heart disease and also the vague and nonspecific symptoms of a heart attack. Periodic depression, sadness, low mood, or "the blues" is often part of life and its inevitable losses. But ignoring a low mood that goes on for more than two weeks can endanger your health.

We know right now you're saying: "Oh, no, here we go again! We Black women always get the worst of everything." But the fact of the matter is that *it does not have to be that way*. We *can* do something about it. We have a great deal more information than our foremothers did about our bodies, and we have ways to stay healthy and prevent illness. A growing body of scientific research suggests that chronic illness is not an inevitable consequence of aging, as our American culture and the medical community long believed. Today, the prospect of living to be a hundred years old is not far-fetched; in fact, it's within our reach.

We as health professionals and African American women are convinced that Black women don't have to die too soon — especially from preventable illnesses. This conviction is the primary reason that we decided to write this book. We are compelled to try to help Black women and other health professionals stem the daily tragedy of African American women dying prematurely. We want you to hear and heed the urgency in this book. We are talking to you as a Black woman — *now is the time to start taking better care of yourself first.* By doing so, you also will help *all* Prime Time African American women in your life live longer and healthier lives, too.

Taking better care of yourself means implementing specific self-care behaviors and also becoming a more informed and active partner with your doctor and other health-care providers. Embracing self-care and forming active partnerships with health-care providers are critical components in preventing disease and illness through routine annual physical exams, ongoing evaluations, and the promotion of good health through adopting a healthful lifestyle.

We know that some of you have had (or know someone who has had) negative experiences with conventional health-care providers and maybe you are concerned about whether you can trust the medical community. However, as health-care providers ourselves, we can say to you that most of our colleagues are well-meaning. And despite the ignorance, racism, sexism, and ageism that is still too commonplace, you can find competent, caring, culturally sensitive, trustworthy health-care providers.

You should also know that the advice and recommendations offered throughout *Prime Time* embrace the healing philosophies of a variety of health-care practitioners. So we authors are not asking you to give up your natural healer, chiropractor, or acupuncturist, because we believe that alternative healers can be an important part of your health-care team. These days, integrating alternative practices with Western medical advances makes sense, since they complement each other in many ways. But to make conventional and alternative treatments work for you, you must inform all the members of your health team about the various interventions that you are using.

# Chapter 3

# THE MIRACLE OF YOU

*I am the light of the world.*
*I am an instrument of the Divine.*
*I am the greatest miracle in the world*
— Iyanla Vanzant, *One Day My Soul Just Opened Up*

We are miracles. Think about it. No, really, think about it! We have within us the divine. Most of us believe in a higher power, a spirit, or a force outside of ourselves. However, what is striking is that no matter what we call this power—God, Yahweh, Jehovah, Christ, Allah, The Buddha, Yemaya (a Yoruba goddess)—believers in every religion profess to be claimed and loved by this power. As Neale Donald Walsch writes in his best-selling book *Conversations with God*: "Every Master, Jesus, The Buddha, Krishna, has had the same message: 'What I am you are. What I can do, you can do. These things and more shall you also do.'"

Christians believe that they are made in God's image. According to Romans 8:17, we are not only God's children, but "joint heirs" with Christ of God's kingdom.

As African American women, we have an ancient spiritual legacy. In Egypt, some of the most important deities were female.

- Isis' healing powers were able to ward off evil and undo destructive acts.
- Sekhnet had priests and priestesses who specialized in medicine.
- Hathor and Serget are the goddesses of fertility and nurturing.
- Maat represented truth, balance, and harmony.

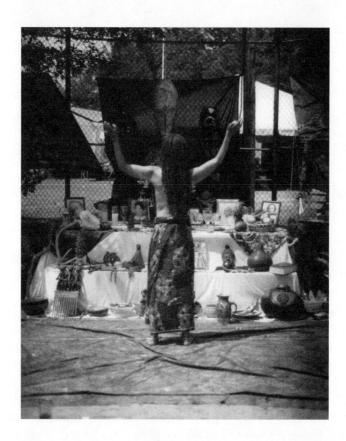

Many Egyptian temples—Hathor's was extremely well known—were early infirmaries or hospitals. Priestesses were often also midwives, providing gynecological and obstetrical care.

Many of the ancient goddesses (or orishas) of West Africa—Eyulie and Lemanya among them—continue to be major influences in several Caribbean religions, including Shango, Vodun, and Santería. *Sangomas* are women in Swaziland who provide both medical and spiritual diagnoses and advice through divination (a process that attempts to determine whether an event has a natural or unnatural cause). Throughout the Caribbean and in many parts of the United States, there are numerous women who continue to function as both priestesses and healers in these traditional religions.

In all of these religions, spirituality and health were and continue to be closely intertwined. It is only when both are in harmony that people are considered to be leading healthy, balanced lives.

Even when Black women did not function as overt physical healers, their ministerial work provided an emotional balm and a powerful motivating voice in their communities. They continued the holistic practice of their ancestors. Christian Black women evangelists, including Sojourner Truth, Jerena Lee, and Rebecca Jackson, made invaluable contributions to the abolitionist movement.

Because of sexism, many women religious leaders were denied ordination in Black churches. However, even without a formal license, they championed various social, educational, and religious causes. Their spirituality and sense of connection to a higher power affected every aspect of their lives. We have benefited enormously from the spiritual gifts of our ancestors.

Most of us have experienced the power of faith directly or through the stories, songs, poems, and prayers of our forebears. We know in our bodies, minds, and souls that our survival across the Middle Passage and triumph over the brutality of centuries of slavery were not arbitrary, capricious acts of nature. **We are part of a greater plan.** Our task today, in these times, is to acknowledge and accept the reality of the miraculousness that surrounds us.

The miracle of being alive is especially apparent in your biology. There never has been and never will be anyone who is exactly like you. Each of us is unique. Our genetic and biochemical makeup and our fingerprints are our own. Even identical twins with identical genetic makeups often have different personalities.

The miracle of our lives is continuously being affirmed and reaffirmed by our religions and our genes, in our spirits and in our bodies. So why is it that we women so often act as if we don't believe we are special? Gayle and her mental health colleagues frequently listen to the stories of loving, caring, responsible women who have accepted years of emotional and sometimes physical abuse from their spouses or partners, boyfriends, girlfriends, children, parents, colleagues, and employers. Many women smoke, overeat, or abuse alcohol to "manage" their stress. Marilyn sees women whose diabetes or hypertension is not being controlled or who are in the last stages of breast, cervical, or lung cancer. Many of these women can afford good health care but did not see to their own needs because they were too busy working or taking care of others.

Why do we ignore our miraculous bodies? Why do we allow others to demean us? Why do we fail to honor and affirm the divine within us? Each of us could probably provide an explanation, from the sublime to the ridiculous, for why we don't consistently honor and care for the miracle of our lives. But we believe that this quote from Nelson Mandela's inaugural address offers a valuable explanation and an invaluable prescription for change:

Our deepest fear is not that we are inadequate. Our deepest fear is that we are powerful beyond measure. It's our light, not our darkness that most frightens us. We ask ourselves, who am I to be brilliant, gorgeous, talented, and fabulous?

Actually, who are you not to be? You are a child of God. Your playing small doesn't serve the world. There's nothing enlightened about shrinking so that other people won't feel insecure around you.

We were born to make manifest the glory of God that is within us. It's not just in some of us; it's in everyone. And as we let our light shine, we unconsciously give other people permission to do the same. As we are liberated from our own fear, our presence automatically liberates others.

Once we confront our fear and accept that we are miracles, our lives are forever changed. And then our work truly begins. As Dr. M. Scott Peck writes in *The Road Less Traveled*, "If we seriously listen to this 'God within us'—we usually find ourselves being urged to take the more difficult path, the path of more effort rather than less."

If we truly believed that we are miracles and contain the divine within us, there is no way that we could smoke. It would be like blowing smoke in God's face. Whatever support groups we had to join, patches we had to wear, cravings we had to withstand, periods of irritability we had to endure, we'd do it.

If we truly believed that we are divine, we could not ignore or minimize unending fatigue, unrelenting sadness, or ongoing insomnia. We'd be racing to find someone—a psychologist, pastoral counselor, social worker, psychiatrist—who could help us develop and implement strategies to gain or regain control of our emotional and physical health so that our divine light could shine through.

If we truly believed that we are miracles, instead of spending so much time making negative comments about our appearance, hair, or size, we would be celebrating our kindness, generosity, wisdom, perseverance, work ethic, thoughtfulness, and ability to love and be loved.

If we truly believed that we are miracles, we wouldn't neglect our temples, our bodies, by "forgetting" to schedule our annual physical checkups or medical tests such as mammograms or Pap smears. These tests are modern miracles themselves—they can help save our lives. We also would ensure (as much as possible) that we work with competent health professionals with whom we have established a positive, trusting relationship.

# **R** PRIME TIME PRESCRIPTION FOR INCREASING SPIRITUALITY

*I am complete,*
*Perfect in God.*
*So I do not*
*covet or*
*envy or*
*resent the*
*reality of any*
*human being.*
*I know my Self.*
*I offer no*
*resistance to*
*the Gift*
*of God*
*in*
*me.*

—Rev. Cecilia Williams Bryant, *Kiamsha—*
A *Spiritual Discipline for African-American Women*

What we're telling you is true. You are a miracle and you contain the divine within yourself. Acting as if we are miracles and developing a strong spiritual base can both provide us with the moral courage we need to make more difficult decisions and lifestyle changes and reduce our rates of morbidity and mortality. Studies from universities and medical centers across the country—Duke, Johns Hopkins, Dartmouth, San Francisco General Hospital—have documented that the prevention of, and recovery from, emotional and physical illness, substance abuse, and surgery are significantly influenced by our level of spiritual connectedness.

• Seriously depressed patients who become more spiritual reduce their depressive symptoms 70 percent more than patients who didn't.
• Weekly churchgoers died 50 percent less often from heart disease, emphysema, and suicide and 74 percent less often from cirrhosis than did infrequent church attendees.
• Women who attended church weekly were one-third less likely to die prematurely from any illness than those who didn't.

• Strong religious affiliation had a greater effect on blood pressure than any other health habit.

• Cardiac patients who were, unbeknownst to them, prayed for were five times less likely to require antibiotics and six times less likely to require artificial ventilation.

To draw on your spirituality and increase your wellness, you might need to assess and develop your conscious practice of faith in daily life. To help you do this, complete the Wellness and Transcending Questionnaire below. It will give you a look at your current spiritual state.

## WELLNESS AND TRANSCENDING QUESTIONNAIRE

This questionnaire can help you assess your perception of your degree of wellness. The higher your score, the greater your sense of wellness.

| Yes | Often | Sometimes, maybe | No, rarely | |
|---|---|---|---|---|
| | | | | 1. I perceive problems as opportunities for growth. |
| | | | | 2. I consider myself to be an integral part of some greater plan.* |
| | | | | 3. I experience synchronistic events in my life (coincidences that appear to have no cause-and-effect relationship but happen more often than chance would dictate).** |
| | | | | 4. I am aware of experiencing miracles in my daily life.*** |

\* Exploration of your views about the universe have considerable impact on how you live your life, and hence your personal wellness.
\*\* Modern physics reveals that the idea of cause and effect may be as limited as Newton's theory of a mechanical universe. It suggests that we must expand our view to see that everything in the universe is connected to everything else. (The word *synchronicity* describes that experience.)
\*\*\* Occurrences that seem to fall outside the realm of causality may be experienced as miraculous, but may just indicate our ignorance of the way things are. They can become everyday phenomena when accepted as a normal part of life.

| Yes | Often | Sometimes, maybe | No, rarely | |
|---|---|---|---|---|
| | | | | 5. I am comfortable about knowing things without understanding precisely how I know them (intuition). |
| | | | | 6. I believe there are dimensions of reality beyond verbal description or human comprehension. |
| | | | | 7. I sing, pray, chant, or meditate with other people, and experience a sense of unity in doing so. |
| | | | | 8. The concept of God has personal definition and meaning to me. |
| | | | | 9. I experience a sense of wonder and awe when I contemplate the universe. |
| | | | | 10. It is okay with me if certain things are unknowable to the mind. |
| | | | | 11. I am aware of a part of me that is greater than my mind, body, and emotions. |
| | | | | 12. I trust and use the part of myself that has a greater wisdom than my mind. |
| | | | | 13. I experience a merging of my consciousness with a larger sense of consciousness (universal mind). |
| | | | | 14. I allow others the freedom to believe what they want without pressuring them to accept my beliefs. |
| | | | | 15. I enjoy practicing a spiritual discipline or allowing time to sense the presence of a greater force in guiding my passage through life. |

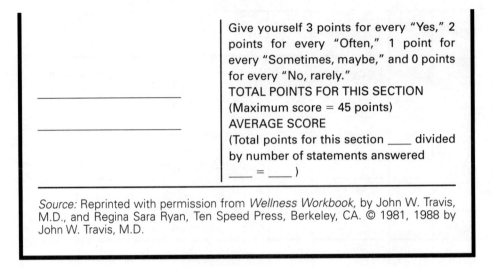

Give yourself 3 points for every "Yes," 2 points for every "Often," 1 point for every "Sometimes, maybe," and 0 points for every "No, rarely."

TOTAL POINTS FOR THIS SECTION (Maximum score = 45 points)

AVERAGE SCORE

(Total points for this section ____ divided by number of statements answered ____ = ____ )

Once you've determined your areas of spiritual strength and vulnerability, follow these steps to enhance your overall spirituality:

• *Pray or meditate at least once a day.* You might start and end each day with at least ten minutes of focused attention on a word or phrase that has spiritual meaning for you.

• *Read daily from a spiritual or religious work.* Try the Bible, the Koran, Cecilia Williams Bryant's *Kiamsha: A Spiritual Discipline for African-American Women,* or Iyanla Vanzant's *Acts of Faith: Meditations for People of Color.*

• *Join a religious or spiritual community.* Participate with a faith group on a regular basis. Learn about the power of prayer and practice it often. Get involved in activities that will help other people, especially those who are less fortunate than you are. Get to know the people in the group.

• *Start writing in a journal to capture thoughts that flow through your mind as you read this chapter.* Use these notes to identify areas of your life that you need to improve. Our advice throughout the book will help you map out strategies to make these necessary changes.

We invite you, as Sisterfriends, to celebrate with us the miracle of being alive, and to use your spiritual power to take charge of your health. You may just decide to take a leap of faith and believe us. Or perhaps this chapter has reminded you of your God-given right and responsibility to take care of yourself. However you choose to celebrate with us, we look forward to sharing this divine experience with you.

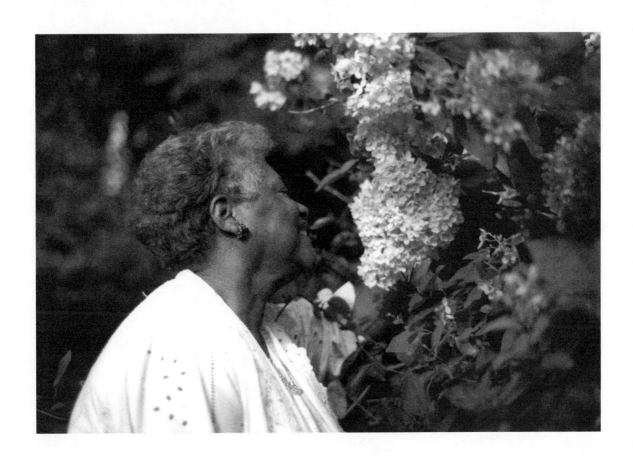

# PART II

# Reframing Your Priorities

# Chapter 4

# NOW YOUR JOURNEY BEGINS

*A thousand-mile journey begins with a single step.*

—Chinese proverb

The first step in taking charge of the Prime Time of your life is to reframe your priorities. To do that, you must first change the way you think. Consider this Yoruba proverb: "For no man can be blessed without the acceptance of his own head."

The power of positive thinking certainly isn't a new philosophy—you've surely heard of this idea before, perhaps in the teachings of Dr. Norman Vincent Peale, who was known to say: "Change your thoughts and you change your world." You may even recall being taught this Bible verse in Sunday school: "For as he thinketh in his heart, so is he" (Proverbs 12:7). You probably remember your grandmother or aunt repeating this old adage: "Thinking is believing."

As a physician and a clinical psychologist, we strongly believe in the power of positive thinking. It's worked in our lives. It will work in yours. Both of us—Gayle and Marilyn—grew up very poor, living in low-income housing ("the projects") at a time when racism and sexism were even more overt and restrictive and there were few to no role models in our future professional fields. (Marilyn's community had a few African American medical doctors, but Gayle didn't meet a Black woman clinical psychologist until she was in college.) Nevertheless, we were taught to believe that we could overcome any obstacles to achieve our dreams.

To become—or continue to be—a healthy, active, optimistic person in your middle years, you must open your heart and mind to examine long-held thoughts and perceptions. Have any of the guiding principles in your life become outdated? Are the perceptions that have influenced your decisions and actions all of your life now *mis*perceptions? These outdated beliefs may be barriers to your enjoying your Prime Time life.

For instance, in our twenties and thirties, most women equated beauty, creativity, intellectual curiosity, vibrancy, and sexiness with youth. Some women still do, but we have plenty of role models today who are in their forties, fifties, or sixties who also represent these qualities. Who would argue that model Beverly Johnson is beautiful, Maya Angelou is creative, Angela Davis is an intellectual powerhouse, Tina Turner is vibrant, or actress Pam Grier is sexy? These are all women in the Prime Time of their lives. They negate conventional ideas about middle age as they live their lives on their own terms.

Just ponder this idea from the late comedian Moms Mabley: "If you keep thinking the same old things in the same old way, then you'll keep doing the same old things in the same old way. And, of course, you'll keep getting the same old things you always got."

So if you think that high blood pressure, a thick waist, and a lackluster sex life are inevitable conditions of your middle years, then you will never buy into the idea that increasing your consumption of fruits and vegetables, exercising, and learning to meditate could prevent these stereotypical signs of aging. But they *can!* Remember, positive change all starts with a thought that something is possible. Better health is possible for you. A vital midlife is possible for you.

> Sow a thought and reap an act,
> Sow an act and reap a habit,
> Sow a habit and reap a character,
> Sow a character and reap a destiny.
>
> —Author unknown

Learning to realign your thinking in positive ways—especially in your time-squeezed middle years—isn't always easy. It sometimes takes practice, and we'll help you with that. The challenges of everyday living—such as a sick parent, a nagging pain, or a looming deadline at work—do have a way of filtering out the joy in your heart, often leaving you feeling exhausted, stressed, and overwhelmed. But taking a little time to reframe your thinking can empower you to make changes that will transform how you feel—physically, emotionally, and spiritually. Reflect on these words of *Essence* magazine editorial director Susan Taylor: "Thoughts have power. And you can make your world or break your world by your thinking."

Keeping Susan's wise words in mind, complete the following exercise:

---

## HOW DO I THINK OF MYSELF?

If the statement reflects your thinking, circle TRUE. If the statement does not reflect your thinking, circle FALSE.

1. I am my number one priority.
   
         TRUE      FALSE

2. I have a positive perception of myself.
   
         TRUE      FALSE

3. I have an upbeat outlook about the middle years of life.
   
         TRUE      FALSE

4. I have a wellness philosophy that guides how I live each and every day.
   
         TRUE      FALSE

---

By the time you finish this book, we hope that you will be able to answer all four of these questions in the affirmative, if you haven't already. If any of these affirmations or beliefs are not true for you now, *Prime Time* will help you reevaluate and change your perceptions and improve your life and your health.

We know that examining and evaluating the way we think about ourselves and how we lead our lives has a way of dredging up painful childhood memories, missed opportunities, mistakes, and bad decisions that shaped our lives. However, the key to successfully reframing your thinking is not to dwell on the negative events in your life. And once you've addressed how you think, you'll see what you need to change.

*It is more blessed to give than to receive, so give to yourself as much as you can, as often as you can.*

—LaVerne Porter Wheatley Perry, quoted in
*African American Wisdom: The Classic Wisdom Collection*

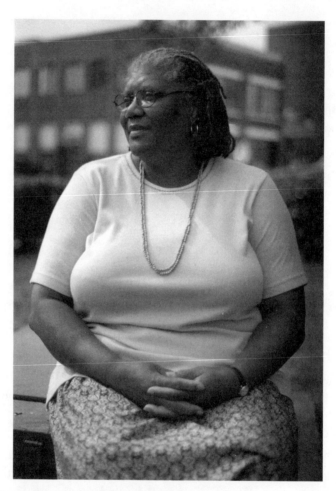

## 1. You Must Be Your Number One Priority

This is the major change we want you to make in your thinking. It sounds simple—so simple that you may think we're overemphasizing it. But stop and really think about how putting your needs before the needs of others would change your life. What comes to mind? How do you feel when you say out loud: "I must be my number one priority?" Do you feel determined, embarrassed, or guilty?

For many women, concentrating on what we want and acting to get what we desire can be quite a difficult concept to accept and accomplish. For African American women in particular, focusing on our own needs may be the most significant challenge we face as we struggle to improve our health and well-being. We grew up watching our primary role models—mothers, grandmothers, and aunts—put everyone else's needs before their own. We learned by their example to do the same. In fact, we were often taught that to think of ourselves first was selfish or even sinful.

By the time we reach our middle years, we have had a great deal of experience trying to please our parents, siblings, spouses or partners, and children. The habit of always cooking, cleaning, and doing for others is deeply ingrained in many midlife Black women. All too often, we attend to the needs of our friends, families, jobs, the church, or others long before we take care of ourselves. We don't even stop and ask ourselves when we're going to do something about our fatigue, our stress, our physical health. Both of us authors understand completely what you are facing; we have faced the same challenge.

We understand that you love and care about your children, parents, spouse, partner, job, and church and that they occupy places of special importance in your life. However, think about this for a minute. Remember the last time you were on an airplane? The flight attendant's instruction on using oxygen masks is always consistent: In case of a drop in air pressure, **put the mask on yourself first, before you help anyone else—even your children!**

A medical fact also demonstrates this point: After blood circulates through the lungs and picks up its valuable load of oxygen, it travels to the heart to be pumped to the rest of the body. But the heart grabs its oxygen *first*, before sending the rest of the oxygenated blood on its way to the other organs and tissues of the body.

The message is clear. We must be in good shape—mentally, physically, and spiritually—before we can ever hope to be of service to others. Therefore, you must take charge of and take care of yourself first! If there is one change we want you to make in your life among all the recommendations in this book, it is to make **your life** your priority.

In fact, probably the most profound directive was given by Jesus when He said, "Love others as you love yourself."

**℞** PRIME TIME PRESCRIPTIONS TO HELP YOU BECOME YOUR NUMBER ONE PRIORITY

*Learn to recognize the cues that prompt you to put the needs of others before your own.* Sometimes the cues are very subtle, such as choosing to drive your daughter to her friend's house or to the movies or to the mall instead of getting to your aerobics class on time. Other times the cues are more overt, such as getting a headache whenever your boss asks you to work overtime as you're walking out the door. Either way, what's most important is that you recognize these cues and change your response to them.

---

## IDA'S STORY

Recently a friend of ours realized why a call from her thirty-five-year-old son always caused her to move into her "mother stance" to help him, take care of him, or do for him. She realized that her triggering cue was when he called her Mom.

This simple three-letter word conjured up memories of her son as a baby and how much he needed her then. She had to break the habit of responding to her adult son as if he were still a dependent child.

Fortunately, Ida's solution was simple. The devoted mother called her son with this special request: "From now on when you phone, please call me Ida instead of Mom."

---

*Establish daily, weekly, and monthly goals.* These will help you change your routines to become more about you and what you need. Some ideas you should consider:

• Every day spend at least thirty minutes enjoying time with just you—no one else—listening to music, reading, soaking in the bathtub, or just daydreaming.

• Every week do something you really enjoy. Attend a support group, go to a movie, check out a museum, or listen to a lecture.

• Every month take 10 percent off the top of your monthly pay and deposit it in a savings account or mutual fund that is just for you. The amount of your monthly income doesn't matter. If your monthly income is $100, deposit $10; if it's $10,000, deposit $1,000. You'd be surprised to know how much having a nest egg of your own can increase your peace of mind.

According to the late African American theologian, modern mystic, and Harvard School of Divinity professor Howard Thurman, quoted in Sam Keen's *Fire in the Belly*, "There are two questions that we have to ask ourselves: 'Where am I going?' and 'Who will go with me?' If you ever get these questions in the wrong order you are in trouble."

## PRIME TIME SELF-CARE SCALE

Use this exercise to estimate the amount of time you spend in an average weekend:

A. Taking care of others as compared to yourself
B. Thinking and worrying about others as compared to yourself

The first step is to complete the table below with the name of the significant people in your life, e.g., parent, child, spouse/partner, and estimate the number of hours each day on the weekend you spend taking care of them (column A) and thinking and worrying about them (column B). Consider twelve hours each day for a total of twenty-four hours for the entire weekend.

Add the total hours (a total of twenty-four for the weekend), and then calculate the total hours dedicated to all others versus the total hours dedicated to you in each column—A and B.

The next step is to show the total hours you spend on yourself in the form of a bar and the total you spend on the others in column A on bar chart A to actually see the time you give yourself compared to the time you give others. Do the same in bar chart B for column B.

Place this chart somewhere you'll see it often as a daily reminder of where you need to change the amount of time you spend on *you*.

| Significant People | Name | A<br>Time<br>(Caring for) | B<br>Time (Thinking and Worrying) |
|---|---|---|---|
| YOU | Your Name | Hours | Hours |
| Spouse/Partner | | | |
| Children | | | |

| | | | |
|---|---|---|---|
| Parents | | | |
| Friends | | | |
| Grandchildren | | | |
| Church | | | |
| Job | | | |
| Add others: | | | |
| | | | |
| | | | |
| | | | |
| | | | |
| Total | | 24 (12 hrs a day, Sat. and Sun.) | 24 hrs (12 hrs a day, Sat. and Sun.) |

Example:

| A | B |
|---|---|
| Hours | Hours |

A

B

| Hours | Hours |
|---|---|

A

B

## 2. You Must Have a Positive Perception of Yourself

As we like to remind you, you are a miracle. Once you truly believe that, it will be easier to put yourself first, take care of yourself, and affirm and honor yourself every day. Just reflect on Oprah Winfrey's advice: "The more you praise and celebrate your life, the more there is in life to celebrate."

You must love yourself with your whole mind, heart, and soul if you are to stay well. Love yourself and you will live longer. If you're a sister with high self-esteem, you will live longer and healthier than someone with low self-esteem.

A study at the University of Wisconsin—Madison suggests that those who think well of themselves are happier with their lives, social relationships, and overall health. Women participants in the study who had a positive self-image were more physically active and reported having lower blood pressure. Conversely, women with low self-esteem were more likely to be overweight and to smoke, drink more alcohol, and expose themselves to dangerous situations. According to psychologist Dr. Duane Hurst, "Our physical health, our behaviors and how we regard ourselves are intertwined. These components contribute to our total well-being. So it's important to take steps that can help you feel better about yourself."

Unfortunately, many women have the habit of negative "self-talk," which often consists of critical comments about ourselves. Do any of these examples sound familiar?

- I should have done this sooner.
- I need to be a better parent.
- My nose is too big.
- I always have a bad hair day.
- I'm too fat.
- I'm not smart enough.
- I can't do that.
- I never do anything right.

Sometimes all this negative nonsense gets translated into a mental and physical message that says, "I'm not good enough." Because thoughts are powerful, what you say becomes what you do and who you are. Since the pattern of putting yourself down often starts in childhood, you must make a conscious effort to stop destructive self-criticisms from influencing your life script. Now is the time to reframe these demoralizing ideas into positive Prime Time Life Scripts.

It's all about how you view yourself in this world. The goal is to become inwardly secure and begin to touch the authentic power of who you are.

**℞** **PRIME TIME PRESCRIPTIONS TO IMPROVE YOUR PERCEPTION OF YOURSELF**

**Assess and change your self-talk.** Complete the following two self-talk exercises to examine your positive and negative inner thoughts. This insight will help you develop a more encouraging Prime Time Life Script.

---

## SELF-TALK EXERCISE #1
## CREATING YOUR PRIME TIME LIFE SCRIPTS

1. List the three most negative things that your parents, other family members, and teachers have said about you in your presence.
   a. _____
   b. _____
   c. _____
2. List the three most negative things that you say about yourself.
   a. _____
   b. _____
   c. _____
3. List the comments that are the same in numbers 1 and 2.
   a. _____
   b. _____
   c. _____

---

## SELF-TALK EXERCISE #2
## CREATING YOUR PRIME TIME LIFE SCRIPT

1. List the three most positive things that your parents, other family members, and teachers have said about you in your presence.
   a. _____
   b. _____
   c. _____
2. List the three most positive things that you say about yourself.

a. _____

b. _____

c. _____

3. List the comments that are the same in numbers 1 and 2.

    a. _____

    b. _____

    c. _____

For many Black women, it's easier to say negative things about ourselves than to make positive statements. As children, we often were told that humility and self-denigration were synonymous and that "pride rideth before a fall." Thus we must take proactive steps to change this habit of self-abasement.

*Adopt an optimistic perspective on life.* Optimistic people have a more positive attitude. Researchers have also found that optimistic people have higher immune cell activity, which helps fight off disease. Using the stress management techniques described in Chapter 13 can help you develop a more hopeful approach to life. To get you started, though, complete the exercise below to assess your level of optimism.

Each morning before Amina, a colleague, leaves the house, she puts her list of five positives in her wallet, and each night before she goes to sleep she takes it out and reads it.

## ARE YOU AN OPTIMIST OR A PESSIMIST?

To use this quiz, vividly imagine yourself in each of the situations described, and choose one explanation. If neither choice seems to fit, choose one anyway. Don't choose the explanation that you believe you should or the one that would seem right to other people. Be yourself, and decide which explanation is more likely to apply to you.

1. You forgot your spouse's birthday.

    a. I'm not good at remembering birthdays.

    b. I was preoccupied with other things.

2. You owe the library a hefty fine for an overdue book.

    a. When I am really involved in what I am reading, I often forget when it's due.

    b. I was so involved in a project at work that I forgot to return the book.

3. You are penalized for not returning your income tax forms on time.

a. I always put off doing my taxes.

b. I was lazy about getting my taxes done this year.

4. You've been feeling down lately.

a. I never get a chance to relax.

b. I was exceptionally busy this week.

5. You lose your temper with a friend.

a. He/she is always nagging me.

b. He/she was in a hostile mood.

6. A friend says something that hurts your feelings.

a. My friend always blurts things out without thinking of others.

b. My friend was in a bad mood and took it out on me.

7. You fall down a great deal while skiing.

a. Skiing is difficult.

b. The trails were icy that day.

8. You gain weight over the holidays, and you can't lose an ounce.

a. Diets don't work in the long run.

b. The diet I tried didn't work.

Give yourself 1 point for every a answer, 0 for every b answer. The lower your total score, the more optimistic you are. A total of 0 points or 1 point means you are extremely optimistic, 3 points or 4 points equates to about average optimism, and anything higher means you're a pessimist!

*Source:* Adapted from Martin Seligman, *Learned Optimism,* 1996.

*Start each day reading something positive such as a favorite meditation, a scripture, or the* **Daily Word.** When you wake up, acknowledge the presence of God. Acknowledge that you are a miracle and a gift to the world.

Look in the mirror and say three positive things about yourself. Focus on your appearance and character. Start each day with this Zora Neale Hurston quote: "Such as I am—I am a precious gift."

*Set two small, manageable goals each week: one personal, one professional.* For example, the personal goal should be something that brings you pleasure, such as a walk through your favorite park or a visit to a museum. The professional goal might just be cleaning off a corner of your desk.

## HOW OPTIMISTIC ARE YOU?

1. List five positive factors in your life.
   a. _____
   b. _____
   c. _____
   d. _____
   e. _____
2. List five negative factors in your life.
   a. _____
   b. _____
   c. _____
   d. _____
   e. _____
3. Every day, take a moment to write out five current positive and negative events that affect your life. You want to acknowledge the events on both lists, but you want to be deliberate in focusing most of your time and energy on the positive ones. Try to resolve as quickly as possible the small negative events and break the larger negative events into smaller pieces.

Even life-altering stressful situations can be helped by positive reframing. For example:

*You've just been given a medical diagnosis that will require an extended hospital stay and aftercare.*

*The first step is to think about the positives that can come out of this experience. Now that you and your medical team know what the problem is, you can start developing an appropriate treatment plan. You have an opportunity to really think about and possibly reassess your long- and short-term goals. You now have additional motivation to change your lifestyle so that you're prioritizing your needs.*

*The second step is to list the things that must be done in descending order of importance and start thinking about who can help with each task. Informing your personal and professional support network of the tasks that need to be done might reveal how you have more support than you knew. This situation can provide you with an opportunity to start eliminating unnecessary responsibilities from your life.*

Again, the key to improving any situation is to recognize that there are multiple ways of assessing it. Make a conscious effort to always look for the best in any situation.

## 3. You Must Develop an Upbeat Outlook About the Middle Years of Life

> *Age is a question of mind over matter. If you don't mind, it doesn't matter.*
> —Satchel Paige

As Black women, many of us grew up with old, tired, negative, or ambivalent thoughts and mental pictures of midlife. We loved and respected our elders, but we laughed at their rolled-up stockings, heavily powdered faces, blue hair, and wigs. To test your perceptions and misperceptions about midlife, take the midlife questionnaire below.

---

### HOW DO YOU FEEL ABOUT BEING A WOMAN AT MIDLIFE?

Have you started thinking about your perceptions of midlife? The questionnaire below will help you sort through your feelings about this important time in your life.

1. I am or was most attractive at age _____.
Why? _____
_____

2. Telling my age is: (circle one)
              EASY       DIFFICULT
Why? _____
_____

3. Coloring my hair is something: (circle one)
    I ALWAYS DO    I SOMETIMES DO    I NEVER DO
Why? _____
_____

4. Growing older is: (circle all that apply)
    WONDERFUL    FRIGHTENING    ANGERING
    HORRIBLE    EXCITING    CHALLENGING
Why? _____
_____

---

5. What is my most significant challenge in getting older?

_____

_____

6. What is my most significant opportunity in getting older?

_____

_____

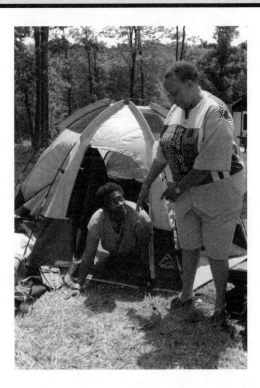

Aging in our community, as in our culture at large, is not considered positive. Middle age is seen as the bridge to old age, a time of gradually diminishing vigor and opportunities, empty nests, stress and worry, poor health, menopause, and crises. Everywhere we turn, we are bombarded with images in print, on television, and in movies that paint a dismal picture of the aging process: wrinkling, graying, thickening. Clinging to the facade of youth, we spend a great deal on cosmetics, dyes, and plastic surgery to mask the signs of growing older. Yet these expenditures have no real influence on the quality or length of our lives. On the other hand, an investment in developing and maintaining a positive outlook and a healthy lifestyle can make a profound and lasting difference.

A recent, large research project by the John D. and Catherine T. MacArthur Foundation Research Network on successful midlife development paints a far different portrait of midlife than that held by most Americans, one that shatters the cultural perceptions of these middle decades. This ten-year study involving eight thousand Americans in midlife found this to be the best time of their lives. The participants described midlife as a time to enjoy stable relationships, financial security, good health, and satisfying, relatively secure work. Less than 10 percent of the participants reported any type of "midlife crisis."

The study also found that although nearly everyone in midlife goes through changes, "most move through it successfully and come out with different aspirations." Because of similar findings in their own work, Cornell University researchers have suggested that the term "midlife crisis" be replaced with a more optimistic phrase such as "turning point." The researchers believe that midlife can signify "a period in time in which a person has undergone a major transformation in views about the self, commitments to important relationships, or involvement in significant life roles, e.g. job, marriage." Evolution, not crisis, is the hallmark of middle age.

The MacArthur Foundation study also found that most of its subjects felt ten to twenty years younger than their chronological age, were more satisfied and happier with their work and marriage than when they were in their twenties and thirties, and felt more in control of their lives.[1]

Based on interviews of hundreds of women in middle life for her book *New Passage: Mapping Your Life Across Time,* author Gail Sheehy found that many women today see midlife as a time of rebirth and regeneration—a time to concentrate on becoming "better, stronger, deeper, wiser, funnier, freer, sexier, and more attentive to living the privileged moments."

Women of all racial and ethnic groups can easily find resonance in the words of one interviewee in Sheehy's groundbreaking book: "I've let the children fly off into their own lives, but even more important, I've left the nest myself."

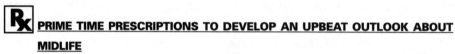

## ℞ PRIME TIME PRESCRIPTIONS TO DEVELOP AN UPBEAT OUTLOOK ABOUT MIDLIFE

*Every day, spend time thinking about the benefits of having lived as long as you have.* Think about how much knowledge and wisdom you've gained over the years. Congratulate yourself on the important things you have accomplished. Consider how much more confident you are now than when you were younger.

*Read books by and about African American women who have accomplished personal and/or professional achievements during their middle years.* To get started, try these compelling books:

- *American Hero* (Barbara Jordan's biography) by Mary Beth Rogers
- *Angela Davis: An Autobiography*
- *I Tina: My Life Story* by Tina Turner
- *I Will Survive* (autobiography) by Gloria Gaynor
- *Lanterns: A Memoir of Mentors* by Marian Wright Edelman
- *Between Each Line of Pain and Glory* (autobiography) by Gladys Knight

*Practice saying positive and grateful statements about aging to yourself and to others.* Here are some statements that might work for you:

- I thank God that I've lived long enough to learn something new.
- I thank God that we've been together long enough to celebrate our thirtieth wedding anniversary.
- I'm so grateful for being healthy enough to play with my grandchildren or help my parents through their transition as senior citizens.

*Celebrate all of your birthdays.* Remember, either you're getting older or you're *dead!* Many cultures celebrate aging and honor the older members of their society for their wisdom and experience.

*Initiate a midlife celebration day in your church, club, and other organization.*

## 4. You Must Embrace a Holistic Wellness Philosophy

As you take charge of your health, we also want you to change the way you think and feel about health and illness. Illness is not inevitable in your life. You have a lot of power over your body and mind, and you can use that to get and stay well. We'll help you become an empowered, informed participant in the creation of your own health. Wellness and health are not merely the absence of illness or disease. You achieve wellness and good health by paying attention to your entire self—your physical, emotional, and spiritual life.

Dr. John Travis and Regina Sara Ryan capture the essence of this lifelong journey to wellness in the introduction to the second edition of their *Wellness Workbook*:

> *Wellness* is a choice—a decision you make to move toward optimal health.
> *Wellness* is a way of life—a lifestyle you design to achieve your highest potential for well-being.
> *Wellness* is a process—a developing awareness that there is no end point, but that health and happiness are possible in each moment, here and now.
> *Wellness* is an efficient channeling of energy—energy received from the environment, transformed within you, and sent on to affect the world outside.
> *Wellness* is the integration of body, mind, and spirit—the appreciation that everything you do, and think, and feel,58
>  and believe has an impact on your state of health.
> *Wellness* is the loving acceptance of yourself.

Our words *health* and *healing* are from an Old English root word meaning "whole." And, of course, *whole* means "integration," "unity of all the parts; completeness." So taking care of your mind, body, and spirit makes you whole and healthy.

The Old English word meaning "whole" is also the source of our word *holy*. Our ancestors knew that healing and wholeness are holy, and in fact,

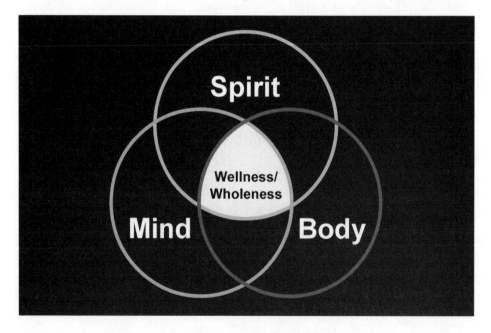

the work of the healers was considered to be a sacred task. The earliest physicians practiced their healing in temples and were thought to be holy men and women, or priests. Somehow, with the growth of modern Western medicine, the spiritual aspects of healing dissipated, and today physical health has its set of practitioners and their places of practice in one corner, with mental health in yet another corner, and the church away from it all.

Living in wellness and health will not only improve the quality of your life now and in the future, it will extend the number of healthy years you will live. Tina Turner's doctor of sixteen years, Dr. Rajendra Sharma, says the dynamic singer may live another sixty years because of her daily regimen of healthy nutrition, exercise, relaxation, and meditation.

To improve the quality of your life, we will help you develop proactive new regimens for preventing disease and illness and promoting health and wellness. Simply reacting to illnesses and treating their symptoms when they occur will not make you truly healthy. Instead, you want to learn to identify the deeper reasons for your mind-body vulnerabilities and turn those vulnerabilities into strengths. For instance, after a pressured time at work, do you always develop a cold? Do you get frequent lower back pain, and does it get worse after arguments with your children or partner over money? Those cold germs and that potential muscle tension are always there, but why do you suppose they take hold in your body only at certain times?

Our parents and forebears grew up in a time when illness was considered unavoidable. It "just happened." And in all fairness, there were elements of truth to that, since many of the illnesses were related to infectious agents and were transmitted through unsanitary and overcrowded environments. Poverty and racism also subjected many African Americans to living and working conditions that compromised their immune systems and made them susceptible to disease.

Now, however, the major killers are not infectious diseases (with the exception of AIDS), but chronic illnesses (such as heart disease, cancer, hypertension, and diabetes), depression, and stress. Today we have much more control over our wellness and can prevent many illnesses. We have more control over how soon we will die and from what.

*These days, good health is about choices.* It's about understanding the choices we're making and the chances we're taking. With choice comes responsibility. You are the one most responsible for maintaining your health. You are the one who will prevent illness from occurring and who will get yourself the right treatments should it occur. You must consider yourself a proactive partner with your health-care provider. No one—not your doctor, your family, or your insurance company—can keep you as healthy as you can. You are in charge.

Taking an active role in your health requires some effort and some common sense. But the payoff is incredible. First, you will be healthier. Second, you won't suffer as much from illness because you will be helping yourself heal. Third, you will reduce the need for necessary hospitalizations and spend less money on treatments. And finally, you will feel more productive and vital, and you'll enjoy a better quality of life.

Your body is a temple of the Holy Spirit. If you truly believe this, you will act differently and revere your body.

> *Or do you not know that your body is a temple of the Holy Spirit who is in you, whom you have from God, and that you are not your own? . . . Therefore, glorify God in your body.*
>
> —1 Corinthians 6:19–20

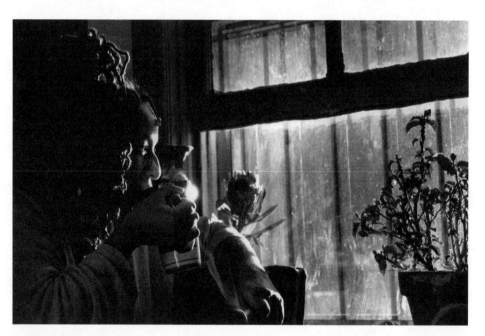

### ℞ PRIME TIME PRESCRIPTIONS FOR DEVELOPING A HOLISTIC WELLNESS PHILOSOPHY

*Learn the major risk factors for the emotional and physical stressors and illnesses to which you are most vulnerable during these middle years.* We will discuss these critical issues in the chapters that follow.

*Develop daily habits of prevention* (e.g., relieving stress, exercising, using proper nutrition). A complete Prime Time Personal Wellness Plan is outlined in Part III of this book: "Putting Self-Care into Action."

*Select the health insurance plan that gives you the best coverage.* You're worth the extra money. Include physical and emotional options and preventive assessments. To learn more about what is covered in various types of health insurance policies, go to Chapter 19: "Become a Smart Health-Care Consumer."

*Find health-care providers who expect you to be active in your self-care and who use a comprehensive and holistic approach.* We'll show you how in Chapter 19.

## TAPPING THE POWER AND STRENGTH OF SISTERHOOD: YOUR PRIME TIME SISTER AND PRIME TIME CIRCLE

As you start your journey toward becoming fully Prime Time, consider enlisting the aid of one of your midlife friends so you can share and help each other through the process. Find someone with whom you enjoy sharing your feelings, someone who is trustworthy, dependable, and willing to be objective, someone who is also making midlife changes. Think of this friend as your Prime Time Sister.

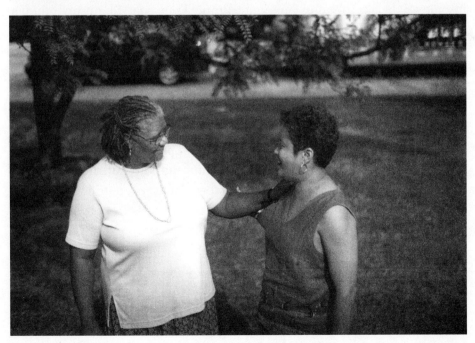

For many African American women, asking for help can be difficult. Embracing the myth of the strong Black woman, we try to fend for ourselves, even when it's obvious that we could use a helping hand. The time to pull out that badge of honor is not when you're trying to make radical, life-altering changes. You *can* make important life changes on your own (with the guidance of this book) if you don't have a Prime Time Sister. However, working with a trusted friend can make the difference between achieving your dream of healthy, happy, satisfying middle years or feeling too overwhelmed to make the necessary changes that will reinvigorate your life.

The secret of a successful Prime Time Sister relationship is identifying a friend who also is determined to make some midlife corrections in her life. That way you can develop a true partnership in this exciting venture. Sharing your thoughts and feelings with a sisterfriend who is having similar experiences, concerns, and doubts is extremely helpful. You can provide each other with emotional support, as well as sound a warning bell when either one of you makes a wrong turn or stumbles. This sure works for us!

In fact, we provide each other with constant support as we travel on our individual journeys. We have agreed to share information and feedback about behaviors—emotional, intellectual, and physical—that we're trying to change. And then we celebrate when we've successfully made a transition. We also sound a warning bell when one of us reverts to old habits—especially if someone breaks the most important Prime Time rule: "I am my number one priority." It's also our job to suggest ways to get back on track. As Prime Time Sisters, we laugh together, pray together, exercise together, and talk seriously about personal and professional concerns and challenges.

To make this partnership work for you, you and your Prime Time Sister should read this book together, discuss it, plan together, and remind each other of goals, timetables, and important dates to keep, such as medical appointments or exercise classes. You will also need to support each other as you break unhealthy habits such as smoking or overeating and substitute healthy behaviors, such as meditation and learning to prepare balanced, nutritious meals.

We also believe in the power of African American sisterhood. In fact, our circle of sisterfriends are often our escape from the stressors we face. One of the most appealing aspects of Terry McMillan's best-selling book-turned-movie *Waiting to Exhale* is the close friendship of the four women and their ability to share important parts of their lives. We find strength and solidarity in the company of other African American women. Sisters seek sisters for celebration, for emotional support, for healing, and to feel connected to ourselves in ways we can't experience with other groups. As Dr. Christiane Northrup writes in *Women's Bodies, Women's Wisdom*: **"When I am with women I am getting a chance to be all of who I am, to say whatever is on my mind. You get a tremendous amount of self-trust because you hear your own words coming back to you, you see your own experience coming back to you, and you don't feel crazy."** That's why we encourage you and your Prime Time Sister to form a Prime Time Circle of Sisterfriends—six to eight African American women in midlife who are willing to provide you with a support network.

Having a diversified mix of concerned and supportive women friends to talk to and share ideas with can help you and your Prime Time Sister face the tough transitions you will make as you work through the advice and recommendations in this book. The women in your circle must be committed to making changes in their lives, and they must be willing to share information, bring in experts to address questions and clarify conflicting advice, and provide a forum for discussion about each other's particular concerns. For instance, our group of sisterfriends meets once a month to go to a play, see a movie, enjoy a concert, view a museum exhibit, attend a lecture, or meet for lunch or dinner at one of our favorite restaurants. We take turns planning the outings and making the arrangements. We also talk about issues with which we are struggling and use each other as sounding boards.

In addition, we all know that a certain special energy is generated when women come together. Psychotherapist Ruth Berlin, cofounder of Inner Source: A Center for Psychotherapy and Healing, located in Annapolis, Maryland, notes that right-brain traits thought of as feminine—such as being receptive, collaborative, and nurturing—are helping to shape a right-brained new culture. Dr. Berlin explains: "The feminine energy, the ability to really honor one's intuition or gut feelings, is becoming stronger. People are coming to understand that on a universal, cosmic level there is enormous power in that feminine energy."

## Choosing Your Prime Time Sister

Traits of a good Prime Time Sister include the ability to listen, supportiveness, and truthfulness. A good Prime Time Sister will encourage you to go for a walk even though you claim you're too tired. She's willing to praise you when you meet your budget or your weight goals. So before you ask someone to be your Prime Time Sister, get a sense of how well she might do by filling out the questionnaire below.

# PRIME TIME SISTER QUESTIONNAIRE

Fill in the name of your potential Prime Time Sister in each blank line, and then circle whether the statement is true or false about her. At the end of the questionnaire, add the points for each true and false answer to determine the score.

1. _____ is someone who could tell me the truth even if I wouldn't like it.

TRUE      FALSE

2. _____ is not trying to make some positive changes in her own life.

TRUE      FALSE

3. If I lost my job, _____ would probably fill my refrigerator.

TRUE      FALSE

4. _____ would insist that I try her Patti LaBelle macaroni-and-cheese dish even though she knows I'm trying to lose weight.

TRUE      FALSE

5. If I were moving at 6 A.M. on a Saturday morning, _____ would be there at 5 A.M. with a cup of coffee.

TRUE      FALSE

6. I could tell _____ the most embarrassing moment in my life.

TRUE      FALSE

|          | Points |       |
| -------- | ------ | ----- |
| Question | True   | False |
| 1        | 5      | 1     |
| 2        | 1      | 5     |
| 3        | 3      | 1     |
| 4        | 1      | 5     |
| 5        | 5      | 1     |
| 6        | 5      | 1     |

If your potential Prime Time Sister scored:
- Between 22 and 28 points, you have a great Prime Time Sister.
- Between 16 and 22 points, reconsider your choice.
- Less than 15 points, find someone else.

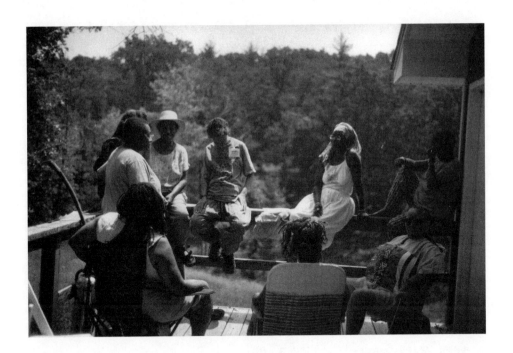

To start your Prime Time Circle of Sisterfriends, ask several friends if they would be interested in meeting on a regular basis to share recreational events and discuss topics that are of particular concern to women in midlife. It's probably best to limit the group to six to eight women who are determined to make some of the changes that we recommend in this book. If you're new to an area or you don't know many Black women interested or willing to focus on change, you can call various Black organizations and institutions, including churches and chapters of the National Black Women's Health Project, to ask if they know of Black women's support groups. You can also find local organizations or groups of women who meet to focus on particular issues from a Black perspective, including sexual preference, parenting, and investing. Look in the Resources section for some contacts to start your search.

Once you've picked your Prime Time Sister, decide what each of you needs to address and how you intend to work together to meet your goals. Before you make the final commitment to help each other, both of you may want to consider agreeing to the principles of the Sisterhood Affirmation, developed by Dr. Sandra Y. Lewis, vice president of the International Congress of Black Women:

## SISTERHOOD AFFIRMATION

*We are Sisters bound by our African ancestry,*
*And our commitment to each other,*
*Our people*
*And by the Creator who brought us into being.*

*Our sisterhood spans generations of women*
*who shared a cup of sugar or flour,*
*took turns sitting with a sick child,*
*or held a Sister's hand in hard times.*

*As reflections of each other,*
*we recognize our Sisters' experiences as our own.*
*We share in our trials and tribulations,*
*our joys and sorrows, and our triumphs.*

*In keeping with our African tradition,*
*we value the power of the spoken word.*
*When speaking of each other,*
*we choose our words carefully.*
*With every word, deed, or thought,*
*we affirm and uplift each other.*
*As we give of ourselves, we reap the benefits of*
*Maat, the spiritual principle of reciprocity.*

*In all things we honor our commitment to each other,*
*resisting any and all forces which may seek to divide us.*

Now that you have a partner to share this life-changing adventure, you need to understand why changing each of the four beliefs that we discussed earlier in this chapter is so essential to the overall success of all the suggestions made throughout this book. Read on.

# Chapter 5

# SELF-ESTEEM: BELIEVING IN YOURSELF

*I love myself when I'm laughing*
*And then again when I am*
*Looking mean and impressive.*

—Zora Neale Hurston, quoted in Diane J. Johnson, ed.,
*Proud Sisters: The Wisdom and Wit of African-American Women*

*One of the nicest realizations that I've come to over the past two years is that*
*I'm finally learning to love all of my selves.*

—Wista Johnson, quoted in Diane J. Johnson, ed.,
*Proud Sisters: The Wisdom and Wit of African-American Women*

How you think about yourself and value yourself as a person affects your ability to reframe your priorities and put your own needs first. You want to act out of your belief in yourself. You want to accept your uniqueness and importance, and celebrate your life. You want to acknowledge the blessings in your life, but sometimes that's difficult to do.

Instead of operating from a frame of mind that we are "miracles of God," many African American women use external gauges to measure their self-esteem. In fact, we talk about our self-esteem as if it were a barometer that goes up or down depending upon whom we're with or how we look: "Girl, when I was with that womanizing so-and-so, my self-esteem was in the toilet" or "Now that she's lost all that weight, I know her self-esteem has improved."

As Prime Time Black women living in America, we need to *run* from any definition of self-esteem that implies or overtly states that our value depends on *any* external condition. From the perspective of a culture that worships youth, thinness, athletic ability, and money, most Black women would be deemed worthless and expendable. Tying your self-esteem to the impression or reaction of others can have a devastating effect, so you as an African American woman must learn to think of yourself positively. Value yourself unconditionally.

---

## RUTH'S STORY

Ruth is a fifty-five-year-old director of a Head Start program. She has been married to Joel for almost twenty-five years. They met in college and were called the "pretty couple." Ruth exercises regularly and is in good health, but she has never regained the flat stomach or lost all of the weight she gained after three pregnancies. Joel frequently makes snide comments about her "sagging breasts." Ruth spends a great deal of time, money, and energy on her appearance—her hair, nails, makeup, and clothes. She is seriously considering plastic surgery to get rid of her wrinkles and to flatten her abdomen.

Joel has always been flirtatious and has gotten more so as he has grown older. He frequently makes sexual comments to or about younger women. Ruth usually laughs or pretends she doesn't hear them, but she suspects that Joel has had an affair or two, especially during her pregnancies. At her fiftieth-birthday party, Joel gave Ruth a blown-up, framed picture of her when she was twenty-five.

He paraphrased one of Moms Mabley's jokes by saying that "the only thing an old woman can do for me is show me where a young woman is." Ruth later told a friend that she was so embarrassed that everyone had seen that picture and realized how old she now looked. Then she told her friend: "My self-esteem was shot to hell."

---

Think about it: Ruth didn't say that she was embarrassed or that her self-esteem was "shot to hell" because she had stayed in a relationship for twenty-five years with a disrespectful, emotionally abusive idiot. She said her self-esteem was compromised because she didn't look the way she did when she was twenty-five. If our self-esteem is so fragile that it's vulnerable to changes in our appearance or other people's perceptions of us, we need to take dramatic steps to change.

This chapter will explore the true meaning of self-esteem and present ways to help you develop and maintain self-esteem consciously, constantly, and unconditionally.

## WHAT IS SELF-ESTEEM AND WHY IS IT IMPORTANT?

In *The Anxiety and Phobia Workbook*, Dr. Edmund J. Bourne defines self-esteem as "a way of thinking, feeling, and acting that implies that you accept, respect, trust, and believe in yourself."

Having self-esteem affects how you function intellectually, emotionally, and physically. Stories like that of Ruth's reaction to her husband's unkind comments as well as formal studies attest to the observable differences in the behaviors of people who have high and low self-esteem.

Women with high self-esteem think well of themselves and are confident of their ability to make positive changes in their lives. They are productive, flexible, and competent. They celebrate their achievements and acknowledge and learn from their mistakes. They operate in their personal and professional lives openly, honestly, and assertively. These women love themselves. Their diet, grooming, and exercise routine indicate that they take care of themselves. They treat others in a loving, respectful, thoughtful manner.

Women who suffer from poor self-esteem are often anxious, depressed, and angry. These women frequently think or make negative comments about themselves and others, such as "I'm ugly," "I'm fat," "She's stupid," "I'm too old," "She's boring," or "I'm unlovable." Low self-esteem often makes them ineffective, unprofessional, and incompetent. Their personal lives are frequently filled with mates and friends who have emotional and behavioral difficulties—such as addictions, poor money management, abusive tendencies, or employment problems—because women with self-esteem problems believe they can attract only this kind of person.

*Self-acceptance* is the critical component in self-esteem—it is our ability and willingness to accept and value ourselves regardless of whether we have made momentous achievements, tragic mistakes, or decisions that have brought positive or negative repercussions into our lives.

In the *Power of Self-Esteem*, Dr. Nathaniel Branden writes that self-acceptance "refers to an attitude of self-value and self-commitment that derives from the fact that I am alive and conscious." Accepting and valuing yourself unconditionally does not mean that you have to approve of all your behaviors. It means that you can differentiate between who you are and what you do or what you possess.

## CLAUDIA'S STORY

Claudia's affair with her husband's business partner was exciting and fun. Without a doubt, she still loved her husband, who was a wonderful spouse and father to their two children, but twenty years of marriage had left Claudia a bit restless. And even though Claudia was a friend of her lover's wife, she saw the affair as being harmless and simply adding "spice to her life."

When Claudia tested positive for syphilis, despair set in. Once she told her husband that he had to be tested for syphilis, she knew that their marriage would probably be over. The news of her affair would also have a devastating effect on his business relationship.

After mentioning thoughts of suicide, Claudia was encouraged to go into psychotherapy. The forty-nine-year-old patient told her therapist that she felt worthless and would never be able to face her children or the rest of her family. She constantly berated herself throughout her initial sessions and refused to even consider the possibility of forgiving herself. After several months of therapy, Claudia was able to forgive herself and then was able to focus on how and why she had made such poor decisions. Only at that point could she start the process of making meaningful positive changes in her life.

Acknowledging and accepting that we are fallible human beings who can sometimes act in a reprehensible manner at a particular moment in time can give us the courage to learn a different way of acting at another moment in time.

*Self-respect* is another important element in self-esteem. Author Nicki Giovanni expresses it this way in *Proud Sisters: The Wisdom and Wit of African-American Women*: "Deal with yourself as an individual worthy of respect and make everyone else deal with you in the same way." And the Staple Singers sang about it in "Respect Yourself." The message, however, is always the same: We have to respect and honor ourselves and treat ourselves with reverence if we expect others to treat us in that manner.

## JEWEL'S STORY

Jewel is everyone's "other mama." Her children and grandchildren all live in different cities. Jewel is sixty-four years old, is retired, and lives on a fixed income. Her next-door neighbor often asks Jewel to baby-sit but never offers to pay or even to send any food with her children. Jewel loves the kids but realizes that they make a real dent in her food budget.

Frequently, whenever any of her family members or their friends come to town, Jewel picks them up from the airport and provides them with free room and board. Jewel enjoys the company, but during the summer months she often laughingly complains to her friends that she feels as if she's running a taxi service and bed-and-breakfast gratis.

Jewel finally became mildly annoyed when her granddaughter, without asking Jewel, suggested that a friend and her cat could stay with Jewel while the friend searched for an apartment. Exasperated, Jewel shared her dilemma with friends. Their response was shocking to her. They all felt that Jewel was being too passive and ignoring her own feelings and needs. Their advice: "Don't get angry, be assertive! Tell your granddaughter that her friend has to find another place to stay."

---

*Self-trust* is another integral part of self-esteem. It allows us to rely on our intuition and to maintain an inner balance and consistency, no matter how much things change around us. We can depend on our thoughts and behaviors to be congruent with one another. Trusting yourself can help you make the right decisions and not compromise your values.

---

## SHARON'S STORY

Sharon, fifty-seven, is the accountant for a medical center that has been having severe financial problems. A major part of the crunch is the exorbitant salaries of the CEO and his administrative team. Sharon has become increasingly concerned about discrepancies between the financial reports that she has seen prepared for the center's board of directors and those prepared for the administrators.

When Sharon expressed her concerns to the financial administrator, she was assured that everything was fine. She was also reminded that her pay increase and bonus were both going to occur in the next few months. Sharon's instincts and experience told her that something was wrong, but she didn't want to cause any trouble and jeopardize her pay raise or possibly her job.

Sharon usually gave the financial report at the board meeting, but as the meeting got closer, she became increasingly distressed. Sharon finally shared her concerns with her husband and her best friend, who both told her that she had to trust her feelings and do what she thought was right.

Sharon told her boss that she would not be able to give the presentation at the board meeting because it was not consistent with what she thought was accurate. He halfheartedly argued with her but finally told her he'd take care of it. Sharon knew that she needed to start looking for another job.

---

Sometimes when you decide to do what you believe is right, you have to make major and often difficult changes in your life. But when faced with such a choice or change, keep in mind the words of *Essence* magazine's editorial director, Susan Taylor, cited *Proud Sisters: The Wisdom and Wit of African-American Women:* "My pain, my changes, have been the major source of my growth. We cut our teeth on our changes; they force us to expand and become the people we are meant to be."

*Self-confidence* is the belief that we have the ability to achieve our goals and the right to fulfill our dreams despite adversity. It is a cornerstone of self-esteem. In fact, African American history is full of women who achieved their dreams despite tremendous odds—Harriet Tubman, Madame C. J. Walker, Mary McLeod Bethune, Maya Angelou, Oseola McCarty, and Oprah Winfrey, as well as many of our mothers, grandmothers, aunts, and friends. Obstacles ranging from slavery and poverty to sexual abuse have not prevented Black women from actively pursuing goals that seemed impossible to achieve. Camille Cosby said it best:

Given the odds, we weren't supposed to stop being slaves.
Given the opposition, we weren't supposed to have an education.
Given the history, we weren't supposed to have families.
Given the blues, we weren't supposed to have spirit.
Given the power of the enemy, we weren't supposed to fight back.
Not only have we achieved victories, we have—despite the powers against us—become our own victories.

Midlife African American women are part of this powerful force. We are continuing the heritage of our formidable foremothers.

## OBSTACLES TO POSITIVE SELF-ESTEEM

Certain childhood and adult experiences can make it extremely difficult for individuals to develop or maintain a sense of authentic, consistent self-worth. But although we can overcome these life events and learn to feel positive about ourselves, we must explore and understand the origins of the negative thoughts and feelings we have about ourselves to make necessary changes.

### Parents Make a Difference

Parents are never a neutral influence on us. Good, bad, or indifferent, their behavior can affect us for a lifetime. For instance, parents who constantly express negative or extremely critical comments such as "You're stupid," "You're too fat," "You're lazy," or "Why can't you be like . . ." can diminish their offspring's ability to perceive themselves as competent, capable adults. On the other hand, children of overindulgent parents often have difficulties accepting appropriate limitations, allowing someone else to be the center of attention, taking no for an answer, initiating and following through on projects, or getting to work on time.

Overly protective parents can diminish their children's willingness to try new things, take risks, or feel safe and secure away from their families. Adult children of smothering parents often turn down opportunities for professional advancement if they must move away from their birth homes, and some are reluctant or unwilling even to go to dinner or a movie alone.

Parents who are rejecting or neglectful can damage a child's expectation that her own needs will be met, and can undermine her sense of security, safety, and even belief in her right to be alive.

Physical, emotional, and sexual abuse by a parent can make it extremely difficult for children to trust themselves or anyone else. Often victims of abuse become abusers themselves, or they unconsciously put themselves in situations where they can be victimized again. Women who are substance abusers or chronic victims of domestic violence or repeat rapes frequently have been abused as children.

Growing up with parents who were substance abusers (including alcoholics) increases a child's risk of being insecure, secretive, and unable to acknowledge his or her feelings. Such children are also at greater risk of being addicted to various illegal drugs and prescription and over-the-counter medications. However, we know that many Black women, including singers Etta James and Natalie Cole, kicked their addiction to alcohol and other drugs, changed their lifestyle, and regained their self-esteem.

## Sexism and Racism

Throughout our lives, Black women are bombarded with racist and sexist comments in movies, television programs, news reports, and music.

### Childhood experiences

Many of us grew up in families where our skin color, hair texture, weight, and features were considered fair game for anyone to discuss. "Big lips," "big butt," "nappy hair," and "ashy skin" were terms often used by our caretakers or other people who we knew cared about us, and these descriptions were usually accompanied with a smile and an admonition to us to not get upset. If we expressed any sadness or anger, we were accused of being thin-skinned, acting like a baby, or being unable to take a joke. When, as children, we were confronted with contradictory messages from people on whom we depended and about whom we cared, it can be difficult for us as adults to trust our assessments of other people.

Separating our innate value and worthiness from our appearance can be difficult, especially if our own families were preoccupied with appearance. One friend remarked that while she thought her mother loved her, she never felt that her mother thought she was okay. She said, "My mother was always fixing my hair, tucking my blouse in, putting Vaseline on my ashy legs, arms, and face. Something was always wrong with me. On the other hand, I knew my father loved and delighted in me because he never cared how I looked."

### Adult experiences

Even if we were fortunate enough to be protected from overt racist and sexist experiences as children, we are inundated with them as adults. Our very absence from television, movies, and plays can have an insidious, negative effect on our self-esteem. Wouldn't you love to see a television program about assertive, diverse Prime Time Black women or a movie about an African American couple in their middle years who have a loving relationship?

Another major strain on African American women's self-esteem is highlighted by psychotherapist Julia Boyd in her book *In the Company of My Sisters: Black Women and Self-Esteem:* "There are so many expectations about Black women that the 'me' in each one of us can get lost in the daily shuffle." Being perceived (in our own minds and in the minds of others) as a strong Black woman, everybody's caretaker, "the mule of the world," and sexy all in one can be exhausting at best, depressing at worst. When we can't do what can't be done but are told that we should be able to do it and that our mamas and grandmamas are/were able to do it—and we believe it—our self-esteem can be devastated.

## LIVING THE SIX PILLARS OF SELF-ESTEEM

Accepting self-worth as part of your birthright as a human being is consistent with the major religious teachings. Certainly in Christianity, God's love and grace are gifts—they are not and cannot be earned.

> *For by grace are ye saved through faith; and that not of yourselves: it is the gift of God: Not of works, lest any man should boast.*
> —Ephesians 2:8–9

Believing that unconditional self-esteem is your right may be easier than accepting that you are responsible for developing your own sense of value or worth. Responsibility can be a frightening prospect. It means that as an adult, you can't blame your lack of self-esteem on any of the following external forces: other people (parents, spouses or partners, children, siblings, extended family, friends, Caucasians, employers, coworkers), your life circumstances (race, sex, age), your appearance (being obese, thin, light, dark, tall, short), or your professional or financial status. None of these things should affect how well you value and treat yourself. Claiming your right to feel good about yourself is more difficult when you've experienced some of the obstacles we mentioned above, but you *can learn* how to value yourself unconditionally.

Unconditional self-esteem does not mean that you have no room for self-improvement. In fact, striving to achieve personal, interpersonal, or professional goals without tying your sense of worth to the outcome can be quite liberating. Sometimes you'll succeed; sometimes you'll fail. The key is to continue trying to improve your skills without linking your overall worth to the success or failure of each attempt. Having the freedom to take risks without judging yourself harshly allows you to be open and honest with yourself and others about your vulnerabilities. It is much easier to accept constructive criticism when you view it not as a condemnation of your entire being, but as information you can use to assess and help change a part of your behavior.

Most of us Black women in midlife were not raised to have unconditional self-esteem, but with persistence and practice, you can learn to accept, respect, trust, and believe in yourself unequivocally. In *The Six Pillars of Self-Esteem*, psychologist Dr. Nathaniel Branden describes six practices that he believes are crucial for developing and maintaining unconditional self-esteem:

1. The practice of living consciously
2. The practice of self-acceptance
3. The practice of self-responsibility
4. The practice of self-assertiveness
5. The practice of living purposefully
6. The practice of personal integrity

## 1. The Practice of Living Consciously

> To live consciously means to seek to be aware of everything that bears on our actions, purposes, values, and goals—to be the best of our ability, whatever that ability may be—and to behave in accordance with that which we see.
>
> —Dr. Nathaniel Branden, *The Six Pillars of Self-Esteem*

Refusing, as Paul Lawrence Dunbar describes it, to "wear the mask that grins and lies" can be very difficult. It requires that we not only stay open to the truth, but actively seek it.

In Chapter 6, "Confronting the Two A's: Attitude and Anger," we discuss our ancestors' need during slavery to distort, hide, and deny their true feelings. As bell hooks writes in *Sisters of the Yam: Black Women and Self-Recovery*, many of us have continued to use denial and lying as a way of negotiating life. Gayle and her colleagues in the health professions see many women (individually and in groups, especially Black women in support groups) who refuse to acknowledge their own self-destructive behaviors. For instance, many of these women won't admit that:

• Their spending patterns are in any way connected to the fact that they're on the verge of bankruptcy ("Saks had this great sale, and I won't have to buy another coat for several years")

• Their lack of positive job evaluations or promotions is in any way connected to their chronic patterns of lateness, unplanned absences, and unfinished work ("Yeah, I'm late sometimes, but she's got her picks")

• Their depression is related to allowing physically healthy adult children, siblings, or friends to live with (and sponge) off them ("Phil's ex-wife took him to the cleaners and he's trying to get himself together. I know it's been five years, but he's my brother")

• Their behavior influences their children's behavior ("I beat her butt when she told me that she lied to the teacher the way she's seen me lie")

• Their refusal to require sexual partners to wear condoms is the source of their sexually transmitted diseases ("I don't know how I got gonorrhea, because neither one of us is playing around")

## Rx PRIME TIME PRESCRIPTIONS FOR LIVING CONSCIOUSLY

Learning to be honest about your actions and feelings requires that you change your behavior.

• *Ask yourself these two questions: What will you gain if you change your behavior in that problem area? What will you lose?*

• *Read self-help books or take classes to help yourself address your vulnerability and overcome or compensate for it.*

• *Join or start a Prime Time support group or go into individual or group therapy.*

• *Affirm your right to love and value yourself every day.*

## 2. The Practice of Self-Acceptance

*In the grand scheme of things, most of the actual failures we will experience are not nearly as harmful as the damage we do to ourselves when we obsess and worry about our failures yet to come.*
—Dr. Daniel Wegner, quoted in *Your Emotions, Your Health: Using Your Mind to Heal Your Body*

Although it's important to accept that love, approval, achievements, mistakes, and deliberate wrongdoing are significant events in your life, *it's wrong to define yourself by any one event or multiple events*. The past does not dictate how you must live your life. To accept and believe this completely, however, you will probably need to change your views about midlife and adopt the positive view of your potential and power that we recommend in Chapter 4, "Now Your Journey Begins." For instance, does either of these statements describe how you feel?

• It is a dire necessity for me to be loved by everyone who is significant to me.

• I must be thoroughly competent, adequate, and successful in all important respects to be considered worthy and worthwhile by myself and others.

If you answer yes to either one of these statements, then you should carefully study the Prime Time Prescriptions below. No one can ever be loved by everyone all the time or be at the top of her form twenty-four hours a day. Having these expectations is unrealistic and should not be the standard by which you judge yourself. You certainly shouldn't base your self-esteem on meeting these expectations.

### $\mathbf{R_x}$ PRIME TIME PRESCRIPTIONS FOR EMBRACING SELF-ACCEPTANCE

*Learn to view mistakes as opportunities for learning.* Doing so will give you the courage to try again. Look at each mistake and try to find the lesson inherent in it.

*Recite the Serenity Prayer daily to help you prepare for the vicissitudes of life and accept them.*

*Read autobiographies and biographies of women* (such as Angela Davis, Gladys Knight, and Shirley Chisholm) whose lives were full of failures and successes to remind you that you are not alone. We all face difficult times, joyous times, and everyday ups and downs.

## 3. The Practice of Self-Responsibility

Accepting responsibility for your life can seem like a double-edged sword, especially for Black women. Deciding that you are responsible for how you treat yourself, how you interact with others, and how you fulfill your dreams means that *you* control your fate—at least as much as is possible. As Black women, we are so tired of being responsible for so many *other* people and so many things that we refuse to acknowledge that it is our responsibility to change our *own* chronic state of unhappiness, sadness, anger, or indebtedness.

Iyanla Vanzant describes, in *The Value in the Valley*, the difficulty that many Black women have in admitting that they had something to do with the situation they are in. In the chapter entitled "Valley of Comeuppance," she encourages readers to assess how their decisions affect the people and situations in their lives: "You know you are in this valley when you find yourself surrounded by negative people, in negative situations, having negative experiences."

In individual and group sessions, Gayle and her colleagues often listen to women complaining that "his [drinking/womanizing/gambling/smoking] makes me so unhappy." Interestingly, these women seem genuinely shocked when the group asks them: "Why do *you* choose to be unhappy or to stay in a situation where you are unhappy?" One woman was enraged when her support group asked her why she hadn't gone to Al-Anon (a support group for family or friends of alcoholics), left her abusive, alcoholic husband, or put him out. Her response: "Why should I have to do anything? He's got the problem." She was astonished when the group explained: "But you're the one who's unhappy."

Unfortunately, many women of every color don't entertain the idea that we are responsible for our own happiness. But it is an absolute truth that the pursuit of happiness sometimes requires us to change our beliefs, our behavior, our surroundings, or our partners. And when all these changes happen at once, as they sometimes do, take comfort in knowing that God or whatever higher being you look toward for guidance had a hand in it, to help us learn a profound lesson.

Vanzant suggests that we must forgive ourselves for not putting ourselves first. We must also forgive others for impeding us. Only then can we eliminate the negative thoughts and emotions that create negative effects in our lives, and get on with putting our needs first.

Accepting responsibility for the quality of your life is the first step in claiming your power to control it. Proactively confronting ideas that can drain you of your emotional strength is the next step. Challenging an irrational belief can also be an important step in becoming more responsible for yourself. An irrational statement such as "There isn't much I can do about my [low self-esteem/anger/sadness/depression] because it is caused by what happens to me and how others treat me" can be countered with "There are things that other people do. I disagree with them and disapprove of them, but I am responsible for how I allow their behavior to affect me."

### ℞ PRIME TIME PRESCRIPTIONS FOR TAKING RESPONSIBILITY FOR YOUR ACTIONS

*Select a specific problem in your life on which to start practicing responsible behavior.* Make a commitment to give immediate attention to changing those areas of your life where you're having difficulty, such as in relationships at work, parenting, or finances. (You'll find more help with these topics in Parts V and VI.) For instance, if you're facing financial difficulties, then schedule an appointment with yourself each week to carefully (and honestly) look at how much you've spent compared to what your budget could handle. Being honest about why you're overbudget is the first step to responsible financial behavior. Getting help, such as financial counseling or reading practical personal financial advice, such as Suze Orman's *The 9 Steps to Financial Freedom* and Brooke Stephens' *Talking Dollars and Making Sense*, is the next step.

*Use your Prime Time Circle to help you stay focused* on accepting responsibility for that problem and changing it by doing what you need to do.

# 4. The Practice of Self-Assertiveness

Expressing your needs and wants in a direct, honest manner and taking steps to ensure that they are met reinforces your perception of yourself as a valuable, worthy human being.

**Rx** **PRIME TIME PRESCRIPTIONS FOR BECOMING MORE ASSERTIVE**

*Practice the assertiveness techniques described in Chapter 6 on attitude and anger.*

*Read books on assertiveness and the "Valley of Courage" chapter in Vanzant's* The Value in the Valley.

*Use your Prime Time Circle to help you challenge irrational beliefs.*

*Read Dr. Edmund J. Bourne's Personal Bill of Rights, from his* The Anxiety and Phobia Workbook, *every day until you have assimilated these principles into your being and feel and act from their truth.*

## Personal Bill of Rights

- I have the right to ask for what I want.
- I have the right to say no to requests or demands I can't meet.
- I have the right to express all of my feelings, positive or negative.
- I have the right to change my mind.
- I have the right to make mistakes and not have to be perfect.
- I have the right to follow my own values and standards.
- I have the right to say no to anything when I feel I am not ready, it is unsafe, or it violates my values.
- I have the right to determine my own priorities.
- I have the right not to be responsible for others' behavior, actions, feelings, or problems.
- I have the right to expect honesty from others.
- I have the right to be angry at someone I love.
- I have the right to be uniquely myself.
- I have the right to feel scared and say "I'm afraid."
- I have the right to say "I don't know."
- I have the right not to give excuses or reasons for my behavior.
- I have the right to make decisions based on my feelings.
- I have the right to my own needs for personal space and time.
- I have the right to be playful and frivolous.

- I have the right to be healthier than those around me.
- I have the right to be in a nonabusive environment.
- I have the right to make friends and be comfortable around people.
- I have the right to change and grow.
- I have the right to have my needs and wants respected by others.
- I have the right to be treated with dignity and respect.
- I have the right to be happy.

*Photocopy the above list and post it in a conspicuous place. By taking time to read through the list every day, you will eventually learn to accept that you are entitled to each one of these rights.*

## 5. The Practice of Living Purposefully

Set short- and long-term personal and professional goals and objectives to demonstrate your self-esteem. Be disciplined, focused, and persistent to achieve them. How many of us have spent more time helping our children or grandchildren with their homework or their college applications than we've spent developing our own professional skills and options?

In *Sisters of the Yam*, bell hooks reminds us, "Learning how to think about work and job choices from the standpoint of 'right livelihood' enhances black female well being." For most Black women, being employed is an integral part of our self-esteem. Thus "right livelihood" means that we find jobs where the work is meaningful, reflects our values, and fully utilizes our skills.

**Rx PRIME TIME PRESCRIPTIONS FOR LIVING PURPOSEFULLY**

*Take a vocational assessment test at a local junior college if you're not certain that you are in a career that suits your personality, interests, or skills.*

*Take time out to relax and rejuvenate,* for as bell hooks warns us, even if we love our jobs, we risk burnout if we don't balance our professional responsibilities with leisure activities.

*Use your Prime Time Circle for reality checks to ensure that your behaviors are consistent with the personal and professional goals you've set.*

# 6. The Practice of Personal Integrity

*This above all: to thine own self be true.*

—William Shakespeare

In *The Six Pillars of Self-Esteem*, Dr. Branden defines integrity as "the integration of ideals, convictions, standards, beliefs, and behavior" and "when our behavior is congruent with our professed values, when ideals and practice match." Many of us refer to this concept as "walking the walk, not just talking the talk."

You express how you value yourself by the consistency of your behavior. Think about it: When you lie (but refer to the fabrication as "just a white lie"), cheat (claiming that "it's just Uncle Sam"), or steal (and assuage your guilt by thinking that "they've got so much they won't even miss it"), the only person you betray is yourself. You also undermine the other principles associated with unconditional self-esteem.

If you practice making small choices in an open, honest way (such as deciding to give a merchant back the correct change), you prepare yourself for making some truly difficult decisions (such as removing a loved one from life support).

You have to accept responsibility for hurting others (whether you intended to or not) and attempt to make amends if you plan to lead a life of integrity. Dr. Branden suggests five steps for assuaging guilt and maintaining integrity:

1. Face and accept the full reality of what you have done.

2. Try to understand why you did what you did. Treat yourself with compassion, but don't dismiss your actions with lame excuses.

3. Be honest about what you did to anyone you've hurt, and explain that you accept the consequences of your behavior as an adult. Acknowledge how others have been affected by your actions and that you accept how they feel about you or what you've done.

4. Try to make amends for or minimize the harm you have done.

5. Firmly commit to behaving differently in the future.

## PULLING IT ALL TOGETHER

How do you know when you have achieved unconditional, positive self-esteem? Your actions—how you treat yourself and others—can be quite revealing. You will be able to:

- Accept appropriate challenges, even if they involve some degree of risk. You will feel comfortable by yourself or with other people.
- Remain flexible and yet set appropriate, healthy limits around yourself and your life.
- Respect your spirit, mind, and body by exposing yourself to books, music, and food that will help you grow and develop in healthy ways.
- Surround yourself with positive, active, loving friends and family members.
- Celebrate small and great achievements.
- See the joy and beauty of life.
- Forgive yourself for mistakes—intentional or accidental.
- Be involved in meaningful professional or volunteer activities.
- Most of all, love, cherish, enjoy, and value yourself.

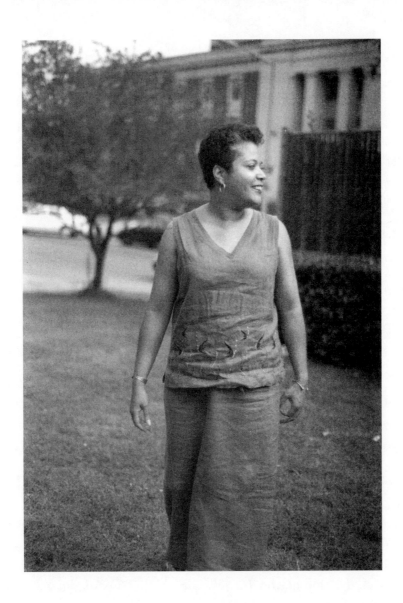

# Chapter 6

# CONFRONTING THE TWO A's: ATTITUDE AND ANGER

*So it's a gorgeous afternoon in the park*
*It's so nice you forget your Attitude*
*The one your mama taught you*
*The one that says Don't-Mess-With-Me!*

> —Kate Rushkin, "The Tired Poem:
> Last Letter from a Typical Unemployed Black Professional Woman"

"Black women" and "attitude" are terms that are so often connected in the minds of African Americans and Caucasians that some people think they're synonymous. Movies and television have reinforced this one-dimensional portrayal of Black women—especially African American women in the middle years. Stereotypical visual images of Black women rolling their eyes, shaking their heads, and telling it like it is in a sarcastic, abrasive, often threatening manner abound in movies and on television. Remember Hattie McDaniel as Mammy in the movie *Gone with the Wind*, or, more recently, Whoopi Goldberg in the movie *Ghost*? What about television's Sapphire on *Amos and Andy*, Florence on *The Jeffersons*, Esther on *Sanford and Son*, and Judge Ephriam on *Divorce Court*?

Even when a middle-aged African American woman is cast as a powerful, often insightful, loving angel, such as Della Reese on *Touched by an Angel*, she must still display a heavy dose of Sapphire, Florence, and Esther. In fact, if you studied the characters played by the only African American women ever to win Academy Awards—Hattie McDaniel in 1939 and Whoopi Goldberg in 1990—you would quickly realize that though their roles were fifty years apart, they shared all of the stereotypical traits that we've been describing.

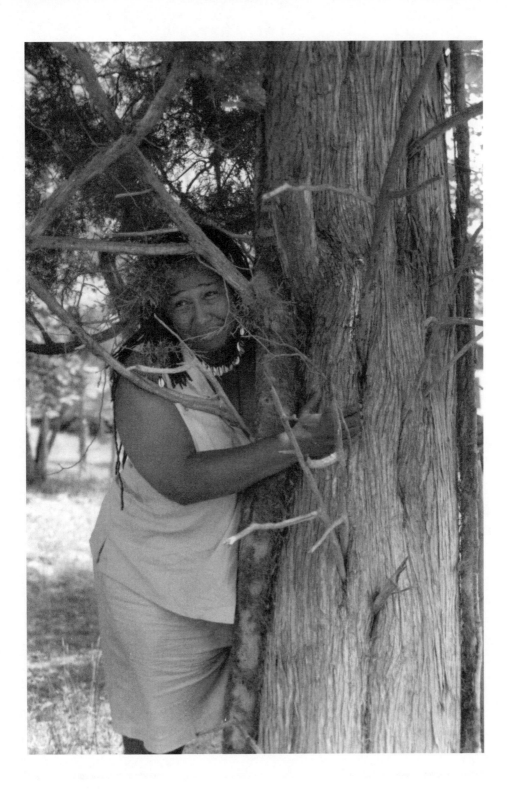

## THE INTERPLAY BETWEEN ATTITUDE AND ANGER

While *anger* is a general term for an emotional reaction of displeasure in any degree of intensity—rage, wrath, or fury—*attitude* is defined in the dictionary as a mental position or feeling toward a fact or situation. For most African Americans, however, the specific feeling identified with attitude *is* anger. When we say, "She's got an attitude," we usually mean that that person is acting angry, probably somewhat abruptly, and even showing some hostility.

For us African Americans, however, having an attitude is not necessarily viewed as a negative. Many Blacks use the word *attitude* as a positive description for someone who "tells it like it is," "doesn't take any stuff," or doesn't suffer any real or fantasized mistreatment or abuse from anyone. African Americans know that our image in the media, filtered through the lens of racism and sexism, has been distorted and even at times caricatured. Yet we Black women often portray ourselves as caustic and domineering, with—as bell hooks describes it—"tongues of fire."

---

## CARLA'S STORY

Carla is a forty-four-year-old paralegal who describes herself as a "Black woman with an attitude." She frequently comments to her colleagues that "I'm not taking no stuff off anybody"—especially her supervisors. Carla has been dating Walter, a night manager for a radio station, for almost two years. Their major arguments often revolve around Carla's attitude.

In late November, Walter told Carla that he would be unable to take her to her company's annual Christmas party, explaining that he couldn't find anyone to cover for him at work that evening. Carla went off. She started rolling her eyes, shaking her head, cursing, and accusing Walter of lying to her. She told him, "I'll bet if your mama wanted you to go someplace, you'd figure out a way to do it—and you know that's the truth." When Walter angrily reminded her that he had arranged for coverage for her birthday—which was two weeks before Christmas—and New Year's Eve, Carla responded that she didn't want to hear it, and stormed out of the house. Walter yelled after her, "I'm tired of you and your attitude."

---

Carla's outburst is the stereotypical response often expected of Black women who are angry, sad, hurt, disappointed, stressed, worried, anxious, frightened, or concerned. When in any of these situations, many women respond with attitude, which includes being quick to anger or being perpetually angry, loud, domineering, touchy, and insulting. Black mothers are depicted in all of these ways as well as "protective" and having "little to no time for verbal or physical affection" on top of it all. We African Americans have even perpetuated this image of Black mothers through our own stories as well as in the humor of many Black comedians, from Moms Mabley to Bill Cosby. Think about it—some of our favorite anecdotal stories are of ourselves, our friends, our colleagues, and certainly our mothers or grandmothers going off, or being tough and demanding.

Much of our literature, especially in books that describe mother-daughter (or mother-surrogate) relationships—such as *Sula* and *The Bluest Eye* (Toni Morrison), *Brown Girl, Brownstones* (Paule Marshall), *His Eye Is on the Sparrow* (Zora Neale Hurston), and *Meridian* (Alice Walker)—feature stereotypical "big bad mama" characters. As a result, our African American literature reinforces the perception that Black women express their anger and assert their authority through the use of coercive commands ("Shut up"), harsh verbal threats ("I'm going to beat your butt"), and physical punishment.

Even when fictional Black mothers are hurt or disappointed, they still only express their anger. For instance, the exchange in Toni Morrison's novel between Sula's mother, Hannah, and her grandmother, Eva, illustrates the limited range of emotional expressions often allowed Black women. Hannah asks her mother: "Did you ever love us?" referring to herself and her two siblings. Eva responds: "You settin' here with your healthy ass self and ax me did I love you? Them big old eyes in your head would a been two holes full of maggots if I hadn't."

In the book, there is a rumor in the community that Eva deliberately put herself in the path of a train (where her leg was severed) so that she could collect the insurance money and support herself and her three children. Although she is clearly angry and hurt by Hannah's question, she is only able to respond with a hostile, somewhat emotionally abusive answer.

It is not only in our personal relationships that attitude is a significant factor, but also in our professional ones. Read Gloria's story.

## GLORIA'S STORY

Gloria, fifty-six, is the CEO and part owner of a successful consulting firm. She and the firm's co-owner, Renee, have been in business for more than five years, but they've lived together as a couple for almost twenty years. Unfortunately, though, as their business grew, their personal and working relationships deteriorated.

Gloria has always been impatient, short-tempered, and sharp-tongued, like her mama, but she is also generous and caring. As the demands of the business have increased, however, Gloria has become more impatient with her staff's imperfections. She believes she has the right to tell them off whenever she deems they need it. While Gloria feels momentary regret for some of her public explosions, she considers herself a tough but fair employer.

Different staff members have complained to Renee about the effect of Gloria's attitude on morale and productivity. Two secretaries quit within six months of being hired; two of the most productive employees are planning to resign. All of the departing staff and most of the remaining employees have expressed their feelings—ranging from discomfort to anger—about Gloria's curt, acerbic, sometimes public criticisms.

Despite Renee's repeated attempts to discuss these concerns with Gloria, her partner refuses to admit she has a problem. In fact, Gloria thinks Renee is too easy on the staff and that their employees take advantage of her good nature and walk all over her. When several customers no longer wanted to work with Gloria because of her abrasive demeanor, Renee realized that she had to confront Gloria about her attitude.

## WHAT'S BEHIND OUR NEGATIVE ATTITUDE?

Why are attitude and anger considered such an integral part of Black women's personalities? Why are anger and attitude so commonly used in place of the range of emotions we so clearly feel? Racism and sexism have certainly played a part in the media's depiction of us as angry women, but why have we ourselves chosen to embrace this portrayal and bequeath it to our daughters, granddaughters, younger sisters, nieces, and mentored children or colleagues?

Dr. Gail Wyatt in *Stolen Women* contends that Black women acquired Sapphire-like traits as a defense against being considered as stereotypes and treated as sexually permissive. Dr. Wyatt writes: "It's not a compliment to be thought of as promiscuous and impulsive. You can only take so many demeaning incidents before you become like Sapphire."

Therapist Audrey Chapman in *Entitled to Good Loving* believes that the exhausting task of trying to always be a strong Black woman in the face of inadequate support may be a factor in our attitudes. Black women expect to be superwomen, and we are expected by others to be superwomen and handle it all. We listen to complaints from Black men about the racism they face, but our experiences of racism and sexism are often minimized or dismissed. The strain of being everyone's caretaker but feeling that we can't depend on anyone or that no one notices or appreciates our own struggle takes a tremendous toll and leaves us angry, hurt, and sad. Yet everyone else just sees a bad attitude or a chip on our shoulder that we dare anyone to knock off.

These explanations offer valuable insights into why so many Black women have an attitude, but questions remain. Since attitude often results from situations in which we feel hurt, sad, and stressed as well as angry, why is it that anger is usually the emotion expressed?

Perhaps the seeds for our inappropriate manner of expressing anger and our inability or unwillingness to express other related emotions—sadness and hurt—were sown and cultivated during slavery. As bell hooks reminds us, our very survival was dependent on our ability to repress feelings: "We were in fact socialized . . . to contain and repress a range of emotions." Expressing anger to the overseers or owners could evoke a life-threatening reaction. Even expressing sympathy or offering support to another slave who was in pain or being punished could elicit reprisals.

Slave owners, parents, and caretakers taught our ancestors as children to be discreet. We learned that our physical and emotional well-being depended on the ability to disguise our true thoughts and feelings. Mothers knew that even normal child behavior—such as crying when hungry, hurt, or angry, and laughing or screaming when playing—were sometimes considered unacceptable and might evoke an enraged, irrational response from slave owners. Children were often beaten, burned, or permanently maimed for accidents or minor rule infractions. This is tragically exemplified in the slave narrative of Delia Garlic, who recounts in *Remembering Slavery* (edited by Ira Berlin, Marc Favreau, and Steven Miller) an incident that occurred when she was a young girl:

One day I was playing wid de baby [her owner's child]. It hurt its li'l han' an' commenced to cry, an' she [the mother] whirl on me, pick up a hot iron and run it all down my arm an' han'. It took off de flesh when she done it.

Slave mothers also constantly worried that their children would be sold to another plantation as punishment for the child's or parent's misbehavior. Thus, these women were willing to take any measures, including beating their children themselves, if it increased the chance that the child would be safe and remain with the family.

Even after formal slavery ended, the psychological and physical intimidation of Blacks continued through Jim Crow laws and race-related beatings, rapes, bombings, and lynchings. The brutal murder of Emmett Till, a fourteen-year-old boy who was killed because he allegedly whistled at a Caucasian woman, reinforced the worst fears of most parents. It encouraged mothers and fathers to become more entrenched in using the methods that they had learned from their owners for controlling behavior—verbal intimidation and corporal punishment.

Habit, multiple responsibilities, and the overwhelming stress of having constantly to battle economic, racial, and sexual oppression helped transform this slave-survival strategy of distorting, minimizing, or denying our feelings into a positive cultural characteristic. This limited emotional repertoire became an accepted, even admired, method for interacting with each other as well as with Caucasians and the larger society.

African Americans now equate stoicism, anger, and having an attitude with being and looking strong. Being perceived as gentle, tender, and verbally and physically affectionate, especially when sad or hurt, is often considered a sign of weakness. Crying unabashedly is denigrated.

In fact, many African American women equate being nonattitudinal with being like "Miss Anne"—a pejorative colloquial expression used to describe Caucasian women who act as if they are entitled to preferential treatment because of their race and social status, and whose behavior is seen as passive and timid. It is also used in a denigrating way to describe Black women who display those same characteristics.

Very few articles, books, television programs, or movies have attempted to explore, in depth, the negative effect on our emotional well-being of having to live up to this image of the angry, sarcastic, tell-it-like-it-is Black woman. But we authors—as Black women and health-care professionals—can tell you that it is emotionally, physically, and spiritually debilitating to constantly defend ourselves against this pervasive image.

According to Debrena Jackson Gandy in *Sacred Pampering Principles*, this self-imposed emotional constriction has negative physical, behavioral, and emotional consequences. When any human being is angry, she is out of balance, and our frequent anger—especially with men—makes us anxious, fatigued, and unable to be interdependent. We are hurting and isolating ourselves, constantly stressing our minds and bodies.

This lack of physical and emotional ease and balance takes a physical toll on our body. Gandy believes that we, as African Americans, are more prone to gynecological problems (such as fibroids and cysts) and cancers of the breast, uterus, and cervix when we are unwilling and/or unable to express a full range of feelings appropriately. Indeed, there is medical evidence for the cellular damage anger and hostility wreak on the heart and other parts of the body.

In *Sisters of the Yam*, bell hooks contends that our ability to give and receive love is compromised by our inability to acknowledge, accept, and express freely and fully all of our emotions, not only anger but sadness and hurt and joy and happiness. She writes:

> Often we replace recognition of inner emotional needs with the longing to control. When we deny our real needs, we tend to feel fragile, vulnerable, emotionally unstable, and untogether. Black females often work hard to cover up these conditions. And we cover up by controlling, by seeking to oversee or dominate everyone around us. The message we tell ourselves is, "I can't be falling apart because I have all this power over others."

Gayle and her colleagues have found, however, that many Black women *are* falling apart under the weight of carrying unexpressed anger or from the burden of inappropriately expressed anger. They feel the strain in their entire being: Emotionally, these women are depressed and anxious; physically, they're more vulnerable to high blood pressure, heart disease, and stroke; and spiritually, they are despairing or hopeless.

## ℞ PRIME TIME PRESCRIPTIONS FOR ANXIETY AND ANGER

*There are two things over which you have complete dominion, authority and control—your mind and your mouth.*

—Molefi Asante

Making a conscious decision to change your attitude can have a profound impact on how you think and feel about yourself, on your overall energy level, and on your personal and professional relationships. To make this transformation, you need to do two things: **change how you assess a situation, and learn to monitor how you express your anger.**

Appropriately expressing any emotions—but especially anger—can be difficult, even frightening for people of any racial and ethnic group. For African Americans, it is even more challenging because we are often positively rewarded for acting like a stereotypical sister with an attitude.

## THE POWER OF A POSITIVE ATTITUDE

Learning how to acquire a positive attitude and assertively—as opposed to passively or aggressively—express your anger are skills that you can learn and master. Here are some suggestions for how you can develop a positive attitude.

*Accept responsibility for your disposition.* Only you can decide whether you want to approach every situation or start each day on an up note (hoping for the best) or on a down note (preparing for the worst). Chances are that if you're reading this, you are not waking up blind, deaf, paralyzed, or homeless, so you're already starting the day luckier than, say, Christopher Reeve or Stevie Wonder, but is your attitude about life as positive as theirs? Every morning, Winnie, a friend of Gayle and Marilyn, listens to the gospel song "It Could Have Been the Other Way," which expresses gratitude to God for allowing us to wake up to another day. What are you doing to celebrate your gifts from above?

*Become the town crier for positive news.* It can be very tempting to be the office gossip, because these folks are often the center of attention. Playing this role not only increases the time you spend immersed in negative thoughts, but often attracts people who have a negative energy and focus. Make certain that most of your conversations are about positive topics. The Hindus and Buddhists call it the practice of "right speech," and it is one of the precepts for spiritual health. You can still talk about very serious subjects in a very serious manner, but reserve the majority of your talk time for topics that are intellectually stimulating and emotionally satisfying.

*Surround yourself with your Prime Time Circle of Sisterfriends.* Acquiring,

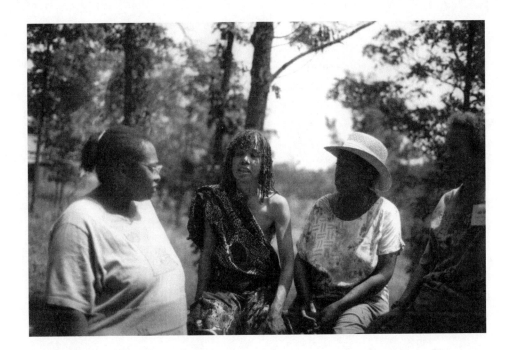

maintaining, and nourishing relationships with optimistic, encouraging people can help you maintain a positive attitude. Unpleasant events occur to everyone, but with a strong support network you can regain your positive outlook and emotional balance more quickly. Studies have shown that people who have a lot of friends live longer.

*Reassess the positive or negative effect that the significant people in your life have on your mood.* Some relationships, even very old ones, can be destructive. If you have relationships like this, you need to end them. Try the following exercise to clarify your thoughts.

## POSITIVE AND NEGATIVE PEOPLE WHO INFLUENCE MY LIFE

List three people who are having a positive influence on your life and three who are having a negative impact.

| POSITIVE INFLUENCES | NEGATIVE INFLUENCES |
|---|---|
| 1. _____ | 1. _____ |
| 2. _____ | 2. _____ |
| 3. _____ | 3. _____ |

Now ask yourself the following questions:
- What are you doing to maintain the positive relationships and to change the negative ones?
- If the negative ones cannot be changed, are you staying in them and feeling like a hurt and angry victim?
- Have you used your Prime Time Circle to help you assess your role in the negative relationships and to give you the support you'll need to either change or leave them?

*Cultivate a positive attitude about work.* Most of us either want to work or have to work or both, and we spend the largest number of our waking hours at work. Thus, if you have negative feelings about work, it's almost impossible not to have them affect your personal life. Your attitude about work not only will affect your job performance, but will also affect how your supervisors and colleagues relate to you. The worksheet below should help assess how you feel.

## WHAT I LIKE AND DISLIKE ABOUT MY JOB

List four positives and four negatives about your job.

WHAT I LIKE ABOUT MY JOB
1. _____
2. _____
3. _____
4. _____

WHAT I DON'T LIKE ABOUT MY JOB
1. _____
2. _____
3. _____
4. _____

Try these four ways to improve your attitude at work.

- For three months, focus exclusively on the positive aspects of your job.
- Treat your job as if it were someplace you really wanted to go.

• Get to work at least fifteen minutes early, drink a cup of tea, and decide what you're going to do to have fun at work (tell a colleague a funny story, have lunch at a new place). Make certain you do it without interfering with your job responsibilities.

• Refuse to participate in negative talk with your coworkers.

If at the end of three months of really trying all of these suggestions and any others that your Prime Time Circle suggests, your attitude about work is still negative, you need to find another job.

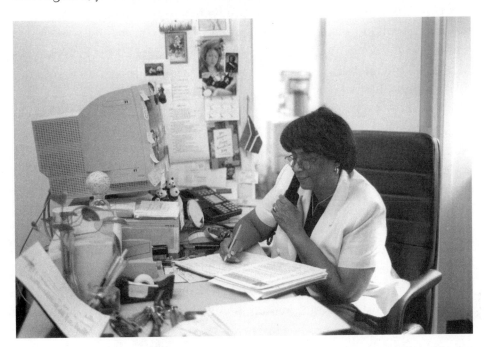

*Prepare for the unexpected.* The best way to cope with the unexpected is always to plan for it. Sometimes things happen over which we have no control, such as a life-threatening accident, illness, or job cutback. Taking steps now to become more prepared will help you have a more positive attitude when negative events occur. Here are some recommendations:

• *Maintain a strong, supportive network of friends and family.* It's easier to call on people during a crisis when they have been there during your "up" time and shared your celebrations.

• *Have regular physical exams.* Developing a relationship with your health-care providers makes it easier for them to respond appropriately to medical emergencies and for you to feel assured that you have a health team you can depend on.

• *Stash away money for a rainy day.* This is an excellent way to reduce the chances of being knocked flat by an unexpected financial setback. Money can't stop unpleasant events from occurring (just look at the Kennedy family), but having a financial reserve, no matter how small, can cushion their impact.

• *Use what you learned from those past life experiences to get you through any future ones.* Remember that you've survived other negative experiences.

• *Have a vision.* Your ability to be productive in the present while always thinking about and planning future goals will help you maintain a positive attitude. Many concentration camp survivors have said that their survival depended on their determination and ability to imagine life beyond the immediate reality of barbed-wire fences.

## ASSERTIVELY EXPRESS ANGER

Having a positive attitude can increase your ability to own all of your feelings and to express them honestly, openly, and appropriately. We know— especially by this age—that the song "Everything Must Change" is an accurate assessment of life. Acquiring the tools to communicate your feelings effectively is an essential step in changing and taking charge of your life.

Anger is a normal emotion, part of our repertoire of human feelings. The literature of Christianity and Judaism includes descriptions of their founders expressing righteous anger. For instance, when Jesus was in the temple, he was angry with the moneychangers, and Moses was angry when the Jews in the desert, after escaping from slavery in Egypt, turned to idolatry. That we mortals become angry is not a problem, but the frequency and intensity of our anger, and the way we express it and use it, can be problematic.

When Carla had the tantrum because Walter couldn't take her to the party, she was not trying to have an open and honest dialogue with him. She wanted to control his behavior and to hurt him, because she felt hurt by what she considered his rejection of her. Carla has never learned how to express her anger appropriately and has been given overt and covert messages from her family and friends that admitting sadness or fear is a sign of weakness or, even worse, "acting like a White girl."

Nonetheless, Carla did have options:

1. She could have repressed her thoughts and feelings and said nothing. (That would have been a *passive* way of handling the situation.)

2. She could have given him indirect hints or done something sneaky to get revenge on him, such as putting water in his gas tank. (This would be considered a *passive-aggressive* response, which is extremely inappropriate, and usually the childish way of responding to anger or frustration.)

3. She could do what she did—attack him and attempt to hurt and humiliate him. (This is considered an *aggressive* response, and we all realize how out of control this reaction was.)

4. She could have expressed to Walter her disappointment and asked him to keep trying to find a replacement, but acknowledged that he had tried to be with her and had made arrangements to get coverage on previous occasions. (This is the type of response we should strive for. It is *assertive* and *positive*, allowing us to express our thoughts and feelings in an open, direct, and honest manner without being verbally or emotionally abusive to someone else.)

## SITUATIONAL PASSIVITY, AGGRESSIVENESS, ASSERTIVENESS

None of us is always assertive, always passive, or always aggressive in all situations. Some women are very assertive with their children but aggressive at work or with their significant others. The first step in determining which areas you need to work at in order to become more assertive requires that you first recognize those situations in which you feel more or less comfortable. Take the quiz below to determine situations in which you're most apt to display a certain type of behavior.

### ASSERTIVENESS QUOTIENT (AQ) TEST

Test your assertiveness quotient (AQ) by completing the following questionnaire. Use the following scale to represent how comfortable you feel when reading each of the situations listed in this test.

Scale

1   Situation makes me very uncomfortable.
2   Situation makes me feel moderately comfortable.
3   I am very comfortable in this situation.

There may be some situations that are not relevant to you or to your particular lifestyle. In such cases, try to imagine how comfortable you might feel if you were involved in the situation.

1. Speaking up and asking questions at a meeting _____
2. Commenting about being interrupted by someone directly to him or her at the moment you're interrupted _____
3. Stating your views to an authority figure (e.g., minister, boss, therapist, parent) _____
4. Attempting to offer solutions and elaborating on them when there are men present _____
5. Entering and exiting a room in which other people are present _____
6. Speaking in front of a group _____
7. Maintaining eye contact, keeping your head upright, and leaning forward when in a personal conversation _____
8. Going out with a group of friends when you are the only one without a date _____
9. Being especially competent, using your authority and/or power without labeling yourself as bitchy, impolite, bossy, aggressive, castrating, or parental _____
10. Requesting expected service when you haven't received it (e.g., in a restaurant or a store) _____
11. Being expected to apologize for something and not apologizing since you feel you are right _____
12. Requesting the return of borrowed items without being apologetic _____
13. Receiving a compliment by saying something assertive, to acknowledge that you agree with the person complimenting you _____
14. Accepting a rejection _____
15. Not getting the approval of the most significant person in your life _____
16. Discussing another person's criticism of you openly with that person _____
17. Telling someone that she/he is doing something that is bothering you _____
18. Refusing to get coffee or to take notes at a meeting where you are chosen to do so because you are a female _____
19. Saying no or refusing to do a favor when you really don't feel like it _____

20. Turning down a request for a meeting or date _____
21. Telling a person when you think she or he is manipulating you _____

22. Commenting to a male who has made a patronizing remark to you (e.g., "You have a good job for a woman," "You're not flighty, emotional, stupid, or hysterical like most women") _____
23. Telling a prospective lover about your physical attraction to him or her before any such statements are made to you _____
24. Initiating sex with your partner _____
25. Showing enjoyment of an art show or concert in spite of others' reactions _____
26. Asking to be caressed and/or telling your lover what feels good to you _____
27. Expressing anger directly and honestly when you feel angry _____
28. Arguing with another person _____
29. Telling a joke _____
30. Listening to a friend tell a story about something embarrassing but funny that you have done _____
31. Responding with humor to someone's putdown of you _____
32. Disciplining your own children _____
33. Disciplining others' children _____
34. Explaining the facts of life or your divorce to your child _____
35. Talking about your feelings of competition with another woman with whom you feel competitive _____

If you scored a 1 on fifteen or more statements, you probably need assertiveness training. Please pay close attention to the pattern of your responses. Try to determine when your level of discomfort is greatest. Is it when you're expressing your opinion in a public forum (questions 1, 3, 6) or interacting in a sexual situation (questions 23, 24, 26)?

## VERBAL AND NONVERBAL CUES OF ASSERTIVE BEHAVIOR

Recognizing signs of passive, aggressive, or assertive behavior is critical to being able to change your behavior. Once you can recognize these behaviors in yourself, it can become easier to share this information with family members, friends, and your Prime Time Circle so that they can help you become more consistently assertive. Read the descriptions listed in the table below and see which one is most characteristic of you.

# VERBAL AND NONVERBAL COMPONENTS OF BEHAVIORS

|  | Passive | Assertive | Aggressive |
|---|---|---|---|
| VERBAL | Apologetic words<br>Veiled meanings<br>Hedging (failure to come to point)<br>Rambling (disconnected)<br>At loss for words<br>Failure to say what you really mean: "I mean," "you know" | Statement of wants<br>Honest statement of feelings<br>Objective words<br>Direct statements that say what you mean<br>"I" messages | "Loaded" words<br>Accusations<br>Descriptive, subjective terms<br>Imperious, superior words<br>"You" messages that blame or label |
| NONVERBAL GENERAL | Actions instead of words, hoping someone will guess what you want<br>Looking as if you don't mean what you say | Attentive listening behavior<br>General assured manner, communicating caring and strength | Exaggerated show of strength<br>Flippant, sarcastic style<br>Air of superiority |
|  | Passive | Assertive | Aggressive |
| NONVERBAL SPECIFIC |  |  |  |
| Voice | Weak, hesitant, soft, sometimes wavering | Firm, warm, well-modulated, relaxed | Tense, shrill, loud, shaky, cold, "deadly quiet", demanding, superior, authoritarian |
| Eyes | Averted: downcast teary, pleading | Open, frank, direct eye contact, but not staring | Expressionless: narrowed, cold, staring, not really "seeing" you |
| Stance and Posture | Lean for support, stooped, excessive head nodding | Well-balanced, straight on, erect, relaxed | Hands on hips, feet apart<br>Stiff and rigid, rude, imperious |
| Hands | Fidgety, fluttery, clammy | Relaxed motions | Clenched, abrupt gestures, finger pointing, fist pounding |

When you respond assertively, you begin by acknowledging your own feelings, and you don't attempt to place them on the other person. This is how you should initiate any discussions about your feelings. Practicing assertive behaviors is the most effective way of learning how to be more consistently assertive in various situations.

Use the examples given below to see if you can develop your own assertive responses.

## ARE YOU ASSERTIVE?

Circle the response you are most likely to choose. In addition, identify each of the responses as being either passive, aggressive, or assertive. Next, devise your own assertive response. Write your response down in the space provided.

*Situation 1*

You have been waiting for forty-five minutes in an open-backed gown in your doctor's office. You are thoroughly chilled and thoroughly angry by the time she or he bursts into the room with a cheery smile and a "Well, how are you today?" You say:

A. "Fine."

B. "How do you think I am after waiting all this time?"

C. "Frankly, Doctor, I'm angry. I've been undressed and in this cold room for forty-five minutes. I would appreciate not having to wait like this again."

Your assertive response: _____

_____

*Situation 2*

You and your husband are selecting a washing machine. The salesperson has handed you the color chart and is explaining how the machine works to your husband. Both of you will use the machine, and you wish the salesperson would talk to you as well as your husband about how it works. You say:

A. Nothing and listen quietly.

B. "Isn't it about time you considered the fact that I might need to know how the machine works, too?"

C. "Excuse me, but I'd appreciate your talking to both of us about the mechanics of the machine. I'll need that information, too."

Your assertive response: _____

_____

*Situation 3*

You are lost. You finally ask directions from a bus driver. He gives them in a condescending way, calling you "honey" and "babe." You resent his tone and his unwarranted familiarity; you feel that he would have responded straightforwardly to a male's request for directions. You:

A. Meekly thank him, grumbling to yourself about his attitude.

B. Explode by saying, "Who do you think you are, calling me 'honey'?"

C. Say, "I appreciate the directions, but I feel very uncomfortable when you call me 'honey' or 'babe.' Please don't do that again."

Your assertive response: _____

_____

*Situation 4*

As part of your job, you are interviewing a local businessman about some research material. He looks you over and says, "Well, well, I sure got lucky to have such a pretty girl interview me." You feel that you are not being taken seriously as a professional. You:

A. Say nothing but feel rotten inside because the remark has taken away your confidence in your own competence.

B. Say, "Look here, Mr. Smith, this is business and I think that's an inappropriate remark."

C. Evaluate the consequences of exploding at this man, smile politely, and say, "You're luckier than you know. I'm also a very good interviewer, and my first question is . . ."

Your assertive response: _____

_____

*Situation 5*

You're over thirty years old and have just returned to college to finish up your degree. When you try to participate in the discussion in one professor's class, he consistently ignores you. You feel frustrated and even more insecure at being in college at "your age." You:

A. Are afraid of a failing grade, so you say nothing.

B. Tell him directly that you don't like being ignored when you have an idea to discuss.

C. Have a conference with him, explaining that you feel out of place in a difficult situation and that you would appreciate his encouragement in helping you to express yourself in class. Specifically, you tell him you want him to call on you when you raise your hand in class.

Your assertive response: _____

_____

## Situation 6

Ever since your husband died, your grown-up children have been treating you like some very fragile object. You are weary of their constant fussing about where you will live and with whom. You want to make your own way, so you:

A. Secretly get a part-time job and quietly resist their attempts to move you from your home.

B. Tell them in no uncertain terms to leave you alone.

C. Explain that you're genuinely touched by their concern but that you have your own plans.

Your assertive response: _____

_____

## Situation 7

You are at a party and are stuck talking to a long-winded person. You're bored by the conversation and want to get involved with other guests.

A. You are so concerned with hurting the person's feelings that you shift from one foot to the other with impatience but say nothing.

B. You interrupt the conversation and say, "Look, there's a friend of mine I want to talk to. See you."

C. When she or he takes a breath, you smile and say something short and appropriate ("That's interesting" or "I never knew that") and quickly follow it with "Let's go over and say hello to John and Mary, shall we?," then take the person's arm.

Your assertive response: _____

_____

## Situation 8

Your spouse did it again. He constantly interrupted your story at a gathering of close friends. It makes you so mad when he does that. When you are driving home in the car, you:

A. Say nothing but are very distant.

B. Yell, "You always tell the punch line of my stories. You're a horrible conversationalist."

C. Say, "You interrupted my story tonight. I don't know if you're aware of it, but you do it a lot. I feel put down by your interruptions, and I wish you wouldn't do that."

Your assertive response: _____

_____

## Situation 9

A man whom you've dated once calls. Your first date wasn't much fun and you don't want to go out with him again. But here he is on the phone asking for another date. You say:

A. "I don't really think that, er, uh . . . Sure, why not?"

B. "Can't take a hint? Bug off!"

C. "John, I don't share your interest in pursuing this relationship."

Your assertive response: _____

_____

*Situation 10*

You plan to attend a meeting, and one of your children comes in late with a request to borrow the car for the evening. The request involves your giving up the car and your meeting. You feel irritated by his or her thoughtless request. You say:

A. "Oh, all right. I guess the meeting wasn't that important."

B. "Can't you ever be considerate? You know I have plans this evening."

C. "This meeting is very important to me and I've already made plans to attend. You'll have to find other transportation tonight. Next time you need a car, let me know a day in advance and we can coordinate our plans."

Your assertive response: _____

_____

*Situation 11*

A friend was to pick you up at 7:30 for a movie that starts at 8:00. It is now 8:30 and your friend has finally arrived, full of apologies, explaining that she or he couldn't get off the phone even though the phone call wasn't important. You feel angry about having been kept waiting. You:

A. Say, "Oh, that's all right. I understand."

B. Grumble, "I hope you're happy now that we've missed the first part of the movie."

C. After taking a calming breath, say, "I'm disappointed that you talked through our date, because we've missed the beginning of the movie. Let's change our plan and go tomorrow night so we can catch the entire show."

Your assertive response: _____

_____

*Situation 12*

You've spent two days completing an art project you're very proud of, and a friend stops by and compliments you on your work. You say:

A. "Oh, this thing. I guess I'm not very talented."

B. "Since when are you the local art critic?"

C. "Thank you. I've spent a lot of time working on it and I'm proud of it. Your compliment really makes me feel good."

Your assertive response: _____

_____

*Situation 13*

You're out shopping for new clothes. You've decided you want a blue blouse. The salesperson insists you choose green by saying, "You look much better in green. Take my word for it: Get green." You're irritated by the unnecessary time this is taking, and you say:

A. "Oh, all right. You probably know best."

B. "Where do you get off being so pushy? I've said twenty times I want blue."

C. "I appreciate your interest. However, I've thought about this and definitely prefer blue. Please ring up my purchase."

Your assertive response: _____

_____

*Situation 14*

You've just been asked for the third straight year to sponsor a charity drive at the office. Although you didn't mind doing it the first two times, you feel it's time someone else took charge. You say:

A. "Okay, but this is the last year."

B. "No, I'm sick and tired of doing the work for the whole office."

C. "No. I've enjoyed the responsibility in the past, but this year it's important to me that someone else take charge."

Your assertive response: _____

_____

*Situation 15*

You've just completed what you considered to be an assertive request to someone in an elevator to put out his or her cigarette. She or he says, "Aren't you being a little too bossy? This is a public elevator." You say:

A. Nothing while reaching for your handkerchief, but mumble to your neighbor.

B. "Wow, talking about being inconsiderate. You take the cake!"

C. "I consider this a fair request. It's a short ride and I'm bothered a lot by cigarette smoke."

Your assertive response: _____

_____

*Situation 16*

A friend who has borrowed your favorite book knows that you refer to it often. She or he has had it for several weeks and you're getting impatient. The next time you see the friend, you say:

A. "Do you still have my book? Oh, well, I'll get it sometime."

B. "Where's my book? I can't believe you're so inconsiderate."

C. "I miss my book. Would you please return it by Friday?"

Your assertive response: _____

_____

## Situation 17

You're at a party. Practically everyone is drinking. You don't object to their behavior but prefer not to join the group. Someone at the party starts to hassle you about your stand. You say:

A. "Gee, I'm sorry, but I just don't feel well tonight."

B. "It's none of your business. Leave me alone."

C. "I'm enjoying the party and I don't want to be hassled about this. I'm not going to change my mind."

Your assertive response: _____

_____

## Situation 18

You're a secretary and you've just spent four hours reorganizing the files. You've very pleased with the results, although you realize that it isn't likely to be noticed. You feel satisfied and say to yourself:

A. "I guess it's too small a job to be very worthwhile. Anyone could have done it."

B. "I've done all this work and now no one will notice. That's the kind of credit I get for my hard work."

C. "It's a small job, but I've done fine work on it and I'm proud of myself."

Your assertive response: _____

_____

## Situation 19

You're walking along the street and someone bumps into you. That person looks at you accusingly and says, "Watch where you're going, stupid."

A. You say, "Oh, gee, I'm sorry."

B. You say, "Who's calling who stupid? I didn't run into you, you ran into me. Watch where you're going."

C. After considering the fact that the person might have had a bad day or is always rude and that saying anything probably won't achieve a positive result, you say nothing and walk on, as it's probably not worth your time.

Your assertive response: _____

_____

## Situation 20

You've been involved in an assertive rap group for several weeks. You're beginning to feel comfortable with yourself and your new assertiveness. Your husband says, "You're really acting strange. I liked you better the old way." You say:

A. Nothing aloud and think, "He's probably right. Maybe I should give it up if he's that displeased."

B. "What makes you think I care what you think?"

C. "I'm sorry you feel that way; this group has really made me feel good about myself. While I want you to feel comfortable with me, I want to feel good about myself. Maybe if you could tell me specifically what you find strange, we could talk about that. However, I am going to continue assertiveness training."

Your assertive response: _____

_____

When you finish circling your responses, go back and study your answers. Look for patterns in the types of situations in which you might find it most difficult to behave assertively. Yes, you're right. The A responses are passive, the B's are aggressive, and the C's are the assertive ones.

You might find it helpful to use these responses as examples of what to say in similar situations, but you are encouraged to devise your own reactions. That will cause you to start integrating assertiveness into your personal style of talking and increase the comfort you'll feel when you actually need to be assertive.

*Join an assertive training group,* where you can practice and receive feedback from other group members about your verbal statements, voice volume and intensity, facial expression, and body stance.

Before you can assertively express your anger and hear other people express theirs, you must become comfortable with the verbal and nonverbal components of anger. You must repeat assertive statements aloud and practice assertive behaviors to have them become part of your intellectual and emotional being. Be patient with yourself. It will take time for this new behavior to become a spontaneous and natural way of responding to various situations.

Give yourself permission and seek the support of your Prime Time Circle to give up the title of Ms. Angry Attitude. As Black women, we have experienced centuries of rage-inducing assaults on our loved ones and ourselves. Like everyone else in our society, though, we also have to go through the everyday annoyances, frustrations, and disappointments that are a part of living. African American women must acquire appropriate techniques for consistently expressing our anger in a manner that reduces the chance of hostility or resentment building up and hurting both our health and our loved ones' health. Becoming assertive will allow you to stand up for yourself and still be warm, compassionate, loving, and sensitive.

# Chapter 7

# THE POWER OF PREVENTION

*"We must realize that our future lies chiefly in our own hands."*
—Paul Robeson

How long we live and the qualities of our lives do lie chiefly in our own hands. African American women don't have to die as early as we're dying, and certainly not from causes that are preventable. For the past four hundred years, African American women have been leaving too soon, but for most of those years we had little to no control over the stressors that contributed to our early demise—lynchings, rapes, forced separations, extreme poverty, poor diets, and no access to any form of health care. Now that we are in the twenty-first century, it's time that we change the picture—*and we can!* Today the prospect of living to the age of one hundred is not far-fetched and is possible for all of us.

We have a great deal more information than our foremothers about our bodies, our health, and ways to promote health and prevent illness. Chronic illness is not an inevitable consequence of aging, as we've long believed. However, these chronic illnesses are the top four causes of death of Black women:

Heart disease
Cancer
Stroke
Diabetes

The major causes of death for African American women compared to Caucasian women are listed in the chart opposite.

## LEADING CAUSES OF DEATH IN WOMEN

| AFRICAN AMERICAN WOMEN | RANK | CAUCASIAN WOMEN |
|---|---|---|
| Heart disease | 1 | Heart disease |
| Cancer | 2 | Cancer |
| Stroke | 3 | Stroke |
| Diabetes | 4 | Chronic lung disease |
| Chronic lung disease | 5 | Diabetes |
| Accidents | 6 | Accidents |
| Chronic liver disease | 7 | Chronic liver disease |
| Kidney disease | 8 | Suicide |
| HIV/AIDS | 9 | Pneumonia and Influenza (flu) |
| Pneumonia and Influenza (flu) | 10 | Infections |

*Source:* National Center for Health Statistics, 1996

Even though Black and White women are dying from basically the same diseases, we really want to emphasize two points. **First, African American women have higher death rates than all other groups of women — Caucasian, Asian/Pacific Islander, Hispanic, American Indian women —** from three of the Big Four diseases: heart disease, cancer, and stroke. Consider Chart A (p. 106).

**Second, for us in our middle years, the risk of dying from breast cancer is high, but our risk of dying from heart disease is higher and increases dramatically in our later years.** To emphasize this point, Chart B (p. 107) shows the major risks of dying from heart disease when compared to breast and lung cancer by age group. Heart disease takes a heavier toll than breast cancer as women pass the age of fifty.

Most African American adults are intimately aware of the Big Four because far too many of us, our relatives, and our friends are struggling with one or more of these diseases. And, sadly, we've all lost one or more of our loved ones to a Big Four illness.

Even though the Big Four are common health concerns in a large

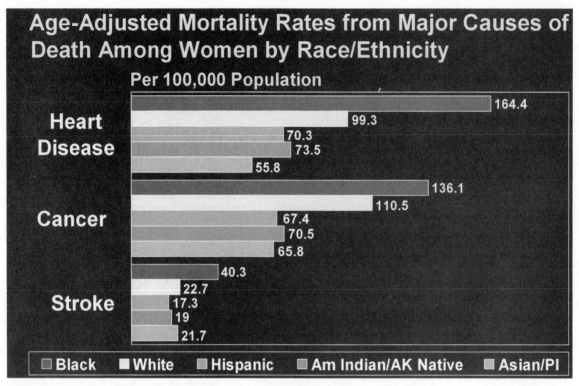

# Age-Adjusted Mortality Rates from Major Causes of Death Among Women by Race/Ethnicity

## Per 100,000 Population

**Heart Disease**
- 164.4
- 99.3
- 70.3
- 73.5
- 55.8

**Cancer**
- 136.1
- 110.5
- 67.4
- 70.5
- 65.8

**Stroke**
- 40.3
- 22.7
- 17.3
- 19
- 21.7

☐ Black ■ White ■ Hispanic ■ Am Indian/AK Native ■ Asian/PI

*Source:* National Center for Helath Statistics, Health United State, 1996.

percentage of African American households, too few of us are well informed about these deadly diseases. For instance, do you know how susceptible you are to developing one or more of the Big Four? And, even more important, if any of these illnesses run in your family, do you know what it takes to reduce the risk factors for it—and are you willing to do it?

Remember: You don't have to leave too soon!

## MAJOR RISK FACTORS FOR THE BIG FOUR DISEASES

A major aspect of preventive medicine is understanding and reducing risk factors—the habits, traits, or personal characteristics—that make you more likely to develop a disease or illness. In this chapter, we want to focus on the six major risk factors that are generally associated with the Big Four causes of death of African American women.

Some risk factors are beyond your control, such as your race, sex, age, and

**Chart B**

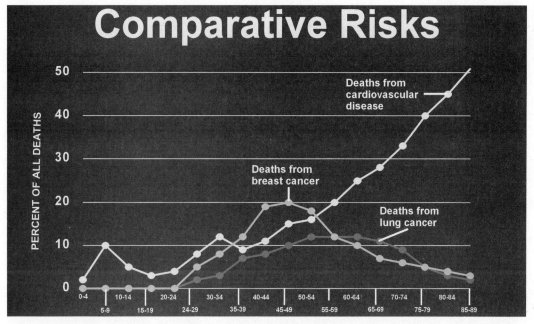

# Comparative Risks

*Source:* From "Putting the Risk of Breast Cancer in Perspective" by Phillips, Glendon, and Knight, from *The New England Journal of Medicine,* Vol. 340, pp. 141–144, January 14, 1999. Copyright © 1999 Massachusetts Medical Society. All rights reserved.

family history. Other risk factors relate to specific lifestyle habits, such as smoking, inactivity, and poor eating habits—and these are definitely modifiable. Identifying your risk factors, even the ones you can't change, and understanding how they affect your health is important for women of all ages. When you reach midlife, though, it is absolutely critical that you make some midcourse corrections. To lower your chances of developing and dying from a Big Four disease, you'll need to adopt a more healthful lifestyle and reduce or eliminate as many harmful behaviors as you can.

Unfortunately, just being a Prime Time African American woman puts you at increased risk for all the Big Four diseases. Ask yourself: How many of your female relatives, church members, or members of your Prime Time Circle who are over forty-five years old suffer from heart disease, have had a stroke, are trying to control their hypertension or diabetes, or have cancer? How many of these women have buried a close family member or friend who died from any of these illnesses? *Why* is the question we need to ask. The answers are varied, but what is often consistent is that our friends and loved ones are smoking, eating improperly, and are overweight, and not fit, and are stressed to the hilt. Each one of these lifestyle habits puts them in jeopardy for developing a Big Four disease. However, many probably don't know the impact of their risk factors on their health.

A good way to start assessing your risk factors for major illnesses is to take an inventory of your family's health history. In fact, we hope you will fill in the Family Health History worksheet that we provide later in the chapter. Once you've traced your family's medical history, you will be able to see any incidences of the Big Four and which of them you are at risk for. To see how your family's medical history can increase your risk for a Big Four disease, check out the table below.

## FAMILY HISTORY IS A MAJOR RISK FACTOR FOR THE BIG FOUR

### CARDIOVASCULAR DISEASE

| | |
|---|---|
| HEART DISEASE | A family history of early heart disease in a mother or sister (diagnosed before age sixty-five) or a father, grandfather, or brother (diagnosed before age fifty-five) increases your risk of heart disease significantly. |
| STROKE | A family history of hypertension and associated stroke increases your risk. |

### CANCER

| | |
|---|---|
| BREAST AND OVARIAN CANCERS | If there is a family history of a mother, grandmother, sister, or aunt with breast cancer (especially occurring before age fifty), you are at increased risk. Scientists have pinpointed two genes—BRCA 1 and BRCA 2—that are linked to both breast and ovarian cancer; however, it is estimated that only 5 percent of all breast cancers are inherited due to this mutated gene. |
| COLON CANCER | A family history of polyps or colorectal cancer also increases your risk for colorectal cancer. Heredity plays a role in more than 20 percent of colon cancer cases. |

### DIABETES

| | |
|---|---|
| DIABETES | If you have one parent with Type 1 diabetes (the type that requires insulin), you typically have a 4 percent to 6 percent chance of developing diabetes. If one parent has Type 2 (the type that does not require insulin), your risk is 7 percent to 14 percent. |

## LIFESTYLE RISK FACTORS THAT YOU CAN REDUCE OR ELIMINATE

Now let's look at the top modifiable risk factors that contribute to the Big Four. These are smoking, inadequate exercise, stress, poor diet and obesity, high blood fat and cholesterol, and hypertension.

The good news is that some of these risk factors are under your control. Still, we cannot emphasize enough how detrimental these risk factors are to your overall health. Here's why:

### Smoking

Cigarette smoking is linked to more than four hundred thousand preventable deaths each year. That's why doctors say cigarette smoking is the number one preventable cause of death. **Smoking by women causes as many deaths from heart disease as from lung cancer.**

Cigarette smoking decreases blood flow and oxygen to your brain and heart cells as well as other vital organs. This contributes to hypertension, heart disease, and increased blood clotting, which can cause a stroke. Smoking also negates the protection that our bodies' natural estrogen gives us in reducing the risk of heart disease. In fact, nonsmoking premenopausal women have a very low incidence of heart disease; nonsmoking women in midlife have a greater incidence, and midlife women who smoke have the greatest incidence. In addition, cigarette smoke actually damages your cells, which can lead to certain types of cancer, including lung, cervical, and uterine.

As soon as you quit smoking, however, your body starts to recover from the damage you've done over the years. (To find out more about quitting, review the Prime Time Eight-Step Smoking Cessation Plan in Chapter 9.)

### Inadequate Exercise

A sedentary lifestyle doesn't give your heart, lungs, and muscles the kind of daily workout they need to stay healthy, keep your blood pressure in check, and allow your blood to flow easily through your arteries. Plus, women who don't exercise and move around a lot usually carry excess weight, which puts additional strain on their heart, blood vessels, and joints. No wonder heart disease is twice as likely to develop in inactive women as in those who are more active.

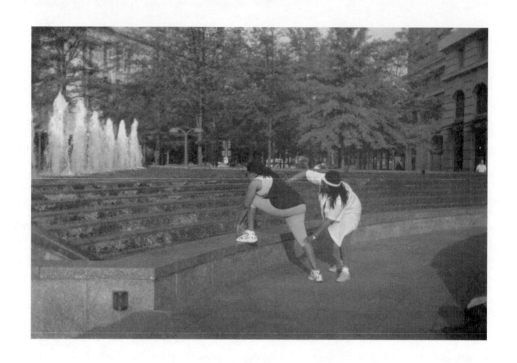

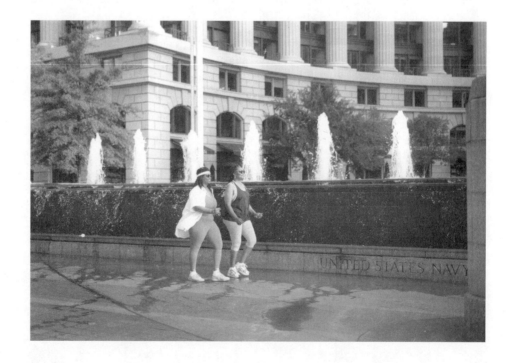

However, as we said before, **inactivity is the number two preventable cause of death.** That's because exercise is an unusually powerful way to alter your risk factors for high blood pressure and coronary artery problems, heart disease, stress, stroke, and diabetes.

Here are some facts to drive this point home:

• Exercise decreases your risk of cardiovascular disease (heart disease and stroke) by 50 percent.

• Exercise decreases the onset of Type 2 diabetes by 30 percent.

• Exercise decreases your risk of developing breast cancer by 20 percent to 30 percent—especially if you are obese.

• Exercise decreases the risk of colon cancer.

• Exercise decreases your chance of developing a hip fracture by 40 percent to 50 percent.

• Exercise improves your mood and decreases stress.

• Exercise improves your sexual pleasure.

(Chapter 9, "Developing Your Prime Time Wellness Plan," discusses a variety of physical activity programs that appeal to women of all ages, sizes, and physical conditions. Finding the right program is key if you are going to make exercise a daily activity.)

## Stress

Some studies show that emotional stress, such as tension, frustration, and depression, more than doubles the risk of a heart attack in patients with existing heart disease. One reason is that stress can keep your blood pressure abnormally high. Stress also prevents your immune system from functioning properly, which can increase your risk of developing cancer and infections. (See Chapter 13, "Stress Can Be Managed," for more information about reducing your stress level.)

## Poor Diet and Obesity

Not only is excess weight unhealthy, but obesity is associated with inadequate exercise and high-fat, high-carbohydrate diets. High-fat diets increase the amount of lipids in the bloodstream, which can lead to clogged arteries. This condition contributes to cardiovascular disease. Overeating also aggravates

# Check Your Weight and Heart Disease
# I.Q.

Prepared by the National Heart, Lung, and Blood Institute • NATIONAL INSTITUTES OF HEALTH

**The following statements are either true or false.**
**The statements test your knowledge of overweight and heart disease.**
**The correct answers can be found on pages 113–114.**

T F **1** Being overweight puts you at risk for heart disease.

T F **2** If you are overweight, losing weight helps lower your high blood cholesterol and high blood pressure.

T F **3** Quitting smoking is healthy, but it commonly leads to excessive weight gain which increases your risk for heart disease.

T F **4** An overweight person with high blood pressure should pay more attention to a low-sodium diet than to weight reduction.

T F **5** A reduced intake of sodium or salt does not always lower high blood pressure to normal.

T F **6** The best way to lose weight is to eat fewer calories and exercise.

T F **7** Skipping meals is a good way to cut down on calories.

T F **8** Foods high in complex carbohydrates (starch and fiber) are good choices when you are trying to lose weight.

T F **9** The single most important change most people can make to lose weight is to avoid sugar.

T F **10** Polyunsaturated fat has the same number of calories as saturated fat.

T F **11** Overweight children are very likely to become overweight adults.

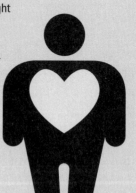

**YOUR SCORE:** How many correct answers did you make?

**10 –11 correct** = Congratulations!
You know a lot about weight and heart disease.
Share this information with your family and friends.
**8 –9 correct** = Very good.
**Fewer than 8** = Go over the answers and try to learn more about weight and heart disease.

**1 True.** Being overweight increases your risk for high blood cholesterol and high blood pressure, two of the major risk factors for coronary heart disease. Even if you do not have high blood cholesterol or high blood pressure, being overweight may increase your risk for heart disease. Where you carry your extra weight may affect your risk, too. Weight carried at your waist or above seems to be associated with an increased risk for heart disease in many people. In addition, being overweight increases your risk for diabetes, gallbladder disease, and some types of cancer.

**2 True.** If you are overweight, even moderate reductions in weight, such as 5 to 10 percent, can produce substantial reductions in blood pressure. You may also be able to reduce your LDL-cholesterol ("bad" cholesterol) and triglycerides and increase your HDL-cholesterol ("good" cholesterol).

**3 False.** The average weight gain after quitting smoking is 5 pounds. The proportion of ex-smokers who gain large amounts of weight (greater than 20 pounds) is relatively small. Even if you gain weight when you stop smoking, change your eating and exercise habits to lose weight rather than starting to smoke again. Smokers who quit smoking decrease their risk for heart disease by about 50 percent compared to those people who do not quit.

**4 False.** Weight loss, if you are overweight, may reduce your blood pressure even if you don't reduce the amount of sodium you eat. Weight loss is recommended for all overweight people who have high blood pressure. Even if weight loss does not reduce your blood pressure to normal, it may help you cut back on your blood pressure medications. Also, losing weight if you are overweight may help you reduce your risk for or control other health problems.

**5 True.** Even though a high sodium or salt intake plays a key role in maintaining high blood pressure in some people, there is no easy way to determine who will benefit from eating less sodium and salt. Also, a high intake may limit how well certain high blood pressure medications work. Eating a diet with less sodium may help some people reduce their risk of developing high blood pressure. Most Americans eat more salt and other sources of sodium than they need. Therefore, it is prudent for most people to reduce their sodium intake.

**6 True.** Eating fewer calories and exercising more is the best way to lose weight and keep it off. Weight control is a question of balance. You get calories from the food you eat. You burn off calories by exercising. Cutting down on calories, especially calories from fat, is key to losing weight. Combining this with a regular exercise program, like walking, bicycling, jogging, or swimming, not only can help in losing weight but also in maintaining the weight loss. A steady weight loss of 1 to 2 pounds a week is safe for most adults, and the weight is more likely to stay off over the long run. Losing weight, if you are overweight, may also help reduce your blood pressure and raise your HDL-cholesterol, the "good" cholesterol.

**7 False.** To cut calories, some people regularly skip meals and have no snacks or caloric drinks in between. If you do this, your body thinks that it is starving even if your intake of calories is not reduced to a very low amount. Your body will try to save energy by slowing its metabolism, that is, decreasing the rate at which it burns calories. This makes losing weight even harder and may even add body fat. Try to avoid long periods without eating. Five or six small meals are often preferred to the usual three meals a day for some individuals trying to lose weight.

**8 True.** Contrary to popular belief, foods high in complex carbohydrates (like pasta, rice, potatoes, breads, cereals, grains, dried beans, and peas) are lower in calories than foods high in fat. In addition, they are good sources of vitamins, minerals, and fiber. What adds calories to these foods is the addition of butter, rich sauces, whole milk, cheese, or cream, which are high in fat.

**9 False.** Sugar has not been found to cause obesity; however, many foods high in sugar are also high in fat. Fat has more than twice the calories as the same amount of protein or carbohydrates (sugar and starch). Thus, foods that are high in fat are high in calories. High-sugar foods, like cakes, cookies, candies, and ice cream, are high in fat and calories and low in vitamins, minerals, and protein.

(continued on next page)

**10 True.** All fats—polyunsaturated, monounsaturated, and saturated—have the same number of calories. All calories count whether they come from saturated or unsaturated fats. Because fats are the richest sources of calories, eating less total fat will help reduce the number of calories you eat every day. It will also help you reduce your intake of saturated fat. Particular attention to reducing saturated fat is important in lowering your blood cholesterol level.

**11 False.** Obesity in childhood does increase the likelihood of adult obesity, but most overweight children will not become obese. Several factors influence whether or not an overweight child becomes an overweight adult: (1) the age the child becomes overweight; (2) how overweight the child is; (3) the family history of overweight; and (4) dietary and activity habits. Getting to the right weight is desirable, but children's needs for calories and other nutrients are different from the needs of adults. Dietary plans for weight control must allow for this. Eating habits, like so many other habits, are often formed during childhood, so it is important to develop good ones.

For more information, write:
**NHLBI Obesity Education Initiative**
**P.O. Box 30105**
**Bethesda, MD 20824-0105**

National Heart, Lung, and Blood Institute
NIH Publication No 83-3034
U.S. DEPARTMENT OF HEALTH AND HUMAN SERVICES
Public Health Service

Type 2 diabetes. Eating too much carbohydrate causes the body to produce spikes of insulin. (Take the Nutrition Quiz in Chapter 9 to find out how much you know about healthy eating habits.)

## High Blood Cholesterol

If you have high blood cholesterol, fat in the blood settles on the inner walls of the blood vessels (especially the arteries) in deposits called plaque, narrowing them and restricting the flow of blood to the heart and brain. This can lead to hypertension, heart disease, and stroke. Cholesterol levels tend to rise sharply at age forty and continue to increase until about age sixty.

Monitoring your total cholesterol count is not enough. You also must keep track of the level of each type of cholesterol (LDL or "bad" cholesterol and HDL or "good" cholesterol) that your body produces. If your HDL is less than 35, the risk of heart disease increases dramatically. On the other hand, if your HDL is 60 or above, you have a lower risk of developing arteriosclerosis (clogged arteries), which can lead to heart disease and stroke. The Framingham Heart Study showed the risk of heart attack to be six times higher in women with the lowest HDL levels.[1] (This was not true in men.) Your LDL level is even more important to watch out for, because LDL promotes the buildup of fatty deposits in the arteries. You want your LDL to be below 130. An LDL above 160 puts you at high risk of developing coronary artery disease. (To learn effective ways to fight high cholesterol, review the Prime Time Prescriptions for nutrition in Chapter 9 and for heart disease in Chapter 10.)

## Hypertension

All five of the modifiable risk factors we discussed above contribute to what we call the "big mama of risk factors" for heart disease and stroke—high blood pressure, also known as hypertension. In fact, hypertension is so prevalent in the Black community that some physicians consider it the number one health problem for African Americans. One out of every three African Americans has high blood pressure, compared to one out of every four Americans as a whole. Hypertension also affects other important organs in the body, such as the kidneys and the eyes. Even if you are taking medication to lower your pressure, a program of exercise and healthy eating should be a critical part of your treatment. (Chapter 10 offers a full menu of ideas on how to address hypertension.)

## HOW YOU LIVE MAKES A DIFFERENCE

### VANESSA'S STORY

We all piled into my car. No one said a word as we pulled away from the funeral home. After a few minutes, the tears started flowing again as we shared our grief and shock over Linda's death at age fifty-five from a heart attack.

Linda had such a full life, working her way up to a supervisory position at a major telecommunications corporation. She was the first member of her family to go to college, and her degree from Spelman College had served her well. She always worked harder and longer hours than anyone else in her office. Although she was dedicated to her family and her church, her job often seemed to be her primary focus. Everyone, including Linda herself, called her a workaholic. Although she insisted that her children and husband keep their medical appointments, Linda never took time to make an appointment for herself.

In many ways, all four of us in the car are very similar to Linda—hardworking and actively involved in caring for our immediate and extended families. I also make certain that my kids, my husband, and my mom get regular medical checkups. I am also happily married, career-minded, and work hard as a teacher.

Even though I know it's a terrible habit, I also try to manage my stress and weight by being a "closet smoker," like Linda. I rarely exercise, and dining out for me is a run past the take-out window at Mickey D's.

As I dropped off my friends and drove home alone, the words of the minister echoed in my head: "Linda was a wonderful woman. It's a shame she could never find the time to take care of herself." Right then and there, I decided to stop smoking, change my eat-on-the-run fast-food diet, and above all, make an appointment for a full head-to-toe physical exam. Fortunately, everything was normal the last time I had gone—five years ago.

As I pulled into my driveway, a picture of Linda's husband's grief-stricken face and the tears in her children's eyes came to my mind, and I vowed not to subject my family to my own premature death—especially since I can do something about it.

---

It took the tragic death of a close friend for Vanessa to take charge of her life. Sound familiar? We've all been there. That's because there are too many Lindas in our African American communities leaving way too soon. These deaths don't have to happen. Don't let it happen to you. Treasuring and protecting your health is a daily activity that **requires you to do two things: prevent disease from entering your life, and promote good health in your life.** The key to achieving both of these goals is to appreciate and nurture your health while you still have it. You can't wait until you are gravely ill or a loved one has died to get serious about your well-being.

One of the greatest achievements of this century is that the average life expectancy of all Americans has risen from forty-five to seventy-five. For Caucasian women, it has jumped from forty-nine to eighty, and for us from thirty-five to seventy-five. The average life expectancy for Asian American women is as high as ninety years! Even though most of us thank medical science for our longer lives, a 1994 report from the Centers for Disease Control and Prevention (CDC) estimates that only five of those additional thirty to forty years can be attributed to new medical diagnostic tools, procedures, and treatments. According to the report, major improvements in nutrition, housing, sanitation, and occupational safety throughout this century deserve the most credit for helping Americans live longer.

Studies also show that lifestyle decisions—from smoking to exercising— have a major impact on how long we live. In fact, according to the CDC, 50 percent of the factors that determine our state of health are related to our behavior! Look at chart C opposite. Lifestyle is more important to our health than any of the three other key factors: the genes that we've inherited (20

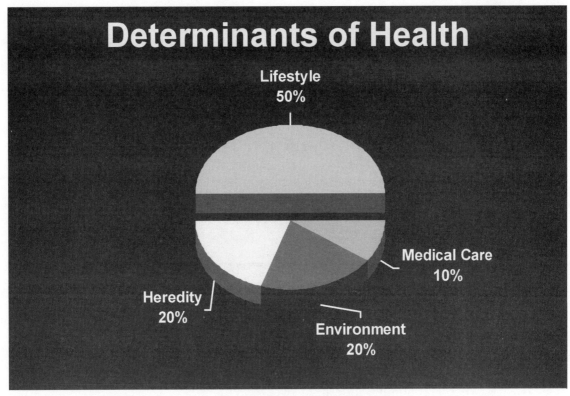

# Determinants of Health

Lifestyle
50%

Medical Care
10%

Heredity
20%

Environment
20%

*Source:* Centers for Disease Control and Prevention, 1995.

percent), environmental influences such as pesticides, asbestos, and work-related issues (20 percent), and the medical care we receive (10 percent).

According to the box below, the top five indicators of health also are based on lifestyle choices. This is good news, because you control your lifestyle. You can choose to exercise. You can choose the foods you eat. You can choose not to smoke, drink alcohol, take drugs, and have unprotected sex. You also can choose good ways to relieve stress.

## THE LEADING HEALTH INDICATORS

The Department of Health and Human Services, as part of the Healthy People 2010 program (www.health.gov/healthypeople), identified the ten major public health concerns in the United States. This list was developed to help Americans more easily understand the importance of viewing health promotion and disease prevention from a holistic point of view.

Developing strategies and action plans to address one or more of these indicators can have a profound effect on the quality of your life and how long you can live.

1. Physical activity
2. Overweight and obesity
3. Tobacco use
4. Substance abuse
5. Responsible sexual behavior
6. Mental health
7. Injury and violence
8. Environmental quality
9. Immunization
10. Access to health care

Your choices in how you live your life can reduce your chances of developing many diseases and chronic long-term illnesses that tend to arise in the middle and later years, such as the Big Four. Your choices also will affect how severe the diseases are if you already have one or more of them and how quickly and fully you can recover from them.

So in this chapter we're going to define and discuss what it really takes to prevent disease and promote health—especially for women at midlife.

## AN OUNCE OF PREVENTION

If we as a country generally and as African American women specifically focused as much time, money, and effort on promoting good health and preventing disease as we do on antiaging products, cosmetics, and dyes to mask the signs of growing older, we could probably extend our lives even longer than the life expectancies we quoted. Making an investment in your health by developing and maintaining a healthy lifestyle will greatly enhance the quality of your life. Prevention works! More than half of all health problems are preventable. And in most cases, prevention is up to you.

Modifying your behavior is not easy. In fact, you'll need to use your new way of thinking about yourself and your health that you developed in reading Chapter 4, "Now Your Journey Begins," to help you. It also requires a decision to make healthy choices every day and to adopt a holistic approach to wellness so that you care for the whole you—your mind, your body, and your spirit.

Yet, like our foremothers, many of us only think about our health or consider seeing a doctor when we don't feel well. Sometimes we don't go until we are already very sick. You've probably even heard older relatives say: "Girl, I'm good and healthy 'cause I don't know when I've had to go see the doctor!"

You don't want to subscribe to this old attitude. Illness shouldn't be your first signal that it's time to take care of yourself or seek medical attention. Illness is a crisis point, and it is preceded by a lot of little red flags that call for your attention. You don't ever want to wait until you get into a full-blown crisis before you get help. Remember the old adage: "An ounce of prevention is worth a pound of cure"? Well, if an ounce of prevention is good, think what a pound of prevention can do!

It's mind-blowing that of the $1 trillion spent on health care in this country, less than 1 percent is spent on prevention! It seems like such common sense to spend more of our health-care dollars on helping people stay healthy. That way, the overall costs of health care and treatment would drop dramatically. But for a paradigm shift of that magnitude to happen, our doctors, nurses, the entire health-care system, Congress, and each one of us would need to embrace the importance and power of preventive medicine. Let's pray and advocate that preventive medicine becomes a top priority in the new millennium, but meanwhile, let's get back to what *you* can do *for you* and your Prime Time Sister. We're going to take you step by step through very practical, very doable ways to prevent illness and boost your own health.

Prevention is daily. Prevention is repetitive. Prevention is continuous, not episodic. Prevention should permeate everything you do. Prevention also requires focus and planning. Let's talk more specifically about the two types of prevention you should practice:

1. **Primary prevention** *means just what it says—taking action to prevent or reduce the occurrence of disease.*

For instance, the best way to prevent HIV/AIDS is not to have vaginal or anal sex, or to practice safe sex by using a latex condom.

A good way to prevent lung cancer is not to smoke. If Americans stopped smoking, we could prevent four hundred thousand deaths each year from heart disease and lung diseases such as emphysema and lung cancer. One of the best ways to prevent heart disease and hypertension is to exercise regularly.

Increasing our physical activity would prevent three hundred thousand deaths each year. That's because **the number one preventable cause of death is smoking!** The number two preventable cause of death is inactivity!

The best way to ensure a healthy, long life is to avoid health problems in the first place. However, if you can't prevent a problem altogether, then the next best thing is to discover it early, when it's easy to treat. That's where secondary prevention comes in.

2. *Secondary prevention means stopping a disease in an early stage from progressing into a more severe stage.*

Having regular medical checkups is the first step in practicing secondary prevention. The way to prevent breast cancer from killing you, for instance, is through routine and regular mammograms, self-exams of your own breasts, and exams by your doctor. All of these interventions increase the probability of detecting the disease as early as possible. With most cancers, the earlier the disease is caught before it spreads to other parts of the body, the greater the chance for a cure.

## THE POWER OF PROMOTING GOOD HEALTH

Now that you have a better understanding of disease prevention, we can explain the importance of *health promotion*. As we've said before, health is not merely the absence of disease; health is also an enhanced state of well-being. In fact, the World Health Organization defines health as "physical, mental and social well-being, not merely the absence of disease and infirmity." We would also add spiritual well-being to this list.

Think of your health as a process that moves along an *illness/wellness continuum*. On one end is premature death, and on the other end is high-level wellness. Your job is to continue moving on the path to good health.

Your degree of health is somewhere on this continuum. (Where do you think you are?) So, you must practice *both* disease prevention and health promotion to avoid getting sick, and also to enhance your current state of health and move even further toward good health. See if you can adopt this positive image of prevention and promotion into your own new paradigm of yourself and your health: Health and wellness is not just about not smoking or avoiding other unhealthy habits; it is also a positive, forward-moving

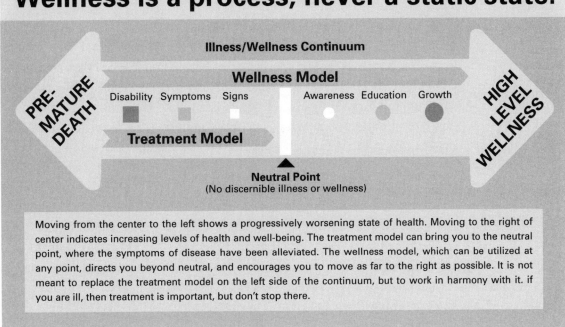

# Wellness is a process, never a static state.

**Illness/Wellness Continuum**

**Wellness Model**

PRE-MATURE DEATH

Disability   Symptoms   Signs

**Treatment Model**

Awareness   Education   Growth

HIGH LEVEL WELLNESS

▲
**Neutral Point**
(No discernible illness or wellness)

Moving from the center to the left shows a progressively worsening state of health. Moving to the right of center indicates increasing levels of health and well-being. The treatment model can bring you to the neutral point, where the symptoms of disease have been alleviated. The wellness model, which can be utilized at any point, directs you beyond neutral, and encourages you to move as far to the right as possible. It is not meant to replace the treatment model on the left side of the continuum, but to work in harmony with it. if you are ill, then treatment is important, but don't stop there.

*Source:* Reprinted with permission from *Wellness Workbook*, by John W. Travis, M.D., and Regina Sara Ryan, Ten Speed Press, Berkeley, CA. © 1981, 1988 by John W. Travis, M.D.

process of adopting positive health behaviors and habits to maximize your health status.

The daily practice of prevention of disease and promotion of health also means enhancing your life with joy, love, and spiritual fulfillment. As Iyanla Vanzant writes in *Acts of Faith*, "Change means identifying what you are doing, recognizing when you are doing it, and gently guiding yourself to do something else." Therefore, you must first examine your risk factors (such as being overweight or being inactive) for developing future problems and illnesses. Then you'll want to minimize these risk factors to prevent or reduce your chances of getting sick. (Throughout this book we'll talk more about risk factors for the major mental and physical illnesses and diseases from which African American women suffer.)

Enhancing your health may involve some difficult lifestyle changes: You will need to **stop doing** things that are not good for you, and **start doing** things that are good for you. We also want you to do things that you enjoy in life, which will improve the quality of your life. Keeping these pointers in mind, here's what we recommend for Vanessa after the death of her friend Linda made her realize she had to focus on her health.

### Rx | A QUICK PRIME TIME PRESCRIPTION FOR VANESSA

First, Vanessa must stop putting everyone's needs before her own and reframe her priorities to start taking care of herself and her health. Second, she must identify the risk factors that are endangering her health. These include smoking, not exercising, not eating the right foods (fast foods are high in fat, cholesterol, salt, and calories), not scheduling regular medical exams, and not managing the stress in her life. Third, Vanessa must develop a wellness plan to address her risk factors and put prevention into her daily life along with health-promoting behaviors.

Vanessa's Prime Time Wellness Plan begins with getting a complete physical exam and a schedule for follow-ups and routine medical tests (such as a Pap smear and a mammogram). Vanessa also must seek help to stop smoking, which will minimize her risk of heart disease and lung disease (bronchitis, emphysema, and cancer), start exercising, stop eating fast foods, and start eating more fruits and vegetables.

Finally, Vanessa must stop working seven days a week and start practicing stress management techniques. She must also start engaging in more activities that bring joy into her life, such as listening to music, spending time with friends, reading, and going to the movies. Praying, meditating, and learning relaxation techniques can dramatically reduce her stress. (For more details on how to develop your own personal Prime Time Wellness Plan, see Part III, "Putting Self-Care into Action.")

See how this stop/start idea works. The exercise below should help you start thinking about how to develop your own Prime Time Prescription for healthy living.

---

### THE STOP/START APPROACH TO HEALTHIER LIVING

Take a few minutes to think about five negative habits you must stop and five good habits that you must start to get on the path to a healthier life.

1. I must stop _____.
2. I must stop _____.
3. I must stop _____.

---

4. I must stop _____.
5. I must stop _____.

1. I must start _____.
2. I must start _____.
3. I must start _____.
4. I must start _____.
5. I must start _____.
If you have more to include, use your journal to continue. The goal is to develop **habits of health** that become second nature to you.

Success in reaching your level of optimal health rests on three things:

1. Your *commitment* to take care of yourself first
2. Your *belief* that you can and must do it
3. Your *determination* to develop and implement plans that will make you a healthier person—now and for the rest of your life

Self-care must become the predominant and most highly prized facet of your identity. In your new paradigm of yourself as an irreplaceable miracle, if you do not value self-care, your attempts to adopt and continue preventive and health-promoting measures are doomed to fail. Remember, *you* can do much more than any doctor to maintain your health and well-being. To get started, find out more about the state of your own health right now by filling out the Prime Time self-checkup worksheet below.

## HOW HEALTHY ARE YOU?

To help you identify some key goals and timetables to get you on the road to good health, answer the following questions.
   1. Did your parents or any of your siblings die before the age of sixty of nonaccidental causes?
                         YES          NO
   2. Do you exercise for at least thirty minutes every day?
                         YES          NO
   3. Do you take vitamin E (400 to 800 IU) every day?
                         YES          NO

4. Are you more than twenty pounds overweight?

        YES        NO

5. Do you floss your teeth every day?

        YES        NO

6. Do you get eight hours of sleep every night?

        YES        NO

7. Do you drink more than two cups of coffee a day?

        YES        NO

8. Are you still cooking with lard and fatback and eating red meat and fried foods regularly?

        YES        NO

9. Are you eating five to seven servings of fruits and vegetables every day?

        YES        NO

10. Do you cook your fish, poultry, or meat until it is charred?

        YES        NO

11. Do you smoke or are you around secondhand smoke on a regular basis?

        YES        NO

12. Do you know your blood pressure and your cholesterol levels and know what they mean?

        YES        NO

13. Do you have a regular physician whom you trust and who treats you with respect?

        YES        NO

14. Do you drink more than one serving of beer, wine, and/or liquor a day?

        YES        NO

15. Do you feel overwhelmed with your family life, financial issues, or work?

        YES        NO

16. Have you been unable to get work done and find yourself procrastinating a lot lately?

        YES        NO

17. Can you shed stress by praying, exercising, meditating, or some other healthy, enjoyable activity?

        YES        NO

18. Do you find joy in your life most of the time?

        YES        NO

19. Have you been sad for more than two weeks?

        YES        NO

## YOUR FAMILY'S HEALTH HISTORY

"Tracing your family's health may be the most important step you ever take toward long life," says geneticist Steven Finch. And we agree. Any disease that runs in your family puts you at risk. For instance, a family history of high blood pressure (hypertension) increases your risk of high blood pressure, heart disease, and stroke. If a disease runs in your family—meaning that several of your relatives (especially parents and grandparents) have suffered from it—then the risk of your developing that disease is quite high. The risk is even higher if your close relative developed the disease at a relatively young age. In that case, your prevention efforts must be quite aggressive.

Just because a disease is not in your family, however, doesn't mean that you are not at risk of developing it. Likewise, if a disease is in your family, it doesn't mean you are doomed to have it. *Some risks stem from habits nurtured by our families, such as our love for rich, fatty soul food.* In fact, lifestyle choices that have passed through the generations can even increase your risk for such illnesses as alcoholism. Studies reveal that up to 25 percent of children of alcoholics are likely to become alcoholics. If excessive drinking is part of your family's history, you must be especially vigilant not to abuse alcohol and encourage your children not to do so as well. So when researching your family's health history, keep this saying in mind: *"Genes cock the gun, but the environment pulls the trigger."*

Tracing your family's health history is critical if you are committed to improving your health and preventing your children, grandchildren, and other relatives from suffering the same fate as some of your older family members.

To help you begin this significant project, fill in the table "My Family's Health History." You can also buy Fran Carlson's medical history kit called *Growing Your Family Medical Tree*. The kit includes a fifty-page booklet, the

# MY FAMILY'S HEALTH HISTORY

| | ME | PARENTS | | MATERNAL GRANDPARENTS | | PATERNAL GRANDPARENTS | |
| | | MOTHER | FATHER | GRAND-FATHER | GRAND-MOTHER | GRAND-FATHER | GRAND-MOTHER |
|---|---|---|---|---|---|---|---|
| AGE AT DEATH | — | | | | | | |
| CAUSE OF DEATH | — | | | | | | |

Health Conditions (fill in YES, NO, or DON'T KNOW)

| | | | | | | | |
|---|---|---|---|---|---|---|---|
| OVERWEIGHT | | | | | | | |
| HEART DISEASE (HEART ATTACK, ANGINA BEFORE 60) | | | | | | | |
| HEART DISEASE (AFTER AGE 60) | | | | | | | |
| ANY TYPE OF STROKE | | | | | | | |
| VASCULAR DISEASE (BLOCKED ARTERY) | | | | | | | |
| ABNORMAL CHOLESTEROL | | | | | | | |
| HIGH BLOOD PRESSURE | | | | | | | |
| DIABETES (ONSET IN CHILDHOOD) | | | | | | | |
| DIABETES (ONSET IN ADULTHOOD) | | | | | | | |
| BREAST CANCER (BEFORE AGE 50) | | | | | | | |
| COLON CANCER | | | | | | | |
| UTERINE CANCER | | | | | | | |

| | ME | PARENTS | | MATERNAL GRANDPARENTS | | PATERNAL GRANDPARENTS | |
| | | MOTHER | FATHER | GRAND-FATHER | GRAND-MOTHER | GRAND-FATHER | GRAND-MOTHER |
|---|---|---|---|---|---|---|---|
| CERVICAL CANCER | | | | | | | |
| OVARIAN CANCER | | | | | | | |
| PROSTATE CANCER (BEFORE AGE 50) | | | | | | | |
| DEPRESSION | | | | | | | |
| ALCOHOLISM | | | | | | | |
| OTHER | | | | | | | |

Prepare additional charts for your aunts and uncles on both your mother's and father's sides of the family. Do an additional chart for your siblings.

Family Deck of Life cards, and color-coded stickers to identify your health risks. (Cost: $14.95 plus $2.50 postage and handling. To order, call (888) 385-KISS, or visit the Web site www.keepitsimplesolutions.com.)

When tracing your family's health history, start with your parents and siblings and then move on to your grandparents, aunts, and uncles. Encourage your spouse to do the same, so you can develop a similar chart for your children, but do your own *first*. Try to find out who was diagnosed with what and at what age. Be as specific as possible about the cause of death and age at death for each of your deceased relatives. Look for patterns of disease within your family. For instance, take note if, say, many of the men on your mother's side of the family have had a stroke or heart attack; that means you are at risk for these illnesses. Also, take into account the mental state of family members. Some types of depression occur often within families — even over several generations. No matter how difficult or uncomfortable you may be, ask your family if any of your relatives suffered from bouts of overwhelming sadness or if anyone attempted or committed suicide.

If many of your older relatives are no longer living, you can send for death certificates or obtain medical records to help fill in your family health picture. For death certificates, contact the state office of vital records or statistics in the state where that person died. The armed services should have records on deceased family members who were in the military.

If this process sounds daunting, please keep in mind that you can't complete this project overnight. Pace yourself, and soon all of the blanks will be filled in. Meanwhile there are other risk factors you can tackle right away to help you move forward on the health continuum.

After you have filled out the charts as best you can, discuss the findings with your family and your doctor. Where there are increased risks for certain diseases, develop your prevention plan of action with your physician, and encourage the rest of your family to do the same. Your family history does not have to repeat itself. Ignoring family illnesses guarantees their place in future generations.

## IT'S NEVER TOO LATE

Despite what you may think, it doesn't matter how old you are when you begin to deal with your risk factors and make significant changes in your lifestyle. *It's never too late!* If you're still not convinced, maybe some encouragement from the sisters Sadie and Bessie Delany, who lived past a hundred years of age and wrote a best-seller, will help. Their story should inspire all of us.

---

### THE DELANY SISTERS' STORY

In the mornings, Monday through Friday, we do our yoga exercises. I started doing yoga exercises with Mama about forty years ago. Mama was starting to shrink up and bend down, and I started exercising with her to straighten her up again. Only I didn't know at the time that what we were actually doing was "yoga." We just thought we were exercising.

I kept doing my yoga exercises, even after Mama died. Well, when Bessie turned eighty she decided that I looked better than her. So, she decided she would start doing yoga too. So, we've been doing our exercises together ever since. We follow a yoga exercise program on the TV. Sometimes Bessie cheats. I'll be doing an exercise and look over at her, and she's just lying there! She's a naughty old gal.

Exercise is very important. A lot of older people don't exercise at all. Another thing that is terribly important is diet. I keep up with the latest news about nutrition. About thirty years ago, Bessie and I started eating much more healthy foods. We don't eat that fatty Southern food very often. When we do, we feel like we can't move!

We eat as many as seven different vegetables a day. Plus lots of fresh fruits. And we take vitamin supplements: vitamin A, B complex, C, D, E, and minerals too, like zinc. And Bessie takes tyrosine when she's a little blue.

Every morning, after we do our yoga, we each take a clove of garlic, chop it up, and swallow it whole. If you swallow it all at once, there is no odor. We also take a teaspoon of cod liver oil. Bessie thinks it's disgusting. But one day I said, "Now, dear little sister, if you want to keep up with me, you're going to have to start taking it, every day, and stop complainin'." And she's been good ever since.

—From *Having Our Say: The Delany Sisters' First 100 Years*

Is it any wonder the Delany sisters lived to be over a hundred years old? Enough said!

# Putting
# Self-Care
# Into Action

# Chapter 8

# THE ULTIMATE CHECKUP

*Let me put my full weight down!*

—African proverb

"Let me put my full weight down" is the English translation of an African saying that means: "Take responsibility for one's life." Part III, "Putting Self-Care Into Action," will help you apply the principles of disease prevention and health promotion that we discussed in Chapter 7. Our goal is for you to develop your own personal Prime Time Wellness Plan—from getting the ultimate physical checkup to developing a fitness and nutrition plan for a healthier life.

Your first step in developing this plan is to assess where you are right now in terms of your health and general well-being, and whether you're ready for Prime Time living.

---

### ARE YOU READY FOR PRIME TIME LIVING?

Answering the following questions will help you get started developing a comprehensive health-care program tailored to your needs as a Prime Time woman.

*YOUR HEALTH TEAM*

    1. Do you have a primary-care physician (trained in internal or family medicine), gynecologist, and dentist?

                      YES          NO

---

2. Do you have regular examinations?

YES     NO

3. Are you comfortable discussing all of your health concerns with these doctors?

YES     NO

*PHYSICAL EXAMS*

4. When was the last time you had the following exams—this year, last year, two to four years ago, or five years ago or longer?

| | |
|---|---|
| Complete physical examination | _____ |
| Gynecological exam | _____ |
| Eye exam | _____ |
| Dental exam | _____ |

5. Do you know what should be covered in these exams?

YES     NO

*MEDICAL TESTS SCHEDULES/RECORDS*

6. Do you keep a schedule of your exams and special tests?

YES     NO

7. Do you keep copies of your latest laboratory test results, such as X rays, mammograms, cholesterol levels, and blood pressure readings?

YES     NO

*FOLLOW-UP VISITS AND ACTION PLANS*

8. Do you review the results of exams and lab tests with your doctors and establish goals and plans for improvement?

YES     NO

*MEDICATIONS*

9. Do you go to one pharmacist to have all of your prescriptions filled?

YES     NO

10. Does the drugstore keep a record of your medications?

YES     NO

11. Does your pharmacist provide information on dosage and discuss other concerns such as the dangers of taking certain medications with alcohol, over-the-counter medicines, and herbal remedies?

YES     NO

ANSWERS

If all of your answers are yes, congratulations! If you've answered no to any question, evaluate what you can do to change the answer to yes.

## GETTING STARTED ON THE PATH TO WELLNESS

Self-care requires you to schedule regular checkups with your primary care physician, gynecologist, and dentist. Your primary care provider will monitor your health closely by taking your medical history, conducting physical exams, scheduling diagnostic tests, and coordinating your care with any specialists you may need. (For more information on working with your doctors and other health-care providers—or for tips on how to find the right doctor for you—see Chapter 19, "Become a Smarter Health-Care Consumer.")

Self-care also requires that you monitor aspects of your health with self-exams (such as breast examinations or blood pressure readings, if necessary) between visits to your health-care professional.

Some African Americans don't schedule regular physical exams because they are afraid of what the doctor may find. Some don't understand the importance of regular checkups in monitoring their health and detecting problems *before* they become major threats. We authors have discovered that a good number of Black women won't go to the doctor because they don't trust the health-care system—that includes the doctors, nurses, and other professionals, as well as the system itself.

We understand that this lack of trust stems from many different experiences, past and present. Many African Americans remember the injustice of the Tuskegee experiments, when Black men were denied treatment for syphilis to allow doctors to study the long-term effects of this illness. You may have known friends or family members who were denied treatment at segregated hospitals or clinics. You probably have read or heard about recent reports on the high number of medical errors in hospitals.

Without a doubt, all of these experiences and injustices are painful to remember and difficult to forget. But despite your fears and distrust, *regular visits to the doctor are one of the best ways to take charge of your health and prevent future problems.*

By monitoring your health and addressing any signs of illness or disease early, you can live a longer and healthier life. Equally important, you must become a smarter health-care consumer and learn how to choose doctors and other health-care professionals who are willing to work with you to address your specific medical needs. You also must learn how to successfully navigate the health-care bureaucracy—from HMOs to insurance claims—to make sure the system works for you. (Turn to Chapter 19 to learn how you can become an informed health-care consumer.)

We also understand that a visit to the doctor can be unnerving, especially when you're concerned that an exam might reveal that you have a medical problem. But trust us: **When it comes to your health, ignorance is not bliss.** If you know, you can do something about it and improve the outcome. Not knowing is absolutely the worst state to be in. If you haven't been to the doctor recently and are uncomfortable going alone, ask your Prime Time Sister to go with you. She can also sit in when you meet with the doctor after your exam to discuss his or her findings.

Since some women postpone going to the doctor out of fear or lack of understanding about why checkups are important, let's review which critical examinations you should have during your middle years, what they should include, and how often they should be performed. (For an at-a-glance table of the exams and how often they should be performed, see the Prime Time Health Calendar at the end of this chapter). This is what you should use to record all your visits and the findings of your physical exam and any tests performed.

## YOUR GENERAL PHYSICAL EXAM

When you reach midlife, you *must* have an annual general physical exam by your primary-care provider, which is usually a doctor trained in internal medicine or family medicine.

You might be asking yourself: "I feel great, no problems, so do I really need a complete checkup every year?" On this point there is no discussion and no compromise! Prime Time women need a head-to-toe examination by a physician every year for three primary reasons:

• To document your baseline health status and monitor the changes in your body that frequently occur during the middle years
• To evaluate your health and review, update, and change, if necessary, your prevention and health promotion activities
• To detect any abnormalities, problems, or diseases as early as possible

Before the physical exam begins, you will be asked to fill out a preprinted questionnaire requesting information about your medical history and the current state of your physical, mental, and emotional health. (Sometimes the nurse or doctor will simply ask you questions from the form.) Some will be medical questions; others will focus on lifestyle issues.

Questions include: *Are you on any prescription or over-the-counter medications? Do you smoke? Do you have allergies? What was the date of your last menstrual period? Do you drink alcohol? If yes, how many drinks do you have each week? Are you worried about anything specifically? Are you sexually active? Do you have multiple sex partners?* The form may even include questions on oral and anal sex. Another section of the questionnaire will ask about your family history. These questions will focus on conditions or illnesses that run in your family.

Although many of the questions may seem intrusive, it is imperative that you answer each one honestly—even the ones that may feel a bit embarrassing. Doctors need all the information they can gather to help you make the right decisions about your health. This is not the time to be concerned about what others think of you.

Expect to give a sample of your urine and perhaps even your blood at the doctor's office. If he or she does not collect samples at the office, the doctor will probably send you to a laboratory for this battery of diagnostic tests. (More on these tests later.)

The next section covers what's included in a routine annual physical examination. If any of the following exams are not done, ask your physician for the reason for their omission. Once the exam is complete, you should meet with the doctor in his or her office to discuss your exam and receive counseling about any risk factors (such as high blood pressure, weight concerns, high stress, or emotional issues) you may have. You should also discuss lifestyle changes that could improve your health or prevent any serious problems from occurring.

Remember, this is your time to talk to your doctor, ask questions, and get more information about yourself and your body. If you don't understand something the doctor says, speak up. Don't be shy. There are no dumb questions when it comes to being absolutely clear about your health. So have a prepared written list of questions about your concerns to make the most of this time with your doctor. (For a sample, see Chapter 19, "Become a Smarter Health-Care Consumer.") If your doctor isn't forthcoming with answers, find a better doctor. You can also ask the nurse for clarification or call any of the many health organizations listed throughout this book for information and advice.

Request copies of the results of all findings on the physical and laboratory tests. (And be sure any specialists you see, such as your cardiologist or gynecologist, send all reports and test results to your primary care physician.) The

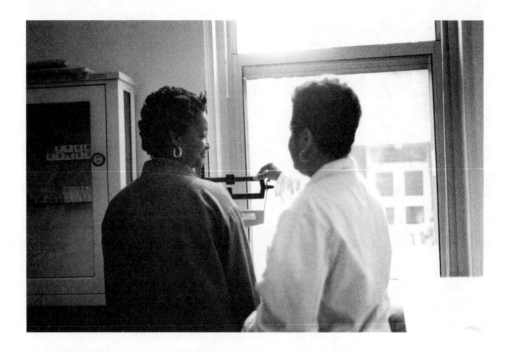

more information your doctors have about the state of your health, the better your care will be. Finally, record all exams and results on the form at the end of this chapter and in your health notebook or journal.

## Checklist for Your Annual Physical Exam

### *Blood Pressure, Pulse, and Weight*

The nurse usually takes these measurements for the doctor. As an African American, you have a one in three chance of developing high blood pressure (hypertension). For white women, the chances are one in five. The longer your high blood pressure goes undetected and untreated, the higher your risk of heart attack, stroke, and kidney damage.

A blood pressure test is quick and simple, but don't worry if a single test turns up high. This may be due to the stress we sometimes feel when visiting the doctor. In fact, this happens so often, it has a name: "white coat hypertension." However, if your blood pressure stays elevated, you may need medical treatment in addition to changing your diet, increasing your physical activity, and starting a program to help reduce your stress. (See the sec-

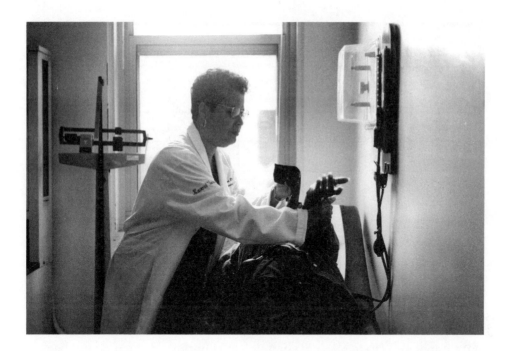

tion on hypertension in Chapter 10 for more information about controlling high blood pressure.)

Blood pressure readings consist of two numbers. The first or top number is the *systolic* pressure, which is the amount of pressure on your blood vessels when your heart beats. The second or bottom number is the *diastolic* pressure, which is the amount of pressure on your blood vessels when your heart is at rest. Your blood pressure is measured in millimeters of mercury (mm Hg).

A blood pressure of 130/80 mm Hg is usually considered normal. However, some experts prefer using a lower reading—120/70—as normal. Nevertheless, if your blood pressure is 140/90 or higher, you are definitely hypertensive. If your blood pressure is high at this reading, have the nurse take it again with you standing up and again after you've rested for a few minutes.

### Eye Exam

The primary-care provider will check for any redness, discharge, or discoloration of the sclera, the white part of the eye. He or she will also shine a

## BLOOD PRESSURE CATEGORIES

| CATEGORY | SYSTOLIC (mm Hg) | DIASTOLIC (mm Hg) | FOLLOW-UP |
|---|---|---|---|
| OPTIMAL | <120 | <80 | Annual checkups are required. |
| NORMAL | <130 | <85 | Annual checkups are required. |
| HIGH NORMAL | 130–139 | 85–89 | Home monitoring and annual checkups are required. Your health-care provider will recommend that you modify your lifestyle by eating better and exercising more. Some doctors start treatments for hypertension in this range. |

light into your eyes to see movement of your pupil and examine the back of your eye—the retina—to see if your blood vessels are narrowed or if any bleeding can be seen, as with high blood pressure or diabetes. A complete exam with special instruments must be completed by your ophthalmologist or eye specialist.

### Ear, Nose, and Throat

The doctor will check all three areas by looking for any types of abnormalities, such as masses, redness or discharge, and signs of inflammation. Periodic hearing tests are advised, since the chances of hearing loss increase after the age of fifty and may go unnoticed.

### Neck and Thyroid

The doctor will feel your neck to see if your thyroid is enlarged or if you have any swollen lymph nodes or other masses in your neck. Every woman over forty should have a blood test to check her levels of thyroid hormone, since at midlife, women have a greater than 40 percent chance of developing hypothyroidism or hyperthyroidism, according to Dr. Ridha Arem, author of *The Thyroid Solution.*

The doctor should also use a stethoscope to listen over the carotid arteries on both sides of your neck for a *bruit*. A bruit is a sound that occurs when blood tries to flow through arteries that are narrowed due to fatty deposits. The carotid arteries lead to the brain, and any narrowing can be a warning sign of a future stroke.

## Breast Exam

Both your primary care physician and gynecologist can perform a clinical breast exam during your annual examination. (A trained nurse practitioner or physician assistant also can perform this exam.) The doctor or clinician will feel both breasts and under the armpit to check for cysts or signs of cancer, including asymmetry (unequal breast size), dimpling, nipple discharge, and abnormal masses. This exam allows clinicians to check the sides of the breasts extending into the armpits, which is an important area that mammograms sometimes fail to screen.

## Cardiac and Lung Exam

The clinician will first feel your chest with his or her hand, check the size of your heart to see if it is enlarged, and also feel for any abnormalities as the heart beats. Then the doctor will use a stethoscope to listen to your heart rhythm and for heart murmurs. He or she will ask you to breathe deeply to check your lungs for any abnormal sounds, such as wheezes.

## Abdominal Exam

During this part of the exam, the doctor gently pokes around your abdominal area to check the size of your spleen (on your left side) and liver (on your right side) and feel for any masses or tender areas. He or she will also feel the middle of your back (over the kidneys) to check for tenderness, which can be a sign of infection.

## Rectal Exam

The doctor will check the outside of your rectum for abnormalities such as hemorrhoids or genital warts and insert a gloved finger into your rectum to check for masses and also feel the size of your uterus and ovaries and placement. The uterus and ovaries are also palpated in the pelvic exam (see "Gynecological Exam," below). He or she will take a small sample of stool to test for hidden blood. (See page 149 for more information on sigmoidoscopy and colonoscopy.)

### Extremities Exam

The doctor will check the pulse in your legs and feet and look for varicose veins, swelling, and discoloration. If you are diabetic, your doctor must regularly examine your feet to check for circulation problems, test your sensation, and look for or monitor sores that are taking a long time to heal. *Although a foot exam is part of your annual checkup, if you are diabetic, you must have your feet examined at least once every year and perhaps more often to prevent any problems from becoming so serious that you must have your leg or foot amputated.*

### Neurological Exam

The doctor will use a rubber hammer to check your reflexes. He or she also will push against your arms or legs to test your strength and look for areas of weakness. The doctor may also use a brush or pin to test sensation in your extremities.

## Gynecological Exam

Your gynecologist will also require you to fill out a form similar to the one at your primary care physician's office; however, it may not be as detailed. The nurse will also take your blood pressure, pulse, and weight. Prior to a pelvic examination, your gynecologist will probably do a breast exam, and may listen to your heart and check your lungs.

The centerpiece of the gynecological examination is the pelvic exam. Your gynecologist will inspect the opening of the vagina (the vulva) for masses, redness, skin lesions, or discharge. Using gloves, the doctor will also insert his or her fingers to feel the size of the uterus and the ovaries and to check for any masses. The doctor then will insert a speculum (a metal or plastic instrument) to check the vaginal wall for changes secondary to menopause and loss of estrogen, and check the cervix for abnormalities, signs of infection, and vaginal discharge. The Pap smear (see below for full description) is done with the speculum in place. If it is performed by a gynecologist, be sure to have the results sent to your primary-care physician.

## The Eye Exam (by an ophthalmologist or optometrist)

Women at midlife should routinely get an eye exam by an ophthalmologist or optometrist every one or two years. The exam should include tests for vision, eye pressure (checking for glaucoma), and cataracts. The doctor will also dilate your eyes to look at the back of the eye (the retina), which is the only place in the body where the blood vessels can be seen directly without cutting into the body. This is one way the physician can check for blood vessel disease, bleeding, or other abnormalities. *If you are diabetic, you should see the eye doctor every year, more often if you are experiencing any problems.*

## The Dental Exam

The dentist will check for masses in your mouth and check for oral cancer; look for discoloration, bleeding, or other abnormalities in your gums; and examine each tooth for cavities. He or she will see how your dentures fit (if you have them) and assess their general condition. X rays will be taken. Your teeth should be cleaned by a dental hygienist every six months.

## EIGHT MEDICAL TESTS THAT WILL SAVE YOUR LIFE

In addition to the blood pressure readings that are taken during your annual checkup (and the monitoring you do at home if you have hypertension), medical experts point to eight other medical and screening tests that could save your life.[1] These are:

1. Mammogram
2. Lipid (fat) profile
3. Pap smear

4. Stool blood test, sigmoidoscopy, and colonoscopy
5. Bone density test
6. Electrocardiogram
7. Fasting blood sugar test and two-hour postprandial test
8. HIV test

These tests are so important that every Prime Time woman must have them at least once in her forties or early fifties to provide a baseline reading or starting point. After the first test, you should then have them as often as your doctor recommends. (See screening guidelines in the Prime Time Medical Calendar on page 153 for suggested schedules.)

Just taking these tests is not enough to ensure your health. You must also discuss the results with your doctor, immediately address troublesome findings, and closely monitor any unusual findings over time. These tests are so vital that if your insurance company won't pay for them or pay as frequently as they are needed (some tests will need to be done more often if something is awry), then you must find ways to pay for them yourself, even if that means a few less visits to the nail salon.

At midlife, most of these exams are annual. One way to help you remember when you're due to get them is to schedule them at the time of your birthday and encourage your Prime Time Sister to do the same. What better way to celebrate your birth, your life, and your health?

Please remember that even though you may only need to see a doctor once or twice a year, you must be committed to improving your health 365 days a year. We hope that once you understand how these early detection methods work and why they are so necessary, you will be committed to getting them and discussing your results with your doctor.

## Mammogram and Clinical Breast Exam

This test can be requested by your primary care physician or gynecologist and can be scheduled at a mammography facility, hospital, women's clinic, or mammography van. Some workplaces offer annual on-site mammography screenings.

For women over fifty, numerous studies have shown that an annual mammogram and a clinical breast exam by a physician or nurse-practitioner cuts the risk of dying of breast cancer by more than 30 percent. The other piece of good news is that the effectiveness of these early-detection procedures increases as we get older because the density of our breast tissue diminishes with age, making it easier to find a tumor. Since this disease kills one out of every thirty women, that's an important edge to have.

A mammogram is a low-dose X ray that can detect a breast lump too small to be felt by you or your doctor. Mammography is able to detect the tiniest of tumors (a fraction of the size of lumps that can be felt during a self-examination) before they become invasive and spread. In fact, health researchers estimate that mammography screening can identify a lump up to two years before it will be found on a self-exam or clinical exam by your physician. This lead time can make the difference between life and death.

New methods of mammography currently under development may eventually lead to improved accuracy. For instance, digital mammography allows the image to be viewed from different angles on a computer. Standard mammography is 80–90 percent effective. Digital mammography has the potential to increase the effectiveness and is the wave of the future. Another test, high-definition imaging (HDI) ultrasound, may reduce the number of biopsies (the removal of cells to view under a microscope) on suspicious lumps by 40 percent.

In recent years, there has been some controversy over when women should start mammography screenings and how often they should schedule this test. For African American women without symptoms or a family history of breast cancer, the National Cancer Institute (NCI), the American Cancer Society, and the National Medical Association all recommend an initial mammography at age thirty-five as a baseline. Some physicians recommend that African American women have annual mammograms beginning at age thirty-five; other women, annually after age forty.

A mammography screening should be done by a qualified radiologist or registered technologist. To take the test, you will need to undress from the waist up and put on a gown with the opening at the front. The clinician will slightly flatten your breast in between two plastic plates to get a clear picture. A mammogram can be uncomfortable if you have cysts in your breasts, so don't have the test the week before your period. You can also take an over-the-counter pain reliever an hour before the test. Do not use talcum powder or deodorant the day of the test because either can show up as calcium deposits on the X ray. You may get the results of the test within fifteen minutes, or the report may be sent directly to your doctor.

Unfortunately, many women still have the misconception that if they do not have symptoms of a problem (such as a lump, pain, or an unusual discharge), they don't need to get screened. Some also believe that unless the doctor recommends mammography, it is not necessary to be tested. The problem is that some doctors don't recommend this test or do not recommend it as early as we Black women need it. Others don't bother to monitor the results. **Therefore, we must take responsibility for ourselves!** If you don't have health insurance or your insurance does not cover mammograms, find a community program that offers low-cost or free breast exams. (Check the resources at the end of this book.)

Some women are simply afraid—of pain, of radiation, or of finding cancer. If you're afraid of the pain or radiation used during the exam, believe us, you don't have anything to worry about. Any minor discomfort from the exam itself goes away quickly after the test is finished. However, the discomfort may last longer if you have fibrocystic disease. And the radiation level is very low and not enough to hurt you in any way.

If you are afraid of finding out your diagnosis—as many women are—ask yourself this: Is it scarier to find out early when something can be done and a cure is 95 percent possible, or scarier to find out later after the disease is severe and spread to other organs in your body and a cure rate is much lower? Don't adhere to the old adage that what you don't know won't hurt you. In this case, not knowing *will* hurt you.

If you are still uncomfortable about scheduling a mammogram, please talk to your Prime Time Sister and Prime Time Circle for support. They can remind you to go for your mammogram and go with you to the exam. You might even want to initiate a Prime Time Circle discussion on breast exams to explore the latest findings and recommendations on breast health.

Since 10 percent to 15 percent of breast cancers don't show up on a mammogram, it's extremely important that you also examine your breasts each month. (See instructions and illustration in the section on breast cancer in Chapter 11.)

Most insurance now covers mammograms, but your policy may not cover this test before age forty or pay for annual exams until you are fifty years old. The average cost is $85, with a range from $35 to $300, depending on where you get them. If you are sixty-five years of age or over, Medicare covers part of the cost. To find mammography facilities certified by the Food and Drug Administration (FDA), call the National Cancer Institute's Cancer Information Center (CIS) at 800-4-CANCER (800-422-6237). Contact your local American Cancer Society, as well as support groups in your area, for information about screening.

## Lipid (Fat) Profile

A lipid profile is part of the routine blood workup that doctors request during annual evaluations. It is performed at a laboratory and is covered by most insurance policies. (Also watch for free screenings in your neighborhood.)

Lipid profiles measure the levels of the two major fats in your blood, cholesterol and triglycerides. High levels of cholesterol narrow the blood vessels, which raises the risk of heart disease and stroke. This test is critical because heart disease is the number one killer of all women, and stroke is the number three killer of African American women.

You must fast for eight to twelve hours before you take a lipid profile. The lab work will measure your total blood cholesterol, which includes high-density lipoprotein (HDL), low-density lipoprotein (LDL), and triglycerides.

HDL is a lipoprotein that is referred to as "good" cholesterol because it helps remove cholesterol from the blood, preventing it from building up in the arteries. If your HDL level is below 35, your risk of heart disease increases dramatically. On the other hand, if your HDL level is 60 or above, you have a lower risk of developing heart disease. According to the Framingham Heart Study, the risk of heart attack is six times higher in women with the lowest HDL levels. (This was not true in men.) Low is not good.

LDL is called "bad" cholesterol because it carries most of the cholesterol in the blood, and high LDL levels can allow fatty buildup in the arteries. You want your LDL reading to be below 130. A level above 160 puts you at high risk of developing coronary artery disease. High is not good.

Triglycerides are fats or lipids that come from two sources: They are absorbed from the foods you eat (particularly high-fat foods, sugar, and alcohol), and they are produced by the liver. You want your triglycerides reading to be less than 200 mg/dL.

| BLOOD CHOLESTEROL LEVELS AND YOUR RISK | | | |
|---|---|---|---|
| | DESIRABLE | BORDERLINE | HIGH RISK |
| TOTAL CHOLESTEROL | <200 mg/dL | 200–240 mg/dL | >240 mg/dL |
| LDL (BAD) CHOLESTEROL | <130 mg/dL | 130–160 mg/dL | >160 mg/dL |
| HDL (GOOD) CHOLESTEROL | >60 mg/dL | 35–60 mg/dL | <35 mg/dL |
| TRIGLYCERIDES | <150 mg/dL | 150–200 mg/dL | >200 mg/dL |

Most women should be screened every one to two years, even if the tests are normal. All insurers pay for these tests. Cost: $12 to $60. Watch for advertisements for free screenings; all communities have them.

## Pap Smear

A Pap smear is performed by the primary care clinician—internist, family doctor, gynecologist, physician assistant, or nurse-practitioner—who performs your pelvic examination.

A Pap smear is a simple but very important test that examines the cells in and around the cervix to detect abnormalities that could lead to cancer. Annual Pap smears help doctors identify changes in the cells at an early stage— and early detection is critical for successful treatment of cervical cancer. Since this test was first introduced, more than forty years ago, deaths from cervical cancer have dropped 70 percent! There is no controversy over the effectiveness of and need for this low-cost test ($10 to $20), and insurers will pay for it.

To perform a Pap test, the doctor will swab a small sample of cells from your cervix (the opening to the uterus) and transfer the cells to a slide that will be examined under a microscope at a laboratory. For the best test results, don't have intercourse, douche, or use vaginal creams, medicines, or spermicidal foams for about two days before the test. Any foreign substance in or around the vagina can rinse away or hide abnormal cells. For the most accurate test, have your Pap smear done twelve to fourteen days after you begin a menstrual period.

A Pap test should be performed annually beginning at age eighteen, even for women who have gone through menopause. Some women mistakenly stop getting Pap smears after menopause even though the incidence of cervical cancer actually increases in older women. In fact, the rate of cervical cancer peaks between the ages of sixty and sixty-nine. If you had a hysterectomy (which is the surgical removal of your uterus and cervix), ask your doctor if you need to continue getting Pap tests.

The Pap test is not 100 percent accurate—but an accuracy rate of 90 percent is pretty darn good. The most common cause of inaccuracies is improper collection or preparation of the sample. Ask your doctor if the lab uses a computer to rescreen smears that did not show any abnormal cells. If you have any symptoms that may indicate a problem (such as bleeding outside your period if you are not menopausal, or bleeding after intercourse) but your test results do not show any abnormal cells, ask your doctor to have you rescreened.

Since one in five abnormalities is missed on standard Pap smears, new, more accurate tests have recently been approved by the Federal Drug Administration (FDA). These include computerized checking systems, called PAPNET and AutoPap 300 QC, which review Pap smear slides by an automated system; then the slides are reexamined by a technologist to confirm any abnormality. These are not currently covered by many insurance companies, although some are starting to pay for them, so check.

The third new option is ThinPrep, which is a Pap test that increases the accuracy of the test and the ability to detect abnormal cells. This is the best test at this time. The cells to be tested are not obscured by mucus or blood and abnormal cells are easier to detect. Therefore, this test is much more accurate than the conventional Pap smear at detecting precancerous cells. It increases the accuracy up to 97 percent. However, this test costs between $40 and $60, and most insurance companies do not currently cover it.

For more information, call the National Cancer Institute's Cancer Information Service at 800-4-CANCER (800-422-6237).

## Stool Blood Test, Flexible Sigmoidoscopy, Colonoscopy

These tests are routine beginning at age fifty, or earlier with signs of a problem or if there is a family history of rectal or colon cancer.

Let's face it: Tests performed to detect cancer of the rectum and colon are no fun, but they truly save lives in people over the age of fifty, who are at greatest risk. Since risk increases sharply with age, you should start getting these screenings at age fifty (age forty if you have a family history of rectal cancer). Here are the three diagnostic tests that are used.

The *stool blood test* requires that you leave a sample of your stool with your doctor or take a sample to a lab. Signs of blood in the stool may indicate any number of things—a gastric ulcer, intestinal polyps, inflammatory disease of the bowel, cancer, or something as simple as hemorrhoids. This annual test is covered by insurance and costs between $20 and $30.

A *flexible sigmoidoscopy* is an outpatient procedure that is usually performed every three to five years on a routine basis, in a hospital or sometimes in a well-equipped outpatient facility. With any indication of a problem or if any of these cancers run in your family, it may be performed more often and started earlier. If you have a family history of problems, you should start getting tested at forty using colonoscopy (see below), not sigmoidoscopy.

To perform a sigmoidoscopy, a hollow, lighted tube is inserted into your rectum and colon to see if any masses or polyps are present. If abnormalities are detected, the doctor will remove the mass during the procedure and examine the tissue under the microscope to see if it's cancerous. This test costs between $200 and $300. Not all insurers cover this procedure. At this time, Medicare doesn't cover this test.

A *colonoscopy* may be necessary to view the entire colon if there is any chance of cancer cells in part of the colon not reached by the sigmoidoscope. (A sigmoidoscopy can view only part of the colon.) Since this is a more complicated procedure that involves the entire colon, you will be sedated.

## Bone Density Screening

You are at risk for developing osteoporosis—where you lose bone mass and your bones fracture easily—after menopause (especially if you don't take estrogen), if you have a parent or sibling with osteoporosis, or if you smoke or drink heavily. In the past, it was commonly believed that African Americans were not really at risk of developing this disease; however, new data indicate that our risk is equal to that of White and Asian women. We're at higher risk than both groups once we reach age seventy. (For more information on osteoporosis, see Chapter 16 on menopause.)

You should have a baseline bone density test at the onset of menopause—about one year after the cessation of your periods. However, if you have a family history of osteoporosis, your baseline should be taken in your early forties.

The most accurate bone density test is called a dual-energy X-ray absorptiometry, or DEXA, which measures the density of your bones at the spine or hip. If your bone density is low, you may need to start estrogen treatment. Your physician must order this test.

Check to see if your health insurance policy covers this important test.

## Electrocardiogram

An electrocardiogram (ECG or EKG) makes a graphic record of the heart's electrical activity as it beats. This test reveals muscle damage, blood flow problems, an enlarged heart, or abnormal heartbeat. Since the ECG measures the electrical activity of the heart muscle, this test may provide the first clue to an abnormality in the functioning of the heart, even when there are no symptoms of a problem. Therefore, an ECG can serve as an early warning of cardiac abnormalities.

This test is often part of a routine physical examination and can be done in the doctor's office or at a laboratory. ECGs are painless, and you and your doctor should determine how often you need one. You probably should get a baseline ECG reading at age forty (to help the doctor track the condition of your heart over time) and a new ECG every two years thereafter. You may need to be tested more often—every year if you have any type of heart problem, such as pain, rapid heartbeat, or any risk factors such as hypertension, obesity, or diabetes.

## Fasting Blood Sugar and a Two Hour Postprandial

The fasting blood sugar test is part of the routine blood workup in annual evaluations and can be done in the doctor's office or at a laboratory.

Elevated levels of sugar after an eight- to twelve-hour fast can signal **diabetes**—the number four cause of death for African American women. Identifying diabetes early reduces the many complications, which is why every adult forty-five and over should be tested for this potentially debilitating disease. Unfortunately, only half of the people with diabetes know they have it. (See Chapter 12, "Dealing with Diabetes," for more information and advice.)

If your doctor sees signs of diabetes or is concerned about your family history of diabetes, he or she will request a two-hour postprandial test or a glucose tolerance test, or both. These tests involve checking the blood sugar levels after you've eaten something sugary to see how your body handles a sudden burst of sugar. With the two-hour postprandial test, a technician will check your blood sugar two hours after you've taken in the sugar. With the glucose tolerance test, your blood sugar levels will be checked at various times over a six-hour period after you ingest the sugar.

## HIV

You must take an HIV test if you have had unprotected sex with a partner (1) whose HIV status you aren't sure of, (2) who has used intravenous drugs or may have had contact with another partner who used intravenous drugs, or (3) who has any other sexually transmitted disease. You must also have this test done if you have shared needles with anyone.

This is an important test because early knowledge of infection allows a woman to take advantage of medications that can prolong her life and improve its quality. Also, knowing your status will keep you from transmitting the virus to your partner if you are infected. The two tests for the HIV infection are the ELISA ($75) and the Western Blot ($30 to $100). Insurers are likely to cover both these tests, but if you're concerned about the confidentiality of your results, you can find an anonymous test site by calling the CDC's National AIDS Hotline at 800-342-2437.

Another test you should know about:

## Thyroid Test

Since women are at higher risk for thyroid disorders than men, another important Prime Time test checks the level of thyroid stimulating hormone (TSH) in your body. This is a reliable, inexpensive blood test used to screen for thyroid disease. The thyroid is a gland in the neck that produces a hormone that affects many bodily functions, including heart rate, respiration, and central nervous system function. It helps control your metabolic rate—the rate at which your body burns energy. Despite the gland's importance, more than 50 percent of thyroid disorders go undiagnosed! If your thyroid is underactive (hypothyroidism), there is too little hormone and you may experience fatigue, weight gain, memory problems, hair loss, depression, a feeling of being cold, constipation, difficulty sleeping, problems swallowing, dry skin, and high cholesterol levels. Hypothyroidism is more common in women over fifty. An overactive thyroid (hyperthyroidism) produces too much hormone, leading to restlessness, irritability, anxiety, mood swings, weight loss, fatigue, and excessive perspiration.

## PRIME TIME MEDICAL CALENDAR

### ANNUAL EXAMS

| EXAM OR PROCEDURE | SCHEDULE | DATE DONE | RESULTS |
|---|---|---|---|
| COMPLETE PHYSICAL EXAM | Every year | | |
| WEIGHT | | | |
| BLOOD PRESSURE* | | | |
| VISION TEST | | | |
| HEARING TEST | | | |
| GYNECOLOGICAL EXAM | Every year | | |
| EYE EXAM | Every 2–4 years (ages 40–65) Every year (after age 65) | | |
| DENTAL EXAM | Every year | | |

### ROUTINE ANNUAL EVALUATIONS

| EXAM OR PROCEDURE | SCHEDULE | DATE DONE | RESULTS | GOAL |
|---|---|---|---|---|
| COMPLETE BLOOD COUNT Hemoglobin, hematocrit (to check for anemia); white blood count (infection); platelets (clotting) | Every 1–2 years | | | |

*If you have high blood pressure, you may need to monitor this yourself at home daily. (See Chapter 10 for instructions.)

| EXAM OR PROCEDURE | SCHEDULE | DATE DONE | RESULTS | GOAL |
|---|---|---|---|---|
| FASTING BLOOD SUGAR† | Every 1–2 years | | | |
| BLOOD SUGAR (2 hours after eating) | Every 1–2 years | | | |
| FASTING LIPID PROFILE† | Every 1–2 years | | | |
| TOTAL CHOLESTEROL | | | | |
| LDL | | | | |
| HDL | | | | |
| TRIGYLCERIDES | | | | |
| URINALYSIS | Every year | | | |
| MAMMOGRAM‡ | Every year | | | |
| PAP SMEAR | Every year | | | |
| STOOL BLOOD TEST | Every year | | | |
| ELECTOCARDIOGRAM | Every year | | | |

### ROUTINE EVALUATIONS (EVERY 3–5 YEARS OR PERIODICALLY)

| EXAM OR PROCEDURE | SCHEDULE | DATE DONE | RESULTS | GOAL |
|---|---|---|---|---|
| SIGMOIDOSCOPY | Baseline at age 50 | | | |
| COLONOSCOPY | Every 5 to 10 years or every 3 to 5 years with risk (family history or positive blood in stool) | | | |
| CHEST X RAY | Perform baseline on advice of your doctor | | | |
| STRESS ECG/EKG | Baseline at age 40 | | | |

†Do not eat or drink anything but water for 12 hours before test.
‡Breast self-exams must be done monthly. (See Chapter 11 for instructions.)

| EXAM OR PROCEDURE | SCHEDULE | DATE DONE | RESULTS | GOAL |
|---|---|---|---|---|
| BONE DENSITY | Baseline at menopause (around age 50) | | | |
| THYROID STIMULATING HORMONE | Baseline at age 50 | | | |

## SPECIAL EVALUATIONS WITH CONCERNS OR ON ADVICE OF YOUR DOCTOR

| EXAM OR PROCEDURE | SCHEDULE | DATE DONE | RESULTS |
|---|---|---|---|
| ECHOCARDIOGRAM | As advised | | |
| THALLIUM STRESS TEST | With concerns on stress ECG | | |
| CORONARY ANGIOGRAPHY | With abnormalities on other heart tests | | |
| VAGINAL AND UTERINE ULTRASOUND | As recommended with history of ovarian cancer, pelvic mass, abnormal uterine bleeding, pelvic discomfort | | |
| HIV | As advised or after unprotected sex | | |

## IMMUNIZATIONS

| IMMUNIZATION | SCHEDULE | DATE DONE |
|---|---|---|
| TETANUS BOOSTER | Every 10 years | |
| DIPHTHERIA BOOSTER | Every 10 years | |
| INFLUENZA VACCINE (FLU)§ | Every year after age 60; varies up to age 60 | |

§You may need to have a flu shot before age 50 if you have lung, heart or kidney disease, diabetes, cancer or HIV.

| IMMUNIZATION | SCHEDULE | DATE DONE |
|---|---|---|
| PNEUMOCOCCAL VACCINE# | One time at age 65 | |
| HEPATITIS B | Once in a lifetime | |

#You may need the pneumococcal vaccine before age 65 if you have lung, heart, or kidney disease, diabetes, cancer, or HIV.

NOTE: You can also use *The Health Diary for Women of Color: Your Personal Log* by Melody T. McCloud, M.D. (New Life Publishing, P. O. Box 3244, Roswell, GA 30077-0344).

# Chapter 9

# DEVELOPING YOUR PRIME TIME WELLNESS PLAN

*My fear of change caused me a lot of anguish and heartache until I learned to accept some simple facts of life: change is the only constant—the trick is to learn to see it as just another opportunity to grow, a chance to transform yourself from the person you are into the person you want to be. When you fear it, you fight it. And when you fight it, you block the blessing.*

—Patti LaBelle, *Don't Block the Blessings*

We know that walking the path to wellness is not an easy journey. It's still difficult for those of us who have been on it for many years. That's because embracing wellness requires making conscious choices about how we live each and every day, sticking with it, and staying motivated over time while keeping our eyes on the goal.

Remember our friend Vanessa, whom we discussed in Chapter 7? When we first introduced her, she was distraught over her friend Linda's death. Understanding how her own unhealthy lifestyle was contributing to risk factors that could cause her own untimely death, Vanessa vowed to get her wellness act together. Over the next three months Vanessa implemented the Prime Time prescription we gave her. Here's how she's doing so far:

## VANESSA'S STORY, CONTINUED

At first the idea of developing and launching a Prime Time Wellness Plan seemed overwhelming, but Vanessa was determined to become a healthier person. The first few weeks were the toughest, as she weaned herself off Mickey D's delicious french fries and set the alarm clock for 6:00 A.M. to do her exercises.

Fortunately, she chose a wonderful Prime Time Sister and developed a Prime Time Circle that has provided love and support during her transition to wellness. They have encouraged her to stay positive and focused even when her thorough physical exam revealed that her blood pressure was slightly elevated. Vanessa's doctor is hopeful that exercise and healthful eating will lower her pressure—and after several weeks, the signs are encouraging. Vanessa joined Smokenders and has been cigarette-free for three months. She's also forced herself not to work late into the evenings at her school or spend entire weekends attending to her family's needs and planning her lessons for the next week. Instead, she is practicing the stress management recommendations we offered, and best of all, she's carving out time to pamper her body and nourish her spirit.

---

You see, anything is possible when you have a sound plan. Now let's look at what it will take to develop your Prime Time Wellness Plan.

Since lifestyle choices make up 50 percent of the determinants of good health, your plan must provide activities that *prevent disease* (which requires you to address your major risk factors) and *promote good health*. You need to especially focus on the following five lifestyle changes that will have the most immediate and long-term positive impact on your health:

1. Manage your stress
2. Start exercising
3. Improve your nutrition and keep your weight within an optimal range for your height and age
4. Stop smoking
5. Nourish your spirit

## MANAGE YOUR STRESS

Managing your stress is so important in your life that we've devoted all of Chapter 13 to this topic. Stress is a major risk factor for just about every physical and mental illness that we discuss in this book, and we consider it an underlying cause of most illnesses and deaths. Learning to deal with everyday stress—from deadlines to deadbeat relatives—also prepares you to

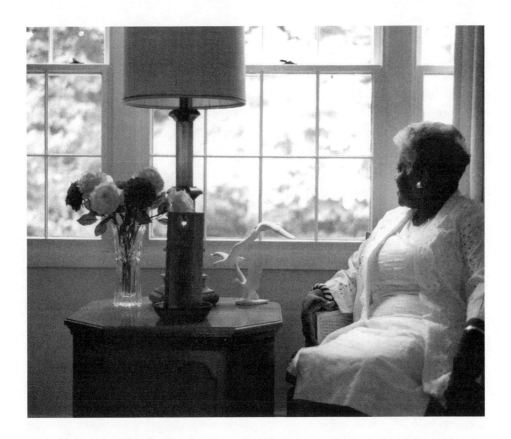

deal with the tragic and traumatic events that happen to every one of us sometime in life, such as the death of a loved one. Chapter 13 is packed with dozens of mental and behavioral strategies that you should incorporate into your life immediately. Once you finish this book, you may find yourself referring to this chapter frequently.

Learning to handle the everyday ups and downs of living is critical if you plan to take charge of your health. Remember, many times you can't control or avoid a stress-inducing event, but you can control your response to it. Life is 20 percent what happens to you, but the other 80 percent is your reaction to it. You also must incorporate strategies for stress reduction, such as relaxation techniques, deep breathing, balancing and prioritizing your time, yoga, meditation, and prayer into your life every day.

You may want to ask your Prime Time Sister and Prime Time Circle to help you develop an appropriate plan for minimizing the negative impact of stressors.

## EXERCISE AND GET FIT

Exercise is one of the most effective magic potions in our lives. If the physiological benefits of exercise could be put in a pill, you would have one of the most powerful health and wellness medications available. Your mind, body, and spirit all respond positively to physical activity. There's no way around it: You must exercise and become physically active if you want to feel better, look better, think better, and be healthier. We discuss the phenomenal benefits of exercise in virtually every chapter of this book.

---

### TWELVE REASONS TO GET ACTIVE

Becoming more physically active will help:

1. Reduce your risk of heart disease and stroke by keeping your blood pressure within the ideal range. If you have hypertension, exercise will help you reduce high blood pressure.
2. Reduce your risk of stroke by increasing blood flow to your brain.
3. Increase your energy levels.
4. Reduce feelings of stress, anxiety, and depression.
5. Improve your sleep.
6. Boost self-confidence by improving your strength, stamina, flexibility, appearance, and sense of control.
7. Reduce risk of colon cancer and constipation.
8. Improve bone density and reduce risk factors for osteoporosis and fractures.
9. Shed extra pounds and abdominal fat, which is the fat most linked to heart disease.
10. Control blood sugar, thereby decreasing your risk of diabetes.
11. Increase HDL ("good") cholesterol and lower triglycerides.
12. Improve sexual satisfaction.

---

The beautiful part is that you don't have to be an athlete or an exercise fanatic to enjoy these benefits of physical activity. As we have said before, *the number two preventable cause of death is inactivity.* So why don't we—especially we Black women—exercise regularly? It's a particular problem for us at midlife. To put it simply: We just don't like it, we are busy, and we don't build exercise into our daily lives.

Studies indicate that regular exercisers work out faithfully because they enjoy what they're doing. The reason that many of us women may not enjoy exercising is because we don't stick with any exercise or sport long enough to learn the routines or work through the soreness that's an inevitable part of increasing our activity level. That's why finding an activity that you enjoy is crucial if you're going to make fitness workouts a part of your daily life. Think about what you like to do: Do you like to dance? Does it feel good to stretch? Are you competitive and enjoy sports? Do you like being with a group? Do you like to be outdoors? Do you get bored doing the same routines and like to try something different every day?

If working out with a crowd will motivate you, consider joining a YMCA or YWCA. Most have excellent fitness programs that offer a variety of different types of exercises and exercise equipment for people just getting started. You can also encourage your church to start an exercise program and hire a fitness instructor to lead classes several times a week.

Before starting any type of exercise program or dramatically increasing your everyday physical activities, discuss your plans with your primary care doctor. He or she will want to examine you if you haven't had a checkup within the last twelve months. Your doctor will probably want to do a stress electrocardiogram to check your heart if you are over forty years old. Discuss fitness regimens that may interest you with your doctor and ask for a recommendation for the one that is best for you. Getting sound medical advice is especially important if you suffer from high blood pressure, heart disease, or have any other type of chronic illness; are very overweight; or haven't been physically active for a long time. For example, if you haven't exercised in a while, you can't jump into something strenuous such as an advanced Tae-Bo workout. You must start slowly and ease into a full-scale, vigorous program.

Set short-term and long-term fitness goals and make a commitment to yourself to hang in for at least a month before you evaluate your progress. According to the Surgeon General's 1996 "Physical Activity and Health Report," a regular exerciser is someone who works out twenty to thirty continuous minutes three times a week at moderate to vigorous intensity. This could include activities such as walking, running, water aerobics, or bicycling. However, only 20 percent of Americans exercise for twenty minutes five times a week, and the numbers drop for women in our age group. Sistergirlfriend, trust us. The best gift you can give yourself is an ongoing fitness plan that becomes part of your lifestyle. Start by taking the fitness quiz on the next page to see where you are right now.

## Check Your Pulse

You should also assess your fitness level by measuring your *resting pulse rate*, which is the average number of heartbeats per minute when you're at rest. As a rule of thumb, a resting pulse of 80 or above suggests that you could definitely improve your fitness. A resting pulse of 70 to 80 suggests that you may need to exercise more. If you are in a fitness program and have an average resting pulse below 70, you are likely to be in good shape.

To measure your pulse, make sure that you are relaxed, then place the tips of your first two fingers inside your wrist below the base of your thumb. Take the number of pulse beats in twenty seconds and multiply that number by 3.

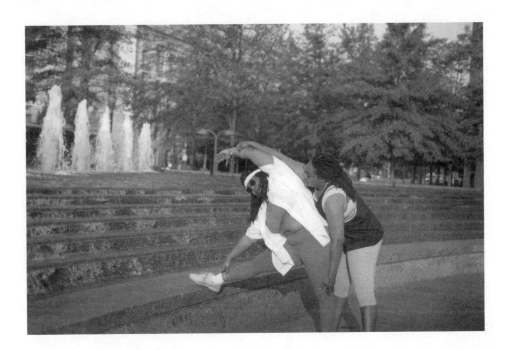

(You can also take the number of pulse beats in 10 seconds and multiply the number by 6.)

## Choosing Exercises that You Will Enjoy

Finding an exercise that suits you will motivate you to do it often. Following are types of exercise that produce wonderful results for your body and your mind. Check in your particular location for specific types of exercise classes, for example, aerobics, Jazzercise, yoga, tai chi. The Y's, churches, academic institutions, and health clubs offer them, or you can practice with television programs.

### Stretching, Yoga, and Tai Chi

Stretching, yoga, and tai chi increase your flexibility and help you relax. These are great exercises for anyone who cannot tolerate stress to the heart because they tone muscles without depleting your energy or interrupting your blood flow. *Stretching* is an important component of the warm-up and cool-down phases in your workout. *Yoga* is thousands of years old and integrates the mind, body, and spirit. Yoga includes body postures, controlled deep breathing, and a focused and positive mind-set. Videotapes, books, and

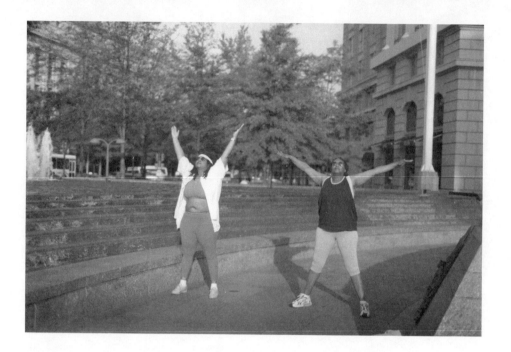

classes are widely available. You may find yoga classes offered on cable television stations early in the morning.

The Chinese believe that practicing *tai chi*, which is an exercise of precise, controlled movements, for twenty minutes each day can rejuvenate your body and prolong your life. Tai chi consists of more than one hundred movements using every part of the body, from the eyes down to the toes. Each movement encourages a sense of peace and emotional stability. The essence of tai chi is *chi*, which means "vital energy." The best way to learn is to take lessons from an experienced practitioner. You can find a local practitioner by checking out the national organizations that we list in the Resources chapter at the end of the book.

### *Walking*

A thirty-minute walk a day helps keep the doctor away. That's because walking can cut the risk of heart disease by as much as 40 percent, which is equivalent to the benefits of jogging or aerobic dance, according to a 1999 study conducted by Dr. JoAnn E. Manson, professor of medicine at Brigham and Women's Hospital, which is affiliated with Harvard Medical School.

Walking is easy, inexpensive, practical, low-risk, and fun, and it provides significant health benefits to Prime Time women. All the equipment you need is a good pair of walking shoes—look for a firm heel cup for stability, a rocker sole to enhance a smooth heel-to-toe motion, and plenty of room for your toes to spread. Take them with you wherever you go. Even though your schedule may seem impossibly tight, you can probably squeeze in at least a fifteen-minute walk.

Start walking for fifteen to thirty minutes at a comfortable pace. Gradually increase your pace until you can walk one mile in fifteen minutes. Then increase the time you walk at that pace until you reach sixty minutes. Each week, write down at least one specific fitness goal, such as walking faster, farther, or longer. Always keep safety in mind whenever you walk: Vary the paths you take, don't walk at night (especially alone), don't walk in a deserted area day or night, and walk with your Prime Time Sister or a walking partner whenever possible.

If the hard pavement of a city street is difficult on your knees or feet, or if the weather is inclement, try using a treadmill at your local gym, health club, or YMCA/YWCA. Have someone show you how to set the machine on the correct speed. A treadmill of your own is super convenient, and you will use it more. However, you must keep your clothes and papers off of it. You can buy one on sale or get a good secondhand one cheaply.

You must try to walk at least five times a week at your target heart rate zone (see box). Schedule your walks in advance—the same time every day is ideal—**and keep this important appointment with yourself.**

---

## TARGET HEART RATE ZONE

Use your age grouping below to find out your target heart rate zone. (You should take your pulse midway during your workouts and again when you finish.)

| AGE | TARGET ZONE |
|---|---|
| 45 years | 88–131 beats per minute |
| 50 years | 85–127 beats per minute |
| 55 years | 83–123 beats per minute |
| 60 years | 80–120 beats per minute |
| 65 years | 78–116 beats per minute |
| 70 years | 75–113 beats per minute |

*Source: Exercise and Your Heart,* National Heart, Lung, and Blood Institute, NIH publication 93-1677

---

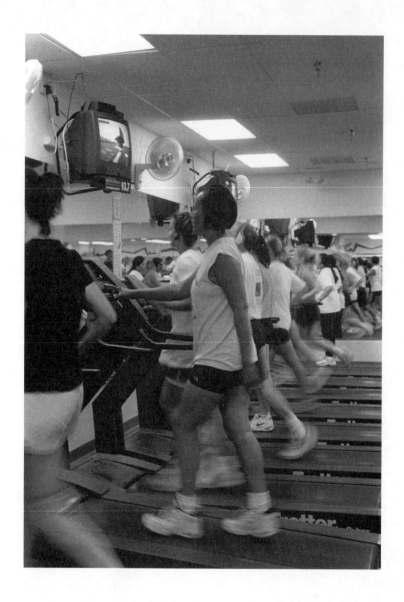

### Aerobic Exercises

Aerobic exercises strengthen and improve how your heart and lungs function. These exercises increase the amount of oxygenated blood carried to muscles and organs and increase your breathing and heart rates. They also burn calories and help firm muscles. You can do aerobic exercises almost anywhere, almost anytime. The activity you choose should raise your pulse and cause you to sweat, but don't overdo it. Discuss any specific physical concerns (such as knee pain or shoulder pain) you may have with your doctor, physical therapist, or exercise instructor before you enroll in a program to see if it's right for you. Here are some activities you might like to try:

At home, jumping rope, jogging, walking on a treadmill, using a cross-country ski machine, and riding a stationary bike are excellent choices. So is working out with exercise videos. For hip-hop, funky, and even gospel workouts, look for videos developed by leading African American exercise gurus: Bonita Perkins, Donna Richardson, Victoria Johnson, and Billy Blanks.

Outdoors, you can go hiking, walking, skating, bicycling, and jogging.

Try a club or class. Aerobics or step aerobics; jazz, tap, African, or hip-hop dancing; or using a rowing machine or a step machine all work up a great sweat.

### Strength or Weight Training

Inactive women in midlife may also start losing muscle and muscle tone. That's why you need to add weight lifting to your routine. Strength training burns fat, builds stronger muscles, decreases muscle loss associated with aging, improves your balance, makes you stronger, increases joint flexibility, firms flab, and increases your metabolism. (It can also help ward off osteoporosis.) Start by lifting small weights (one to two pounds) two or three times a week. The goal is not to build big muscles (the main muscle to worry about is your heart muscle) but to tone and increase strength in your muscles. Trainers at fitness centers, wellness and community centers, gyms, and your local YMCA/YWCA can help you develop a program. Some gyms provide trainers for free; some charge an hourly rate to develop and monitor your workouts.

**R**<sub></sub> **PRIME TIME PRESCRIPTION TO LAUNCH YOUR FITNESS PLAN**

*Phase 1: Begin your journey to fitness by making some simple, everyday changes listed on the Activity Pyramid on page 169.*

*Park on the outskirts of the parking lot whenever possible* (especially if safety isn't an issue) instead of trying to find the closest spot. We call those close spots "killer spots."

*Take the stairs instead of the elevator as often as you can.* You can burn one calorie every five steps.

*Stretch while standing and waiting in line.* This can help improve your flexibility.

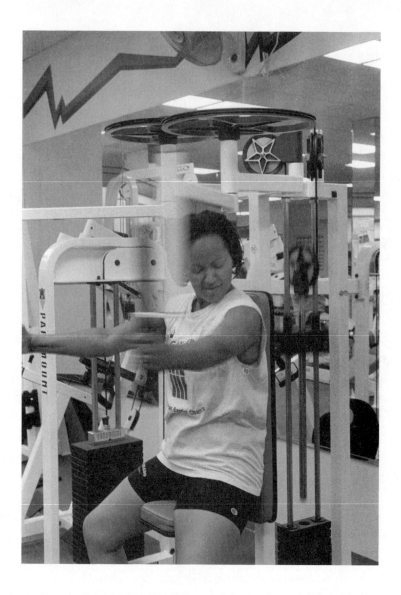

*Throw away your television remote control.* That will keep you moving. (Laughter is also good exercise, and we know that's what you're doing right now at this suggestion.)

*Walk whenever you can.* Even just a few trips around the house or yard burns calories.

*If you have a dog, walk the dog more.* If not, think about getting one. Walking the dog is a good motivator to get out.

**Use the Pyramid to develop a comprehensive weekly exercise and activity program, which includes stretching, aerobics, and strength training.**

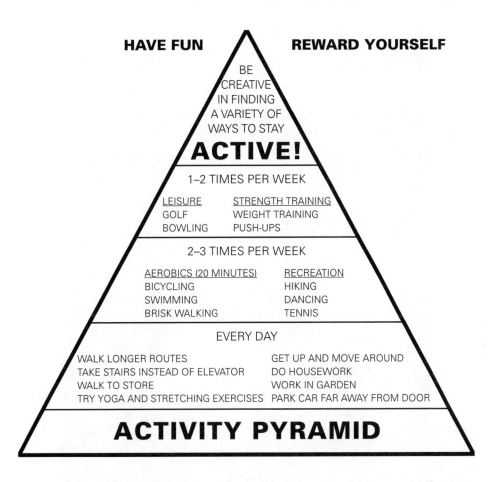

**HAVE FUN**     **REWARD YOURSELF**

BE CREATIVE IN FINDING A VARIETY OF WAYS TO STAY

# ACTIVE!

1–2 TIMES PER WEEK

| LEISURE | STRENGTH TRAINING |
|---------|-------------------|
| GOLF | WEIGHT TRAINING |
| BOWLING | PUSH-UPS |

2–3 TIMES PER WEEK

| AEROBICS (20 MINUTES) | RECREATION |
|-----------------------|------------|
| BICYCLING | HIKING |
| SWIMMING | DANCING |
| BRISK WALKING | TENNIS |

EVERY DAY

| | |
|---|---|
| WALK LONGER ROUTES | GET UP AND MOVE AROUND |
| TAKE STAIRS INSTEAD OF ELEVATOR | DO HOUSEWORK |
| WALK TO STORE | WORK IN GARDEN |
| TRY YOGA AND STRETCHING EXERCISES | PARK CAR FAR AWAY FROM DOOR |

# ACTIVITY PYRAMID

## Phase 2: Develop a workout you will stick with.

*First, find the exercises that you like.* If you love to dance, do that. To stay motivated, you must enjoy what you do and find fun in it.

*Figure out what type of exercise environment suits you.* Do you need to join a gym? Should you hire a trainer? Or can you convince your Prime Time Sister to work out with you? (The buddy system really works.) Would you enjoy doing aerobics with a group of sisters? Or would you rather enjoy the solitude of a long walk alone or buy a treadmill or bicycle to exercise in the privacy of your home? Only you know what turns you on. You can even exercise while you watch your favorite TV programs or listen to your latest CD. Another option is to get an exercise videotape. There are so many great ones to choose from, featuring the music you love—gospel, hip-hop, golden oldies, disco, you name it. Earlier we listed some leading exercise gurus whose videos you should consider.

*Set aside the same time every day to exercise,* even if that means waking up

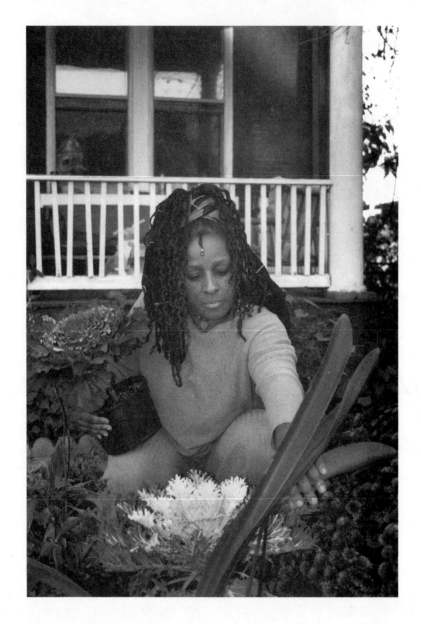

an hour earlier. The morning is a good time to work out, because you have more energy at the beginning of the day and exercising will increase your metabolism throughout the day. Daily gardening is a light workout.

*Get the right footwear and clothing for your workout.* They don't have to be fancy, but they must be comfortable and cool in the summer or warm in the winter. However, if dressing up in a cute exercise outfit motivates you, go on, girl, and get something that really turns you on.

*Start slowly and build up your endurance.* You want to slowly increase how far, how long, or how hard you exercise each session. If you decide to walk for exercise, start by walking fifteen minutes; next, go to thirty minutes; eventually build up your workout to forty-five minutes to one hour. If you are doing strength training, you'll want to start out with light weights and a few repetitions and build up to a more vigorous session.

*Staying motivated is the real challenge!* However, you must keep going for a long enough time so you can actually see results. The real goal is to make it part of your life from now on. If you miss a few days here and there, don't panic, get frustrated, and stop altogether. Instead, get back to your routine as soon as you can.

*Set small, realistic goals that you can reach.* Stay away from overly broad goals such as "I'm going to lose weight and get more fit." Don't set a goal of losing fifty pounds. Instead, aim to lose five to ten pounds over the next month or two.

*Devote a section of your heath journal to record each workout.* Include the intensity of the workout (strenuous, moderate, or light), how long you exercised and the numbers of repetitions you completed (if you're working out with weights). Jot down your pulse rate during and after your workout. Finally, set goals for the next session.

## IMPROVE YOUR NUTRITION

Improving your dietary habits in midlife or even later can significantly enhance your health. Scientific research clearly shows that nutrition and health are dramatically linked. In fact, age-related body changes make it even more important to pay attention to the foods you eat and the nutrients they contain.

---

### HOW HEALTHY IS YOUR DIET?

Circle true or false for each of the statements below.
1. I nearly always drink skim or 1-percent milk.
          TRUE     FALSE
2. Breakfast typically includes fresh fruit or fruit juice, along with cold cereal or whole-grain bread.
          TRUE     FALSE

---

3. My breakfast is seldom something like a sweet roll, a buttery crois-sant, bacon and eggs, or an egg sandwich.

TRUE         FALSE

4. I make sure that every day I have a bowl of a low-fat dairy product such as yogurt or cottage cheese.

TRUE         FALSE

5. Usually the sandwiches, burritos, and pizzas I eat have either cheese or meat (chicken or turkey) but rarely both.

TRUE         FALSE

6. I prefer sandwiches made with whole-wheat or multigrain bread; I rarely eat white bread.

TRUE         FALSE

7. Whenever I have chicken, I make sure the skin has been removed or I take it off myself.

TRUE         FALSE

8. I always eat a multicolored salad, cut-up red or green bell peppers, or carrots for lunch.

TRUE         FALSE

9. My morning and afternoon snacks are more likely to be fresh fruit, raisins, or juice than potato chips, candy, or soft drinks.

TRUE         FALSE

10. Half the dinners I eat each week contain little or no meat.

TRUE         FALSE

11. At dinnertime there's always something dark green, bright orange, or deep red on my plate.

TRUE         FALSE

12. I use vegetable oil or tub margarine, rarely butter or stick margarine.

TRUE         FALSE

13. When I order pizza, I always ask for veggies instead of pepperoni or other meats, and I tell them to go easy on the mozzarella.

TRUE         FALSE

14. When I go to a restaurant, I tend to order grilled fish or shrimp.

TRUE         FALSE

15. I usually don't have dessert.

TRUE         FALSE

16. At fast-food restaurants, I typically pass up the hamburgers and fries in favor of grilled chicken-breast sandwiches.

TRUE         FALSE

17. I make a point of eating several meals each week made with beans, such as chili, split pea soup, or three-bean salad.

TRUE      FALSE

18. I usually have salads made with spinach, romaine lettuce, cabbage, arugula, or other flavorful, colorful greens.

TRUE      FALSE

19. Dessert in my household is more likely to be fresh fruit or sorbet than cookies, cake, or ice cream.

TRUE      FALSE

**Total number of true answers circled: _____**

Scoring:

14 or more true—You're eating better than most Americans. Be sure to get some daily exercise, and you can feel proud of your health habits.

8 to 13 true—Not too bad, not exactly great. If nothing else, try to bypass some of the artery-damaging animal fat. Choose skim milk, veggie pizzas, and turkey sandwiches.

7 or fewer true—Your eating habits could use a tune-up. Read this section carefully.

*Source: Woman's Health Guide.*

As Vanessa learned, changing to live in wellness involves stopping certain habits but also starting others. Her nutrition plan is a good example. In developing her daily nutrition plan, Vanessa used the Food Pyramid for Older Adults on the next page as her guide.

At a glance you can see that water is an essential and major part of our diets, *eight to ten 8-ounce servings* every day. You can also see that meat is not the foundation of a healthful diet, and it certainly doesn't need to be the centerpiece of every meal, which is what many of us learned as we grew up. Grains, vegetables, and fruits should make up the bulk of your diet. Nutritionists recommend that we reduce the amount of fatty meat we eat and get the bulk of our protein from fish and dried beans, as well as poultry, lean meats, eggs, and nuts. While not omitted from healthful eating, fats, oils, and sweets are the smallest food group in the pyramid, and low-fat foods from the meat and milk groups are to be eaten in only moderate amounts. The flag represents the addition of dietary supplements to the basic food pyramid.

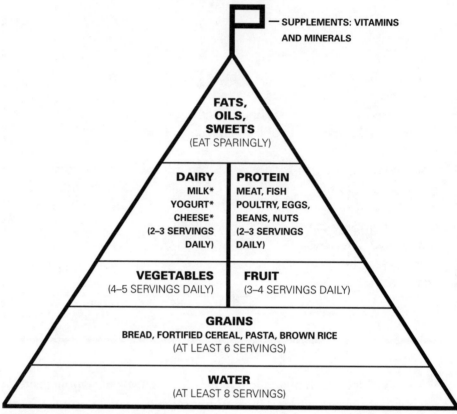

# FOOD PYRAMID
# FOR OLDER ADULTS

— SUPPLEMENTS: VITAMINS
AND MINERALS

**FATS,
OILS,
SWEETS**
(EAT SPARINGLY)

**DAIRY**
MILK*
YOGURT*
CHEESE*
(2–3 SERVINGS
DAILY)

**PROTEIN**
MEAT, FISH
POULTRY, EGGS,
BEANS, NUTS
(2–3 SERVINGS
DAILY)

**VEGETABLES**
(4–5 SERVINGS DAILY)

**FRUIT**
(3–4 SERVINGS DAILY)

**GRAINS**
BREAD, FORTIFIED CEREAL, PASTA, BROWN RICE
(AT LEAST 6 SERVINGS)

**WATER**
(AT LEAST 8 SERVINGS)

*Midlife and older African Americans have a higher incidence of lactose intolerance, and therefore many of us need to limit our food choices listed in the dairy section of the pyramid. If dairy products make you feel bloated or give you gas, you may be lactose intolerant, so you should choose lactose-reduced milk, milk with lactase added, low-fat hard cheeses, and yogurt.

*Source:* U.S. Department of Agriculture.

Using this food pyramid as a guide, here is a five-point food plan to help Vanessa become a healthier eater. It will also work for you.

*1. Drink at least eight to ten 8-ounce glasses of water every day.* The amount of water you need can vary with your level of activity and the temperature outside. You will also need more water if you are drinking dehydrating beverages such as caffeinated coffee, tea, and colas throughout the day; alcohol is also dehydrating. Drink an extra cup of water for every cup of these beverages. Don't rely on getting your water requirement from juices and other liquids. You must drink water. To get your daily dose of water,

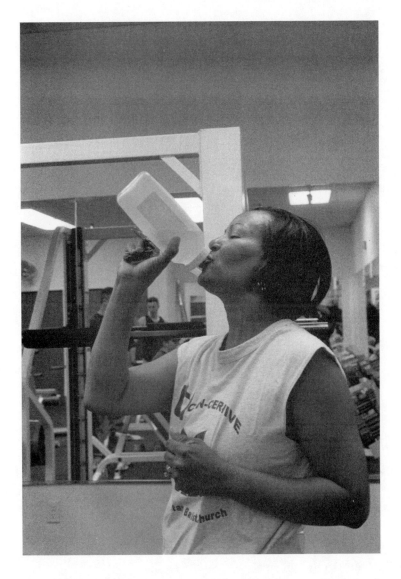

keep a full pitcher or bottle by your bed at night; have a drink in the morning, at bedtime, and during the day with meals; and keep a water bottle handy during the day. Drink distilled water when possible.

**2. *Increase your dietary fiber.*** Researchers have found that a high-fiber diet lowers your risk of heart disease, high blood pressure, colon cancer, and diabetes.

Here is what some studies have found:

• Women who ate 25 grams of fiber a day were 25 percent less likely to develop high blood pressure than women who ate only 10 grams daily.

• High fiber intake reduces the risk of developing diabetes by 22 percent.

• Foods or supplements that contain soluble fiber (found in some breakfast cereals and fiber supplements such as Metamucil) reduce the risk of heart disease.

Despite the recent controversy surrounding the benefit of fiber in preventing colon cancer, Dr. Edward Giovannucci of the Harvard Medical School reported in the January 1999 issue of the *New England Journal of Medicine* that a high-fiber diet can decrease the risk of colon cancer by speeding the passage of fecal material through the colon, thus reducing the colon's exposure to carcinogens in the diet.

On average, Americans consume about 11 to 13 grams of fiber per day; however, nutritionists recommend eating 25 to 35 grams daily, with the bulk coming from grains, including wheat bran. An adequate daily diet contains plenty of fruits and vegetables, whole-grain cereals, and legumes. This will provide you with both insoluble fiber (from bran, whole-grain cereals, whole-wheat bread and crackers, bulgur) and soluble fiber (from oats, barley, legumes, and fruits.) For fiber to be effective, you must drink plenty of water.

To add fiber to your diet, switch from:

• White bread to whole-grain breads
• Fruit juice to fresh fruit
• Fried or mashed potatoes to baked, roasted, or mashed potatoes with the skin
• Creamy soups to bean, lentil, or pea soups or chili
• Corn chips or potato chips to pretzels or hot-air-popped popcorn
• White rice to brown rice
• Iceberg lettuce to mixed greens

---

## MEASURING FIBER INTAKE

**13.5 g of wheat fiber** = 1 serving (½ cup) of a cereal very high in bran, such as All-Bran with Extra Fiber, Fiber One, or Bran Buds
**1.5 g of fiber in fruit** = 1 serving (1 cup)

---

## PRIME TIME GUIDE TO HEALTHY GRAINS

The only sure way to know if the product you buy contains whole grains is to read the label. Here are some tips for finding whole grains.

* *Whole-grain foods are made of whole wheat, oats, brown and wild rice, whole-rye flour, barley, natural bran, and wheat germ. Refined grains, such as white rice and white flour, have been stripped of their bran and germ and thus have lost most of their fiber and many of their nutrients.*

* *Although oats are always whole-grain foods, oatmeal bread does not contain whole oats and therefore does not provide the same level of nutrients as, say, oatmeal cereal.*

* *Do not be fooled by the following words:* enriched, unbleached, bromated, stone ground, granulated, 100 percent wheat, rye, pumpernickel, multigrain, seven-grain, semolina, *or* organic. *These products may contain little or no whole grains. You can find whole grains in many products, including crackers, breads, pasta, rice mixes, and hot and cold cereals.*

* *Other foods high in fiber are nuts (including almonds, peanuts, pecans, and walnuts), seeds (including pumpkin and sunflower), fruits (including apples, pears with skin, dates, figs, prunes, blueberries, raspberries, and blackberries), beans (including chickpeas, lentils, black, lima, and pinto), and vegetables (including broccoli, cabbage, cauliflower, artichokes, parsnips, pumpkin, squash, and rutabaga).*

---

**3. *Load up on fruits and vegetables.*** Eating seven to nine helpings of fruit and vegetables every day can literally save your life. Fruits and veggies contain antioxidants that protect against disease, provide fiber, and give you essential vitamins and minerals. They are virtually fat-free and help control your weight. They also promote healthy bowel function. Numerous studies demonstrate that fruits and vegetables can help lower high blood pressure; vegetarians have lower blood pressure than meat eaters, and switching to a vegetarian diet will lower your blood pressure. According to a report in the October 1999 issue of the *Journal of the American Medical Association*, fruits and veggies also protect against the risk of stroke.

Fruits and vegetables provide a variety of nutrients. Some are excellent sources of carotenoids, which form vitamin A in the body, while others may be rich in vitamin C, folic acid, or potassium. Dark green leafy vegetables and deeply colored fruits are especially rich in many nutrients.

Fresh vegetables and fruits are the most nutritious; frozen ones are next best, and canned are the least nutritious. Eat fresh fruits and veggies within two days of purchase, and eat them immediately once you cut them. Wash them with a brush thoroughly before eating (but don't use soap) to decrease your chance of ingesting pesticides. Peeling is also a good idea. Strawberries contain the most pesticides, so buy organic.

Eating fruits and vegetables raw is the healthiest choice, since nutrients are lost during cooking. Microwaving and steaming are the best cooking methods to preserve the nutritive value of vegetables. If you must boil your vegetables, use very little water. Also, try to cook vegetables with the skin on to preserve the nutrients; you can take the skin off when you eat them.

## A SERVING OF FRUITS OR VEGETABLES CONSISTS OF:

1 medium fruit or 1 cup small or cut-up fruit
¾ cup (6 ounces) of 100 percent fruit juice
¼ cup dried fruit
1 cup raw, leafy vegetables (lettuce or spinach)
½ cup cooked beans or peas

Studies are indicating that certain vegetables and fruits are important in preventing cancer. These include broccoli, BroccoSprouts, brussels sprouts, kale, cabbage, cauliflower, tomatoes, berries (blueberries, strawberries, raspberries, blackberries), and currants.

**4. Dramatically reduce the amount of fat in your diet and be careful about the type of fat you consume.** Your daily fat intake should only be 25 percent to 30 percent or less of your daily total calories. If you are overweight, that range should be 20 percent to 25 percent.

Since new studies indicate that the type of fat is as important as the total amount of fat you consume, take an inventory of the types of fats you eat and use to cook.

**Saturated fat** is solid at room temperature. (For a listing of foods and cooking oils with saturated fat, see the table "What You Should Know About Fats in Foods," page 180.) Foods that contain large amounts of saturated fat raise the risk of coronary artery disease more than foods with high cholesterol (found in foods such as eggs and certain shellfish such as shrimp). Because of the dangers to your heart, **keep saturated fat intake to 7 percent to 10 percent of your calories or less.**

Meats, lard, fatback, poultry skin, and whole-milk dairy products contain the most saturated fat. Limit red meat (beef, pork, and lamb) to two or three servings per week, choose lean cuts, and eat small portions (about 3 ounces cooked). Remove the skin from chicken and turkey. Have several meatless meals during the week. Eat less whole-milk cheese—it contains more saturated fat than red meat. Instead, use low-fat dairy products.

*Unsaturated fats* do not raise blood cholesterol and they lower the LDL level. There are two types of unsaturated fats: *polyunsaturated fat* and *monounsaturated fat.* Half of your total fat intake should come from monounsaturated fats, which lower LDL (bad) cholesterol but leave the beneficial HDL level intact, which is exactly what you want. This fat is found in foods such as olive oil, canola oil, almonds, and avocados. Use only olive oil that is labeled "extra virgin," which guarantees that the oil has been cold-pressed from freshly harvested olives and does not contain chemicals. Use olive oil in cooking, salad dressings, and sandwiches. Polyunsaturated fats lower both LDL (bad) cholesterol and HDL (good) cholesterol levels. It's good to lower LDL, but you want your HDL level to be high. Vegetable oils (such as corn, soybean, and cottonseed) and many nuts are good sources of polyunsaturated fats.

**Have at least one serving per week of omega-3 fatty acids.** Fish has a type of polyunsaturated fat, called omega-3 fatty acids, that not only lowers cholesterol, but may have other protective properties for your heart, such as possible protection against abnormal heart rhythms. Studies show that this fat may slow the onset of arthritis, boost the immune system, prevent some forms of cancer, and affect memory and stress levels. Even though canola and flaxseed contain omega-3, experts say fish oil is still the best source. Fatty fish such as salmon, sardines, herring, and tuna contain the highest amount of omega-3 fatty acids.

**Eliminate trans fats from your diet.** Trans fats are formed when food manufacturers add hydrogenate fats or hydrogen to unsaturated fats so the fats won't become rancid as quickly. Trans fat is converted to saturated fat in the body and increase lipid levels; some studies suggest that trans fats may increase the risk of breast cancer. Trans fats are found in many fried foods, packaged baked goods, and margarine (hard or stick margarines has more trans fat) than soft or tub kinds; look for the word *hydrogenated* on the label and avoid these as much as possible.

We know how hard it is to rid your diet of harmful fats; Marilyn and Gayle

## WHAT YOU SHOULD KNOW ABOUT FATS IN FOODS

| FATS | IMPACT ON LDL AND HDL | FOODS | OILS |
|---|---|---|---|
| **DRAMATICALLY REDUCE OR ELIMINATE THESE FATS FROM YOUR DIET:** | | | |
| SATURATED FAT | Increases LDL | Beef, butter, whole milk, cheese, ice cream | Coconut, palm, palm kernel |
| TRANS FAT OR HYDROGE-NATED FAT (usually found in packaged foods) | Increases LDL | cakes, pies, cookies, candy bars, crackers, frozen dinners, some breakfast cereals, fried fast foods | Margarine, Crisco |
| **REPLACE THE FATS ABOVE WITH THESE HEALTHIER ALTERNATIVES:** | | | |
| MONOUNSATUR-ATED FAT (YOUR BEST BET) | Decreases LDL, does not affect HDL | Fish, nuts, vegetables | Olive, peanut, almond, avocado |
| POLYUNSATUR-ATED FAT | Decreases both LDL and HDL | Fish (salmon, mackerel, tuna, sardines, shellfish) walnuts and other nuts | Corn, sunflower seed, safflower |

have been working on this for years. We have finally stopped using fatback in our greens and started flavoring them with smoked turkey, spices, and herbs. We drink skim milk, eat low-fat cheese and ice cream, and use soft low-fat margarine. We always remove the skin from poultry and trim off the fat. We now eat several meatless meals each week, and we've increased our fiber intake, which helps us excrete fat more rapidly and control our LDL cholesterol. We purchased inexpensive steamers and steam all our vegetables. We started baking or grilling our meats instead of frying them, and we use non-stick sprays, broth, or orange juice when we cook. Plus, we make our own salad dressing with olive, canola, or sunflower oil (at least some of the time); we also use our juicer a lot more.

Remember, these recommendations need not be followed precisely for each meal or even on a daily basis. Even out your fat intake over the course of a week. For example, if you eat a high-fat lunch, you can compensate by eating a low-fat dinner or less fat over the next several meals.

**5. *Don't forget your vitamin and mineral supplements.*** Here's a look at some of the most important vitamins and minerals for Prime Time women:

***Vitamin E.*** There's evidence that vitamin E promotes heart health by reducing the oxidation of LDL (bad) cholesterol and serving as an anticoagulant. Studies from Harvard report a 40 percent reduction in heart disease risk in those who took vitamin E supplements. This vitamin is also a powerful antioxidant, guarding cells against free radicals, which can damage cells. The recommended supplement dose is 400 to 800 IU per day. If you have a choice, buy natural vitamin E (look for "d-alpha tocopherol" and/or "mixed tocopherols" on the label).

***Vitamin C.*** Many good studies show that vitamin C lowers your blood pressure and guards against cancer, heart disease, cataracts, and other disorders. We recommend a diet rich in fruits and fruit juice (get that juicer out) and a daily supplement of 500–1,000 mg of vitamin C.

***Vitamin D.*** This nutrient helps the body absorb calcium and may help prevent arthritis, osteoporosis, and certain cancers. Calcium won't do you much good unless you also get enough of this "sunshine vitamin." Vitamin D is found mainly in milk, butter, egg yolks, and fortified breakfast cereal. We recommend a supplement of 400 IU of vitamin D up to age seventy. Women older than seventy need to up their intake to 600 IU.

***B vitamins.*** Many people over age fifty don't get enough B vitamins in their diets. Without B vitamins, you may face increased risk of heart disease, stroke, certain cancers, depression, dementia, and overall mental decline. Folic acid and vitamins $B_{12}$ and $B_6$ can protect our hearts and keep us mentally sharp as we age. Folic acid is important in reducing *homocysteine*, an amino acid in your blood that is linked to increased risk of heart disease. Vitamin $B_{12}$ is important for preventing a form of dementia in older people that may be mistaken for Alzheimer's. A decline in the ability to absorb vitamin $B_{12}$ can leave older people susceptible to a deficiency. A daily multivitamin will supply these B vitamins.

***Calcium.*** We need plenty of this mineral to reduce our risk of osteoporosis. The dose is 1,000 mg for women up to age fifty and 1,500 mg for ages fifty-one and older.

***Chromium.*** This mineral helps stimulate the metabolism of carbohydrates and fats. Since a chromium deficiency impairs the functioning of insulin, this is a critical mineral for diabetics. Dose: 200 mcg.

***Magnesium.*** This is vital for bone and dental health. Dose: 300–400 mg.

## WOMEN'S DAILY RECOMMENDED DOSAGES OF VITAMINS

| VITAMIN | PREMENOPAUSAL | POSTMENOPAUSAL |
|---|---|---|
| $B_1$ | 5 mg | 2.5 mg |
| $B_2$ | 5 mg | 2.5 mg |
| $B_3$ (niacin) | 100 mg | 100 mg |
| $B_6$ | 4 mg | 3 mg |
| $B_{12}$ | 20 mcg | 40 mcg |
| Beta-carotene | 25,000 IU | 25,000 IU |
| Biotin | 210 mcg | 300 mcg |
| Folic Acid | 300 mcg | 400 mcg |
| Pantothenic Acid | 30 mg | 30 mg |
| C | 500 mg | 500–1,000 mg |
| D | 400 IU | 400 IU |
| E | 400 IU | 400–800 IU |

## WOMEN'S DAILY RECOMMENDED DOSAGES OF MINERALS

| MINERAL | PREMENOPAUSAL | POSTMENOPAUSAL |
|---|---|---|
| Calcium | 1,000 mg | 1,500 mg |
| Copper | 2 mg | 3 mg |
| Chromium | 200 mcg | 200 mcg |
| Magnesium | 300 mg | 400 mg |
| Manganese | 2 mg | 5 mg |
| Molybdenum | 50 mcg | 50 mcg |

| MINERAL | PREMENOPAUSAL | POSTMENOPAUSAL |
|---------|---------------|----------------|
| Selenium | 200 mcg | 200 mcg |
| Zinc | 15 mg | 15 mcg |
| Iodine | 150 mcg | 150 mcg |
| Potassium | 860 mg | 860 mg* |

*Authors recommend obtaining 3,000–4,000 mg of potassium *in your diet* daily.

*Source: Look 10 Years Younger, Live 10 Years Longer: A Woman's Guide* by Dr. David Ryback.

## Important Dietary Additions

There are a number of herbs, spices, and other natural substances that many healthy older people have made a part of their diet. Doctors and nutritionists now recommend that we all eat more of the following items:

*Herbs and spices,* such as rosemary, sage, thyme, oregano, ginger, and cumin, add flavor to foods and may act as antioxidants and anticancer agents.

*Garlic* and other members of the garlic family may lower blood pressure, benefit the heart, and decrease the risk of cancer. The garlic family includes garlic, onions, shallots, leeks, chives, and scallions. Eat garlic raw to get the most benefit since cooking decreases its effect.

*Soy foods,* including tofu, soy milk, soybeans, and soy protein, contain substances that are converted to a type of estrogen in the body that can help relieve the hot flashes of menopause and protect against cancer. Studies point to the phytoestrogen content of soy for its positive effects. Eating 25 to 50 grams per day of soy decreases your risk of heart disease by decreasing your LDL and total cholesterol without decreasing your HDL. This is a lot of soy. The richest source is powdered soy protein; next are tempeh, tofu, and soy milk.

Increasing your consumption of whole soy seems to be more effective than taking soy isoflavone supplements. Mix up a soy shake with soy protein and fresh fruit. Stir-fry tofu with fresh vegetables. Boil whole fresh soybeans in salted water for about five minutes and then pop the beans out of the pod into your mouth. Drink a cup of delicious soy milk. Try dry-roasted soy nuts.

*Green tea,* according to new research, may reduce the risk of many cancers and has positive effects for your cardiovascular health. Oolong tea may also provide some benefits.

# VITAMINS

*Fat-soluble vitamins can be stored in the body and need not be consumed daily.*

| Vitamin | Its Functions | Good Dietary Sources | Signs of Deficiency | Signs of Overdose |
| --- | --- | --- | --- | --- |
| Vitamin A | Helps maintain skin, hair, nails, gums, bones, teeth; helps ward off infection, promotes eye function | Dairy products, green and deep yellow or orange vegetables, deep yellow or orange fruit | Night blindness, reduced growth in children | Headache, blurred vision, fatigue, diarrhea, joint pain |
| Vitamin D | Helps build and maintain teeth and bones; helps body absorb calcium | Egg yolk, liver, tuna, cod-liver oil, fortified milk | Rickets in children, bone diseases in adults | Calcium deposits, fragile bones, hypertension, high cholesterol, diarrhea |
| Vitamin E | Helps form red blood cells, muscles, and other tissues; preserves fatty acids | Poultry, seafood, seeds, nuts, vegetable oils, wheat germ, fortified cereal, eggs | Rare in humans | Blurred vision, headaches |
| Vitamin K | Aids blood clotting | Made by intestinal bacteria. Spinach, oats, wheat bran | Excessive bleeding, liver damage | Jaundice in infants |

## Water-soluble vitamins are stored in smaller amounts than fat-soluble vitamins and need to be consumed more frequently.

| | | | | |
| --- | --- | --- | --- | --- |
| Thiamin (Vitamin B1) | Enhances energy, promotes normal appetite and digestion | Pork, fortified cereals and grains, seafood | Anxiety, hysteria, nausea, Extreme cases: beriberi | |
| Riboflavin | Metabolism of foods, release of energy to cells | Organ meat, beet lamb, dark meat of poultry, dairy products, fortified cereals, dark green leafy vegetables | Sores around nose and mouth, visual problems | |
| Pantothenic Acid (Vitamin B5) | Needed to convert food to energy, aids digestion | Found in nearly all foods | Weakness, irritability | |
| Niacin (Nicotinic Acid) | Helps release energy from foods, aids nerve function, digestion | Poultry, seafood, seeds, nuts, potatoes, fortified grains and cereals | Extreme cases: pellagra, a skin disease | Skin flushing |
| Pyridoxine (Vitamin B6) | Aids protein metabolism and absorption, and carbohydrate metabolism | Meat, fish, poultry, grains, cereals, potatoes, bananas, prunes | Depression, confusion, and convulsions in infants | Extreme cases: sensory nerve destruction |
| Cobalamin (Vitamin B12) | Builds genetic material needed by cells; helps form red blood cells | All animal products | Deficiency rare except in strict vegetarians, the elderly, and those with malabsorption disorders | |
| Biotin | Metabolism of glucose, essential for many bodily processes | Made by intestinal bacteria. Meats, poultry, fish, eggs, nuts, seeds | Rare except in infants: scaling skin, fatigue, pain | |
| Folic Acid (Folate Folacin) | Manufacture of red blood cells and genetic material | Poultry, liver, dark green leafy vegetables, legumes, fortified whole-grain bread and cereal | Anemia, diarrhea, bleeding gums, weight loss, stomach upsets | |
| Vitamin C (Ascorbic Acid) | Helps bind cells together, strengthens blood vessel walls, helps resist infection, speeds healing of wounds | Citrus fruits, strawberries, cantaloupe, sweet potatoes, cabbage, cauliflower | Bleeding gums, loose teeth, easy bruising. Extreme cases: scurvy | |

# MINERALS

**Because the body needs relatively large amounts of these three minerals, they are called macro- (Greek for "large") minerals.**

| Mineral | Its Functions | Good Dietary Sources | Signs of Deficiency | Signs of Overdose |
|---|---|---|---|---|
| Calcium | Helps build bones and teeth, promotes proper muscle and nerve function | Milk and milk products, canned salmon with bones, oysters, broccoli | Rickets in children, bone diseases in adults | Kidney stones, lethargy, pain |
| Phosphorus | With calcium, helps build bone and teeth | Dairy products, egg yolks, meat, poultry, fish | Deficiency is rare | Lowers blood calcium |
| Magnesium | Helps release energy in body, promotes bone growth | Green leafy vegetables, beans, fortified whole-grain cereals and bread | Muscle weakness, cramps | Nervous-system disorders; overdose can kill people with kidney disease |

## Trace minerals, which perform a wide range of functions, are needed in very small amounts.

| Mineral | Its Functions | Good Dietary Sources | Signs of Deficiency | Signs of Overdose |
|---|---|---|---|---|
| Iron | Essential for healthy blood | Meat, liver, legumes, fortified breads & cereals, green leafy vegetables | Weakness, fatigue, headache, iron-deficiency anemia | Toxic buildup in liver, diabetes, liver disease |
| Zinc | Essential to digestion and metabolism | Beef, liver, oysters, yogurt, fortified cereal, wheat germ | Slow wound healing, loss of appetite, slow growth | Nausea, vomiting, abdominal pain, gastric bleeding |
| Selenium | Helps avoid breakdown of fats and body chemicals | Chicken, seafood, whole-grain breads and cereals | Unknown in humans | Nausea, abdominal pain, diarrhea, irritability, death |
| Copper | Stimulates iron absorption, helps make red blood cells and nerve fibers | Lobster, organ meats, nuts, legumes, prunes, barley | Rare in adults | Liver disease, vomiting |
| Iodine | Essential to thyroid gland | Iodized salt, seafood | Goiter, cretinism in infants | Disturbed thyroid function, goiter |
| Fluoride | Promotes strong teeth and bones | Fluoridated water, tea | Tooth decay | Mottling of tooth enamel |
| Manganese | Contributes to tendon and bone structure | Tea, coffee, bran, legumes | Unknown in humans | Nerve damage |
| Molybdenum | Needed for metabolism | Legumes, dark green leafy vegetables, whole-grain breads and cereals | Unknown in humans | Joint pain |
| Chromium | Aids glucose metabolism | Whole-grain breads and cereals, brewer's yeast | Diabetes-like symptoms | Unknown for food chromium; chromium salts toxic |
| Sulfur | Helps make hair and nails | Wheat germ, legumes, beef, peanuts, clams | Unknown | Unknown for food sulfur; sulfur salts toxic |

## Electrolytes are minerals essential to proper body chemistry.

| Mineral | Its Functions | Good Dietary Sources | Signs of Deficiency | Signs of Overdose |
|---|---|---|---|---|
| Potassium | With sodium, helps regulate body's fluid balance | Bananas, citrus fruit, dried fruit, potatoes, legumes | Muscle weakness, cardiac arrhythmias, irritability | Nausea, diarrhea, cardiac arrhythmias |
| Sodium | Helps maintain body fluid balance | Salt, processed foods, milk, water in some areas | Deficiency is rare in the United States | High blood pressure, kidney disease, heart failure |
| Chloride | Helps maintain acid-base balance | Same as sodium | Deficiency is very rare | Upset in acid-base balance |

*Note:* Remember to discuss with your primary-care physician what vitamins, minerals, herbs, and other supplements you're taking, because they can sometimes have a negative effect on the body or interact with your other medications. Always check the dose with your doctor. Don't think that if a little is good, a lot is better. Some vitamins, minerals, and other nutrients are dangerous at high doses.

## Be Smart About Your Weight

Shedding as little as five to ten pounds can lower blood pressure, improve your lipid profile, and reduce your blood sugar. Doesn't that sound encouraging? So if you are overweight, don't focus on the twenty-five pounds you may need to lose to be at the recommended weight for your height; rather, start with a realistic goal of losing one to two pounds a week and getting fit. Think about it: At that rate you will lose twenty pounds in just ten weeks. And by combining healthy eating with exercise, those will be pounds you'll keep off.

Diets that include all the food groups are also easier to stick to than a diet based on a wacky plan that lets you eat only one type of food or a plan that restricts you to a dangerously low amount of calories. Even if you need to

# BMI by Height and Weight

Without calculating your **BMI (Body Mass Index)** you can use this chart to see whether you are at your ideal weight. Find your height in the left-hand column, then read to the right. The middle column shows how much you would weigh if you had a BMI of 25 (overweight); the right-hand column shows your weight with a BMI of 30 (obese).

| HEIGHT | BODY WEIGHT IN POUNDS | |
| --- | --- | --- |
|  | BMI=25 | BMI=30 |
| 4'10" | 119 LBS | 143 LBS |
| 4'11" | 124 | 148 |
| 5'0" | 128 | 153 |
| 5'1" | 132 | 158 |
| 5'2" | 136 | 164 |
| 5'3" | 141 | 169 |
| 5'4" | 145 | 174 |
| 5'5" | 150 | 180 |
| 5'6" | 155 | 186 |
| 5'7" | 159 | 191 |
| 5'8" | 164 | 197 |
| 5'9" | 169 | 203 |
| 5'10" | 174 | 207 |
| 5'11" | 179 | 215 |
| 6'0" | 184 | 221 |
| 6'1" | 189 | 227 |
| 6'2" | 194 | 233 |
| 6'3" | 200 | 240 |

lose a lot of weight, your primary goal should be to get healthy by eating balanced, nutritious meals. Eating smaller meals six times a day combined with exercise is a strategy that offers tremendous benefits.

If you need help staying motivated or putting together a nutritious low-fat, high-fiber meal plan, consider working with a nutritionist or joining a reputable weight-reducing program such as Weight Watchers, which incorporates all the food groups into its meal plans.

If you want to go it alone, follow these guidelines:

*Every day select an appropriate number of servings from each of the food groups in the pyramid.* Choose the middle of the servings range if you want to maintain your weight, the low end (except for vegetables) if you are trying to lose weight. If you don't normally stock these foods in your house, take this book with you so you can refer to the food pyramid while you shop. If you dine out, know what food groups you need to include in your meal to follow a healthy eating program.

*Watch your portion size.* We all need to do this better. For instance, a 3-ounce serving of cooked meat is about the size of a deck of cards. Don't forget to read what's considered the recommended serving size on the food label. Be sure you know how many calories, total fat, cholesterol, sodium, total carbohydrate, protein, and vitamins and minerals are in one serving. And take note: Sometimes even small packages hold two or more servings.

---

## GUIDELINE FOR ONE SERVING

- BREAD GROUP: 1 slice of bread, ½ small bagel or muffin, ½ cup cooked cereal pasta or rice, ½ to 1 cup ready-to-eat cereal
- VEGETABLE GROUP: 1 cup raw vegetable, ½ cup cooked vegetable
- FRUIT GROUP: 1 medium fresh fruit, ½ cup cut or canned fruit, ¾ cup fruit juice
- MILK GROUP: 1 cup milk or yogurt
- MEAT GROUP: 2–3 ounces cooked, trimmed, boneless lean red meat, skinless poultry, or fish, 4 ounces tofu, ½ cup cooked dried beans, 1 egg, 2 tablespoons peanut butter
- FATS, OILS, AND SWEETS: 1 teaspoon butter, margarine, sugar, or jelly, 1 tablespoon mayonnaise or salad dressing, 2 tablespoons sour cream, 1 ounce cream cheese

---

# Check Your Smoking

# I.Q.

## AN IMPORTANT QUIZ FOR OLDER SMOKERS

*If you or someone you know is an older smoker, you may think that there is no point in quitting now. Think again. By quitting now, you will feel more in control and have fewer coughs and colds. On the other hand, with every cigarette you smoke, you increase your chances of having a heart attack, a stroke, or cancer. Need to think about this more? Take this older smokers' quiz. Just answer "true" or "false" to each statement below. The correct answers are on the next page.*

T F **1** If you have smoked for most of your life, it's not worth stopping now.

T F **2** Older smokers who try to quit are more likely to stay off cigarettes.

T F **3** Smokers get tired and short of breath more easily than nonsmokers the same age.

T F **4** Smoking is a major risk factor for heart attack and stroke among adults 60 years of age and older.

T F **5** Quitting smoking can help those who have already had a heart attack.

T F **6** Most older smokers don't want to stop smoking.

T F **7** An older smoker is more likely to smoke *more* cigarettes than a younger smoker.

T F **8** Someone who has smoked for 30 to 40 years probably won't be able to quit smoking.

T F **9** Very few older adults smoke cigarettes.

T F **10** Lifelong smokers are more likely to die of diseases like emphysema and bronchitis than nonsmokers.

*Source: Prepared by the National Heart, Lung, and Blood Institute Smoking Education Program*

**1. False.** Nonsense! You have every reason to quit now and quit for good — even if you've been smoking for years. Stopping smoking now will help you live longer and feel better. You will reduce your risk of heart attack, stroke, and cancer; improve blood flow and lung function; and help stop diseases like emphysema and bronchitis from getting worse.

**2. True.** Once they quit, older smokers are far more likely than younger smokers to stay away from cigarettes. Older smokers know more about the short- and long-term health benefits of quitting.

**3. True.** Smokers, especially those over 50 years old, are much more likely to get tired, feel short of breath, and cough more often. These symptoms can signal the start of bronchitis or emphysema. Stopping smoking will help reduce these symptoms.

**4. True.** Smoking is a major risk factor for four of the five leading causes of death including heart disease, stroke, cancer, and lung diseases like emphysema and bronchitis. For adults 60 and over, smoking is a major risk factor for six of the top 14 causes of death. Older male smokers are nearly twice as likely to die from strokes as older men who do not smoke. The odds are nearly as high for older female smokers. Cigarette smokers of any age have a 70 percent greater heart disease death rate than do nonsmokers.

**5. True.** The good news is that stopping smoking does help people who have suffered a heart attack. In fact, their chances of having another attack are smaller. In some cases, ex-smokers can cut their risk of another heart attack by half or more.

**6. False.** Most smokers would prefer to quit. In fact, in a recent study, 65 percent of older smokers said they would like to stop. What keeps them from quitting? They are afraid of being irritable, nervous, and tense. Others are concerned about cravings for cigarettes. Most don't want to gain weight. Many think it's too late to quit — that quitting after so many years of smoking will not help. But this is not true.

**7. True.** Older smokers usually smoke more cigarettes than younger people. Plus, older smokers are more likely to smoke a high-nicotine brand.

**8. False.** You may be surprised to learn that older smokers are actually more likely to suceed at quitting smoking. This is more true if they're already experiencing long-term smoking-related symptoms like shortness of breath, coughing, or chest pain. Older smokers who stop want to avoid further health problems, take control of their life, get rid of the smell of cigarettes, and save money.

**9. False.** One out of five adults age 50 or older smokes cigarettes. This is more than 11 million smokers, a fourth of the country's 43 million smokers! About 25 percent of the general U.S. population still smokes.

**10. True.** Smoking greatly increases the risk of dying from diseases like emphysema and bronchitis. The risk of dying from lung cancer is also a lot higher for smokers than nonsmokers: 22 times higher for males, 12 times higher for females.

## How did you do?

**10 correct:** Congratulations! You could have written this quiz. As you already know so much about the effects of smoking in older adults, share this information with your family and friends. If you smoke, you should also know enough to quit — today.

**8 – 9 correct:** Excellent. If you got at least eight right, then you have at least eight good reasons to stop smoking — or never start. Ask your doctor or nurse for more information.

**Fewer than 8 correct:** Take your time to review the facts in the quiz. Then, talk to your doctor or nurse soon about the ways of stopping smoking.

*For more information, write:*
*NHLBI Smoking Education Program*
*4733 Bethesda Avenue, Suite 530*
*Bethesda, MD 20814-4820*

*NIH Publication No. 91-3031, October 1991*

*U.S. DEPARTMENT OF HEALTH*
*AND HUMAN SERVICES*
*Public Health Service*
*National Institutes of Health*

## STOP SMOKING

Getting tobacco and nicotine out of your life is essential because *smoking is the number one preventable cause of death*. Giving up smoking will reduce your risk for developing so many health problems—from heart disease to lung cancer—that just trying to list the benefits of not smoking would take up a whole chapter.

You *can* stop smoking. Today the results are much more encouraging, and you can double and triple your odds of breaking the habit. Seventy percent of folks who want to quit smoking will be successful. Be patient, though. It usually takes four or five tries before you successfully quit. But it is one of the best things you can do for yourself—*and you are worth it*.

### Prime Time Eight-Step Smoking Cessation Plan

A majority of smokers try to go "cold turkey," which is the least successful method, according to scientific studies. Like most smokers, you'll probably need support to help you quit the habit. Our plan should help.

*Step 1: Examine your motivation to stop.* The questionnaire below, "Why I Want to Quit Smoking," will help you identify some common reasons why smokers smoke. Please feel free to add your personal reasons as well. Use the results of this questionnaire to keep you motivated when the going gets tough. You may need to review your reasons for quitting again and again and again.

---

### WHY I WANT TO QUIT SMOKING

Check all that apply.

_____ I will greatly lessen my chances of having a heart attack or stroke.

_____ I will greatly lessen my chances of getting lung cancer, emphysema, and other lung diseases.

_____ I will have fewer colds or bouts of the flu each year.

_____ I will climb stairs and walk without getting out of breath.

_____ I will have fewer wrinkles.

_____ I will be free of my morning cough.

_____ I will have better smelling clothes, hair, breath, home, and car.

_____ I will have more energy to pursue physical activities I enjoy.

_____ I will have more control over my life.

---

| | |
|---|---|
| _____ | I will _____ |
| _____ | I will _____ |
| _____ | I will _____ |
| _____ | I will _____ |

*Source:* Prepared by The National Heart, Lung and Blood Institute, National Institutes of Health

*Step 2: Set a target date for stopping.* Put the date on a piece of paper and have your Prime Time Sister sign the paper with you. This is your contract. Ask your Prime Time Sister to give you special support in your efforts to quit. Talk with her regularly and have her participate frequently as you move forward.

*Step 3: Examine when and why you are smoking.* Are you continuing to smoke because you're afraid of gaining weight if you stop? If so, please dismiss this as a reason. First, the enormous risks of smoking far outweigh a little extra weight. The average weight gain for ex-smokers is only about five pounds, and you can prevent even this by snacking on veggies and increasing your physical activity level. **Weight control is not a benefit of smoking.** There are many overweight smokers.

Examine your "triggers," which are situations and feelings that bring on the urge to light up, such as eating a meal, drinking coffee, talking on the phone, driving or being stressed. Once you identify your triggers, try not to respond to them by smoking. When possible, find alternative behaviors for each trigger. For instance, instead of drinking coffee, try tea. If you feel stressed, stop, take slow, deep breaths, and count to ten. It's hard to quit smoking, but *you can do it if you hang in there*!

Use this form to write down your triggers and some more appropriate responses that you would like to try.

## WHAT TRIGGERS YOUR SMOKING?

Write down some activities or situations that make you more likely to smoke. Then think of what else you can do instead of picking up a cigarette. (See below for some suggestions.)

| TRIGGER SITUATION/FEELING | ALTERNATIVE BEHAVIOR |
|---|---|
| _____ | _____ |
| _____ | _____ |

| TRIGGER SITUATION/FEELING | ALTERNATIVE BEHAVIOR |
|---|---|
| _____ | _____ |
| _____ | _____ |
| _____ | _____ |
| _____ | _____ |

Consider these healthier responses to your triggers:

- To keep your hands busy: draw, write, read the paper, work crossword puzzles, polish your nails, knit or crochet, _____ (you fill in the blank.)
- When you feel stressed out, find different ways to relax: take a deep breath, walk away, go outside, listen to music, meditate, read, drink some herbal tea.
- After meals, brush your teeth, call a friend, or drink tea if coffee is a trigger for smoking.

*Step 4: Ask your doctor for help.* There are many free or low-cost programs to help you stop. Check with the American Lung Association, the American Cancer Society, and your employer. Remember, you can't do it alone.

*Step 5: Check out the slew of smoking cessation aids.* Nicotine chewing gum and nicotine patches are available over the counter and account for more than 90 percent of the nicotine-replacement market. These substitutes still deliver nicotine to your bloodstream, but more slowly than smoking does and at a lower dose. If you have a heart problem and/or high blood pressure, don't use nicotine substitutes except under the supervision of your doctor.

Prescription nicotine treatment include a potent nasal spray and an inhaler that resembles a cigarette. In addition, Zyban (bupropion), an antidepressant, has been approved for smoking cessation treatment. Patients who take Zyban tend not to gain weight when they quit smoking. Don't take it if you have seizures or have had a head injury or a stroke.

*Step 6: Consider alternative treatments.* Hypnosis can be used to change those messages about smoking in your head. Only a one-hour session may be needed. Contact the American Society of Clinical Hypnosis at 847-297-3317.

Acupuncture helps in the short term. However, there is very little research on its effectiveness. One study from Norway, reported in the March 1997 issue of *Preventive Medicine*, reveals that electrified needles in the body and regular needles in the ears hold hope for people trying to quit smoking.

Home remedies work for many people. For instance, you may want to try chewing pieces of dried pineapple mixed with honey.

The herb acorus (sweet flag) supposedly decreases desire for nicotine, according to a study released in the journal *Chinese Herbal Medicine*; however, this treatment needs further study.

*Step 7: Ask for support from your Prime Time Sister, Prime Time Circle, a self-help group, and your family.* Support at this time in your life is essential, so don't be shy about reaching out. It really made a difference for Marilyn.

*Step 8: Don't get discouraged.* Remember, it takes multiple attempts before success. Keep trying. If you slip, don't go back to smoking. One slip doesn't mean you're a smoker again. Keep thinking of yourself as a nonsmoker. You are one.

---

## COMBINING CESSATION STRATEGIES MAY WORK BEST

A recent study has demonstrated that the most effective method to date is a combination of three approaches: the nicotine patch, Zyban, and supportive group counseling (tailored counseling to explore the reasons why you smoke). Dr. Linda Ferry, chief of preventive medicine at Veterans Affairs Medical Center in Loma Linda, California, reports that a year after four thousand smokers tried the new three-part program, 40 percent to 60 percent remained smoke-free. This is a dramatic improvement over previous data.

---

## NOURISH YOUR SPIRIT

As we emphasized in Chapter 3, "The Miracle of You," celebrating your uniqueness and enhance your spiritual life are critical components of wellness. Not only can an active spiritual life make you feel better about yourself and the world around you, studies are reporting that spirituality can help you heal faster. The fact that patients committed to religious beliefs have better hospital outcomes and have shorter hospital stays, decreased depression, and less anxiety is probably because spiritual activities decrease stress and increase activity in the temporal lobe of the brain, which is important in enhancing the immune system.

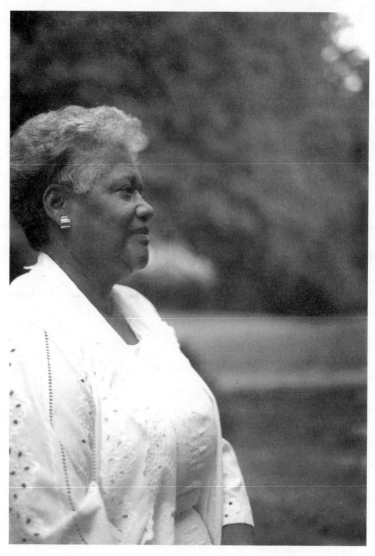

℞ **PRIME TIME PRESCRIPTION TO NOURISH YOUR SPIRIT**

*Read the prescriptions on meditation in Chapter 13.*

*Consider going back to church, if you have stopped, or joining another type of organized religious or spiritual group.* Group worship and prayer is a wonderful way to warm your soul.

*Become more active in your church or temple, or volunteer for a community program.* Helping others less fortunate than you are will encourage you to appreciate your own life.

*Try prayer walking or walking meditation.* Prayer walking, which is simply "taking a stroll with your soul," has been practiced by poets, philosophers, and holy people from many religious traditions for centuries. There is no wrong way to do it. Ideally, it is done outdoors to experience the divine presence of nature—the wind, the trees, the birds in flight, the beautiful formation of the clouds. But it can be done whenever and wherever you exercise.

The beauty of prayer walking is that it gets you moving and exercising while you focus on relaxing and slowing down your mind. To achieve this state, you must repeat (aloud or silently) a word, sound, or prayer while you walk or run. The goal is to breathe consciously and time your breaths and chants with your steps. Don't let your mind wander, though. Keep your mind in the present to enjoy the peace and joy you will feel once you get the hang of this practice.

If you want to learn more about the power of prayer walking, check out these three works by Linus Mundy: *Taking a Prayer Walk* and *Prayer Walking*, pamphlets that he published in 1992, and *The Long Road Turns to Joy*.

## PLANNING YOUR PRIME TIME DAY

We realize that important, lifesaving lifestyle changes cannot be made overnight. So, again, start slowly, but start right now, and believe that in time you can make these major life-enhancing changes. Be patient. False starts or returns to your old patterns of behavior are part of learning and acquiring new skills.

Here is an example—and that's all it is—of how you can incorporate the different recommendations that we have made into a health-promoting, disease-preventing Prime Time day.

### MORNING

- *Get eight hours of sleep so that you can wake up rested.*
- *Start the day with a prayer of thanks and/or meditation.*
- *Schedule time to exercise for at least thirty minutes—and make sure you stick to your plan. If you can exercise first thing in the morning, great. That way nothing will prevent you from completing your workout.*
- *Eat a healthy breakfast that includes fruit, fiber, supplemental vitamins, minerals, and water.*
- *Set a positive personal or professional goal.*

- *Make a conscious decision to treat yourself and others in an assertive, loving manner.*
- *Spend your day—whether at home, at work, volunteering, or on vacation—engaged in satisfying, affirming, useful, productive activities.*
- *Take a break during the morning for a snack such as fruit or yogurt. Don't forget to drink your water.*

## LUNCH/MIDDAY

- *Make sure your lunch includes vegetables, fruit, and water.*
- *Take a few moments of personal time to do some relaxation exercises, meditation, or deep breathing. (You might prefer to exercise before lunch.)*
- *Floss teeth.*

## AFTERNOON

- *Eat a nutritious snack, such as a piece of fruit or vegetable sticks. Don't go for the cookies, candy, or caffeinated cola. And remember, drink some water.*

## EVENING

- *Listen to music, try some yoga stretches, or take a soothing bath to transition from your day activity to have a relaxing or enjoyable evening.*
- *Eat a healthy dinner with plenty of vegetables and water.*
- *Spend time with family or friends, even if it's a phone call or sending an e-mail message.*
- *Have a soothing cup of tea before you get ready for bed (you can find suggestions for relaxing teas in the Prime Time Prescriptions in Chapter 13). Be sure you go to bed early enough to ensure you'll get eight hours of sleep.*
- *Say a prayer of thanks, or express gratitude for all the positives that happened during the day (and there are always some).*
- *Forgive yourself and possibly others for mistakes or hurts.*

We know that not every day, every week, every month, and every year will go smoothly, because to paraphrase Dr. Scott Peck, life can be difficult. However, we hope that you will focus on the beauty, joy, and amazing grace of life. We also hope you truly believe that *now is your time to take charge of your spiritual, emotional, and physical health.*

# PART IV

# You Can Save Your Own Life

# Chapter 10

# CONTROLLING CARDIOVASCULAR DISEASE: HEART DISEASE, HYPERTENSION, AND STROKE

## AISHA'S STORY

Aisha, a forty-five-year-old computer programmer, had started her day as usual, with a long walk with her dog. After lunch, though, she felt nauseated, and her back started to hurt. At first Aisha tried to ignore these symptoms. When her discomfort increased, she took an antacid and vowed never to return to the restaurant where she'd eaten lunch. An hour passed, but she still had no relief.

Concentrating on a major project that was due the next day was getting increasingly difficult for Aisha, as the nausea and back pain had intensified. When she mentioned how she felt to a colleague, he tried to reassure her that it was "just stress." Aisha still was uncomfortable, so she called her Prime Time Sister June for advice. June encouraged her to go immediately to a hospital emergency room. There Aisha was diagnosed as having a heart attack. June saved Aisha's life because she knew the symptoms of a heart attack.

The number one cause of death in this country for everyone—men and women, Black and White—is heart disease. Are you surprised? Most women are, because we often think that cancer, especially breast cancer, is our greatest health threat. In fact, only 8 percent of women surveyed by the American Heart Association (AHA) named heart disease or stroke as a disease they should worry about.[1] But the reality is that women are three times more likely to get heart disease than breast cancer.

The AHA survey also revealed that 50 percent of women believed that men are more likely than postmenopausal women to have heart attacks. Wrong! **The truth is that heart disease kills more women every year than men.** Forty-nine percent of women who have heart attacks die within one year, as compared to only 31 percent of men. The major reason for the increased incidence of heart disease deaths in women may be that women and health-care professionals tend to minimize the symptoms and signs of heart problems in women. It is still considered a "man's disease."

The symptoms of heart disease in women are also different from men's symptoms. Women report symptoms of indigestion, upper back pain, and being very fatigued, *not* the crushing chest and left arm pain that men report. Many women and even many physicians don't realize that the symptoms are different.

Another reason that we African American women have poorer outcomes can be found in a recent study of physicians that documented how sexism and racism affect the quality of medical evaluations of patients for heart disease. Caucasian men received the most thorough evaluations, with African American men next in line. All women, Black and White, received the most superficial evaluations, if they received them at all. However, African American women were the least well evaluated and had the least complete treatment of the four groups studied. African American women were evaluated minimally and treated less aggressively. For instance, doctors ordered a heart catheterization, the gold-standard diagnostic test, on Black women only 40 percent of the time when it was clinically indicated.[2]

This lack of proper evaluation is one major reason why heart disease in women, especially African American women, often goes inadequately treated until the condition becomes severe. Another reason is that when a heart attack does occur, women are also more likely to delay calling 911 for help. Women who have heart attacks typically take an hour longer than men to get to the hospital. When we arrive, we are not treated as aggressively as men, which is why we are more likely to die in the hospital. Women are less likely to receive lifesaving drugs for heart attacks. The study mentioned above reported that clot-busting drugs went to 59 percent of the White men diagnosed as having a heart attack, 56 percent of the White women, 50 percent of the Black men, and 44 percent of the Black women.

It's important that you understand that heart disease is not just a White male thing! According to the American Heart Association, when it comes to heart disease, probably no group is more susceptible than African American women.[3] The National Center for Health Statistics reports that heart disease accounts for 45 percent of deaths in African American women. We die from heart attacks at twice the rate of other women, and we die from heart disease earlier than our Caucasian peers. From ages thirty-five to seventy-four, our age-adjusted overall death rate is 71 percent higher than the rate for White women, according to the American Heart Association.

So what does this mean for you? These findings scream to all of us that we must take charge of our lives and our medical care to make sure we get the appropriate evaluation and therapy. Therefore, if you suspect a problem, or if you're having problems and you don't feel like you're getting the care you need, *demand a second opinion!*

Do we have your attention now?

---

## WHAT'S YOUR RISK OF A FIRST HEART ATTACK?

Fill in the correct points (listed in parentheses) for each risk factor.

POINTS

AGE:                                                                          _____
- Less than 41 (0 points)
- 42 to 44 (1 point)
- 45 to 54 (2 points)
- 55 to 73 (3 points)
- 74 or older (4 points)

FAMILY HISTORY: My family has a history of heart
disease or heart attacks before the age of fifty-five. (2 points)      _____

INACTIVE LIFESTYLE: I rarely exercise or do anything
physically demanding. (1 point)                                              _____

WEIGHT: I'm more than twenty pounds over my ideal
weight. (1 point)                                                            _____

SMOKING: I'm a smoker. (1 point)                                             _____

DIABETIC: (2 points)                                                         _____

TOTAL CHOLESTEROL LEVEL:                                                     _____
- Less than 240 mg/dL (0 points)
- 240 mg/dL to 315 mg/dL (1 point)
- More than 315 mg/dL (2 points)

HDL LEVEL:                                         _____
- Over 60 mg/dL (minus 1 point)
- 39 mg/dL to 59 mg/dL (0 points)
- 30 mg/dL to 38 mg/dL (1 point)
- Under 30 mg/dL (2 points)

BLOOD PRESSURE:                          _____
- I don't take blood pressure medication; my blood pressure is _____.
(Use your systolic, or top, blood pressure number.) _____
  - Less than 140 mm Hg (0 points)
  - 140 mm Hg to 170 mm Hg (1 point)
  - Greater than 170 mm Hg (2 points)
- I am currently taking blood pressure medication. (1 point)

TOTAL POINTS (see below)                 _____

SCORING: If you scored 4 or more points, you could be at above-average risk of a first heart attack compared to the general adult population. The higher the score, the greater risk you have.

*Source:* Developed by the American Heart Association.

## WHAT IS HEART DISEASE?

Heart disease occurs when the blood supply from the coronary arteries to the heart muscle is severely restricted. This happens when fatty deposits along the inner wall of the arteries narrow the arteries and reduce the blood flow, a condition called *atherosclerosis*. Atherosclerosis can progress and completely block your arteries. If the blood flow is completely cut off, muscle cells in the heart will die from a lack of oxygen and nutrients. This is what is commonly referred to as a *heart attack*.

## WARNING SIGNS FOR A HEART ATTACK

An easy way to remember the warning signs is to know your ABCs of a heart attack:

A *Angina:* chest pain or tightness in the chest that may radiate down the arm or up into the jaw (this may feel like heavy pressure, squeezing, or burning in the chest, back, neck, arms, jaw, or shoulders)

B *Breathlessness:* unusual shortness of breath that may even cause you to wake up breathless at night

C *Chronic fatigue:* feeling unusually tired to the point that you're over-whelmed by fatigue

D *Dizziness, lightheadedness, blackouts*

E *Edema:* swelling that occurs particularly in the ankles and lower legs

F *Fluttering, rapid, or irregular heartbeat*

G *Gastric upset:* nausea, vomiting, and gas pains

H *Heavy pain in your upper back on exertion or at rest*

I *Indigestion*

*Source:* Adapted from the Washington Hospital Center.

Women's heart attack symptoms are not as clear as the classic symptoms experienced by most men. For women, the pain of a heart attack may travel into the neck, jawbone, or back, and unlike in men, this pain doesn't necessarily increase with exertion. Women also experience shortness of breath, indigestion, or a vague feeling of anxiety or doom.

If you notice any of these warning signs, contact your doctor or get to an emergency room immediately, because when you suffer from a heart attack, you must get help right away. It is essential to get the proper medications into your system quickly, to minimize damage to the heart muscle.

## Are You at Risk for Heart Disease?

When you reach midlife, **your age** becomes a risk factor for heart disease. Although heart disease can strike women of any age, your chances increase significantly after menopause. In fact, 90 percent of the problems associated with coronary artery disease happen to postmenopausal women.

A **family history** of early heart disease, especially if your mother, father, or sibling died before age fifty-five, increases your risk of developing this disease. Also, recent research suggests that women's hearts may be different from men's hearts and hence more vulnerable to heart disease. For instance, there are areas in the heart where estrogen (a female hormone) can bind to the heart tissue and affect it in ways that are not fully understood. Also, we may be more prone to clotting, which increases the risk of heart attack. Finally, **diabetic women** have a higher risk of developing heart disease than diabetic men. According to the Nurses' Health Study, there was a sevenfold increase in cardiovascular events in women with diabetes.[4]

Surprising as it may seem, **smoking** by women in this country causes almost as many deaths from heart disease as from lung cancer. *If you smoke,* *you are two to six times more likely to suffer a heart attack than a nonsmoking woman.* Only three to five cigarettes per day increases your risk for heart disease, and the risk rises even more with the number of cigarettes you smoke each day. In the first year after stopping smoking, the risk of heart disease drops sharply, and it will eventually return to the same level as that of a nonsmoker. No matter what your age, quitting will lower your chances of developing heart disease. Smoking also boosts the risk of stroke.

## Risk Factors for Heart Disease

As we have mentioned, the top six modifiable risk factors for heart disease are *smoking, high blood pressure (hypertension), high blood cholesterol levels (especially high LDL cholesterol, and low HDL cholesterol), inadequate exercise, obesity,* and *stress.* Inactivity doubles your risk of heart problems.

Not only does obesity contribute to heart disease, your body shape can also increase your risk. "Apple-shaped" women, with extra fat around the waistline, may have a higher risk than "pear-shaped" women, with heavy hips and thighs.[5]

Having more than one risk factor increases your chance of dying from heart disease. For example, if you smoke and have high blood pressure, you boost the risk of developing heart disease to eight times that of women who have no risk factors. Because we tend to have a combination of risk factors, Black women are particularly at risk for heart disease.[6] In fact, according to National Heart, Lung, and Blood Institute research, we are more likely to have high blood pressure, be obese, consume high-fat and high-cholesterol diets, and not exercise.

**Rx** **PRIME TIME PRESCRIPTIONS TO REDUCE YOUR RISK OF HEART DISEASE**
Modifying your risk factors can prevent coronary heart disease and reverse this disease if maintained over time, so carefully check out the following Prime Time Prescriptions. Many of our recommendations may be easier than you think.

*Get a thorough checkup, including the appropriate tests for heart disease.* (See the box "Critical Tests and Procedures for Heart Disease," below.)

## CRITICAL TESTS AND PROCEDURES FOR HEART DISEASE

As we discussed in Chapter 8, "The Ultimate Checkup," routine tests to check for any signs of heart disease are critical if you want to reduce your risk of a heart attack. In fact, these tests can actually save your life. Depending on your risk level and current state of health, here are seven tests and procedures you should know about.

**Electrocardiogram (ECG/EKG).** This is the old workhorse in cardiac evaluations and the one test cardiologists rely on the most. It is one of the eight tests that could save your life and should be performed at age forty to serve as a baseline reading. After age fifty, an ECG should be included in every annual exam. This test is valuable in detecting abnormal heart rhythms and new heart attacks and areas of previously damaged heart muscle. A normal resting ECG does not eliminate the possibility of decreased blood flow to the heart muscle, which may occur and cause chest pain during increased physical activity. Therefore, other tests are required if heart disease is suspected.

**Stress test.** If a resting ECG is normal in the face of symptoms and suspected heart disease, the next step is an exercise stress test. You take this test by exercising on a treadmill or stationary bike while hooked to an ECG machine. Unfortunately, stress tests aren't very accurate, especially for women. More than 33 percent of women who take a stress test show a problem when there isn't one, or do not show a problem when there are other indications of heart disease. That's why you should always question your doctor regarding the results of a stress test and push for further tests if you feel there is a problem.

**Thallium stress test.** If the routine stress test shows some indication of heart disease, then the next step in an evaluation may be a thallium scan to check the blood flow into the heart. The thallium stress test is more accurate than the standard exercise stress test in determining the extent and localization of heart damage from coronary heart disease and in predicting the likelihood of future heart attacks. Here's how the test works: Thallium is injected into your bloodstream, and then you exercise on a treadmill or bike. A scanning camera records how much of the thallium is absorbed by the heart muscle.

**Echocardiogram.** Abnormal findings during your physical exam or ECG may prompt your doctor to order an echocardiogram. This test bounces sound waves off the heart and converts them into images on a video screen that show the heart's structure (i.e., size and shape) and how well it is functioning (i.e., how the heart moves and the volume of blood being pumped when the heart contracts). This detailed information will help your doctor make an even more complete assessment of your risk for a heart attack. Although most insurers will pick up the cost of an ECG, many insurers don't routinely pay for a screening echocardiogram. The cost is anywhere from $40 to $90.

**Exercise echocardiography.** With this test, you take the echocardio-gram *after* you have exercised. This test has been shown to be very specific and the best diagnostic tool in women.

**Coronary artery scan.** This involves a special type of X-ray scanner that is superfast. The scan helps determine the presence and extent of any calcium deposits in your coronary arteries, which may indicate disease or narrowed coronary arteries. The main advantage of this superfast CT scan is that it may detect calcified plaques *before* they actually clog arteries. The thallium scan and exercise stress tests can only find abnormalities once blood flow is obstructed. It may also be useful to determine if the level of calcium decreases with treatment by drugs to lower lipids with this test. However, the accuracy, effectiveness, and interpretation of results of coronary artery scans are still being researched.

**Magnetic resonance imaging (MRI).** This test lets doctors visualize a patient's *actual* coronary artery plaque.

**Coronary artery angiography.** At the present time, coronary angiography is the gold-standard method for determining the status of the coronary arteries. It is most often performed when an exercise stress test or thallium stress test is abnormal. This is a painless procedure in which dye is injected into the coronary arteries so that doctors can see them. The dye helps your doctor see and determine if the arteries have narrowed or if they are blocked. If there is a problem, the next step is to perform an angioplasty to unclog the artery.

**Angioplasty.** In this procedure, a tube with a tiny collapsed balloon at its tip is threaded through the artery to the point at which there is plaque or a narrowing. The balloon is inflated to open the blockage and a stent (a small tube) may be inserted in the artery to keep it open. If this doesn't work, the next option is *bypass surgery*, where the obstruction in the coronary artery is bypassed by a graft from a normal blood vessel.

*Commit yourself to the Prime Time Wellness Plan.* (See Chapter 9.) This plan will help you reduce or eliminate the six leading risk factors for heart disease.

*Control your cholesterol.* Since high LDL cholesterol readings are a particularly strong risk factor for heart disease, we're going to spend some time in this section discussing ways to reduce this problem. Remember, you can have high total cholesterol and not need treatment if your LDL (bad) cholesterol is normal and your HDL (good) cholesterol is high. (See the table

"Cholesterol" in Chapter 8 for optimal levels.) However, if your LDL level is high, work with your doctor to set a target LDL level that is best for you. Your ideal LDL depends on the number of risk factors you have. For example, being middle-aged—say, fifty years old—with high blood pressure constitutes two risk factors, which means you must get your LDL cholesterol level down below 130.

## LDL CHOLESTEROL GOAL

| RISK GROUP | GOAL |
|---|---|
| No heart disease; less than two risk factors for heart disease | <160 mg/dL |
| No heart disease; more than two risk factors for heart disease | <130 mg/dL |
| Heart disease | <100 mg/dL |

*Take the fat out of your diet.* See Chapter 9 for a full explanation of fat and the health risks associated with it. The elimination of saturated and trans fats lowers your risk for heart disease. The fats you should be eating and cooking with are *unsaturated* fats, of which there are two types: *polyunsaturated fat* and *monounsaturated fat*. (See the table "What You Should Know About Fats in Foods" in Chapter 9.) Increasing evidence suggests that reducing total dietary fat is less important for lowering coronary risk, however, than *replacing* **harmful fats with healthier ones.**

We know how hard it is to rid your diet of harmful fats—both Gayle and Marilyn have been working on this for years. To help ourselves, we started flavoring our greens with smoked turkey and spices and herbs instead of fatback. We also try to drink skim milk and eat only low-fat cheese and ice cream. We've had good success with the Mediterranean Diet, outlined in the box on the next page. The Mediterranean Diet contains plenty of unsaturated fat, found primarily in olive oil and fish, and an abundance of fruits and vegetables, and has significant heart benefits. Here are some other tips that can help reduce artery-clogging fats in your diet:

- *Remove the skin from poultry and trim off the fat.*
- *Increase your number of meatless meals each week.*

• *Increase your fiber intake.* Fiber helps you control LDL cholesterol and excrete fat more rapidly, so aim for 25 to 30 grams of fiber each day. Water-soluble fiber, in particular, can help control coronary heart disease by lowering blood cholesterol levels. Foods containing water-soluble fiber should be included in the diet each day. Regular use of products that contain soluble fiber from psyllium seeds—such as Metamucil—can lower cholesterol levels by 5 to 10 percent. The fiber found in oats, bran, and vegetables is especially helpful. Stick to fresh foods as much as possible; processed foods won't give you enough fiber. For example, ½ cup bran cereal supplies 13 grams of fiber; 1 cup of oatmeal supplies 4 grams; one pear supplies 4.6 grams.

• *Stop frying.* Broil, bake, steam, or grill your food. Use nonstick sprays when cooking, and broth or orange juice to provide flavor.

• *Drink one to two cups of green tea a day* to block the absorption of cholesterol. It may also strengthen your blood vessels. Use decaffeinated.

• *Add garlic to your food.* Data suggest that garlic also lowers cholesterol. Allicin is the most potent compound in garlic, and taking a supplement that provides 600 to 900 mg of allicin potential daily (equal to one or two cloves of fresh garlic) can lower blood pressure by 8 percent in one to three months. Garlic also helps to prevent blood clots.

## THE MEDITERRANEAN DIET

Years ago, researchers noticed that people who lived in Mediterranean countries—Greece, Italy, and Spain—had low rates of coronary artery disease and cancer despite a high total fat intake. At this time, many researchers are recommending the Mediterranean Diet for people who are at risk for coronary disease.

Following this diet involves more than simply cooking in olive oil, even though the main source of fat in this diet is olive oil. Vegetables, fruits, grains, and legumes are staples of the Mediterranean Diet, supplemented by yogurt, fish, nuts, and small amounts of cheese. Meat, especially red meat, is consumed infrequently, and butter is never used. Here's the diet:

• *Eat more bread, whole grains (such as barley and brown rice), and whole-grain cereals.*

• *Increase your servings of fruits, especially oranges and grapefruit, and vegetables to five to seven per day. Some nutritionists recommend eight to ten servings of fruit and vegetables a day.*

- Eat much more fish.
- Limit your red meat. Eat poultry instead.
- Eat legumes such as chickpeas, kidney beans, and navy beans two or three times a week.
- Use extra-virgin olive oil.
- Eat nuts several times a week.
- Make dairy products a regular part of your daily meals, but choose low-fat versions.
- Stay away from packaged products made with partially hydrogenated oils, as they contain unhealthy trans fats.

*Increase your physical activity.* Regular exercise has many advantages. It controls your body weight, raises your HDL cholesterol, reduces your blood pressure, releases the stressors from your life, and improves the heart's work capacity. All of these improve your heart's health. Remember, as we stated, in postmenopausal women walking thirty to forty-five minutes a day, three times a week, reduces the risk of a heart attack by 50 percent! See Chapter 9 for exercise suggestions. First and foremost, get advice from your doctor before proceeding on your exercise program.

*Weight Control.* A low-fat diet combined with regular exercise will help you maintain an appropriate weight or lose weight. Weight loss is the most effective way to lower triglyceride levels, help raise HDL cholesterol, and prevent Type 2 diabetes. A weight loss of as little as five to ten pounds may lower blood pressure enough to make antihypertensive drugs unnecessary.

*Discuss with your doctor medications that lower cholesterol and fight heart disease.* If three to six months of eating a low-fat, low-cholesterol diet and exercising fail to lower your cholesterol levels, you may need medication, especially to lower your LDL. There are several types of lipid-lowering drugs available; of these, the statins (all of their names end in *statin*) are well tolerated and are the most effective agents for controlling cholesterol. Statins can help you lower your LDL by about 30 percent to 40 percent, increase your HDL by 10 percent, and reduce your triglyceride levels by about 10 percent to 20 percent. These drugs are especially effective in women with diabetes. In addition to their positive effect on blood lipid levels, they also appear to improve the tone of artery walls and help them open up to increase blood flow during exercise.

The statin drugs are Lipitor (atorvastatin), Baycol (cerivastatin), Lescol (fluvastatin), Mevacor (lovastatin), Pravachol (pravastatin), and Zocor (simvastatin).

Because these drugs are relatively new, long-term effects have not been established. Stomach and intestinal symptoms or reversible liver injury with a rise in liver enzymes occurs in 1 percent to 2 percent of patients who take high doses of these medications. Therefore, if you take any statin drugs, you need to have your liver enzymes monitored regularly. You can have this tested at the same time you have your cholesterol levels checked, which should be about every six months if your cholesterol is high enough to require medication.

You may want to consider red yeast rice, a traditional Chinese food that works like the statins—especially lovastatin (Mevacor)—to reduce cholesterol and triglycerides. A red yeast rice product called Cholestin is a natural way to lower moderately elevated cholesterol levels (200–240 mg/dL). However, no long-term studies have been done on this product.

*Discuss aspirin treatments with your doctor.* Aspirin reduces heart attack risk in two ways: It stops the blood cells from clumping, and it acts as an anti-inflammatory agent. Aspirin provides both primary prevention (prevents the first heart attack from happening) and secondary prevention (prevents more attacks after the first one).[7] Therefore, talk to your doctor about taking one baby aspirin every night to decrease the potential for clotting and inflammation.

*Release your stress and anger.* Psychological stressors in African Americans and type A behavior (being aggressive, impatient, easy to anger, and competitive) are linked to heart disease. Studies show that emotional stress, such as tension, frustration, and sadness, more than doubles the risk of a heart attack, and actually decreases blood flow to the heart. New research suggests that a mental stress test might predict your risk for heart attack as well as the standard exercise test can.

Of all the emotional stressors, anger heads the list. Anger increases your risk not only for a heart attack, but also for a stroke. According to medical studies, holding on to anger increases your chances of a heart attack threefold, and it also increases your blood pressure and risk for cancer.[8] Forgiveness and letting go of anger will lower your blood pressure and heart rate. (For more on anger-reducing techniques, see Chapter 6, "Confronting the Two A's: Attitude and Anger.")

Remember, laughter heals the soul and also may keep your heart healthy.

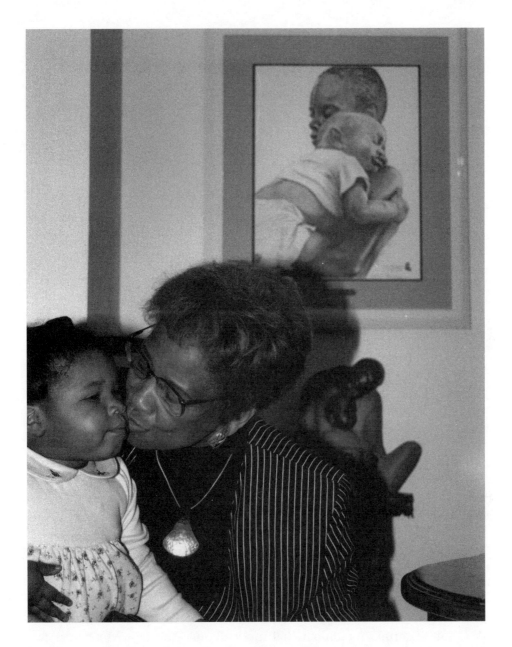

Laughter is good medicine for our hearts and our immune systems, and probably in other ways not yet studied.

Remember, also, to get all the love, hugs, and kisses possible. Grandchildren are just the ticket.

## Less Common Risk Factors for Heart Disease

### Depression

A landmark study by researchers at Johns Hopkins, based on forty years of medical data, demonstrated the link between depression and heart disease when all other risk factors are controlled.[9] The researchers found that both men and women with depression are twice as likely to have a heart attack or develop heart disease than peers who aren't depressed. Not only can depression trigger the onset of heart disease, it can also complicate the disease once you get it. The exact mechanism of action is not clear, but some researchers speculate that it is somehow tied to the level of serotonin in the brain. Depressed individuals may also be more prone to blood clots, which can cause a heart attack when the clot occurs in the coronary artery.[10]

Your heart needs more than a healthy diet and regular exercise. Our hearts need also to find peace. Dean Ornish believes our hearts also need intimacy, a spiritual life, to learn how to forgive, and to be committed to others.[11] (See Chapter 15 for Prime Time Prescriptions for depression.)

### Alcohol

Women who drink heavily on a regular basis have higher rates of heart disease than either moderate drinkers or nondrinkers. Several recent studies show that moderate drinkers (those who consume one to two drinks a day) may be less likely to develop heart disease than people who don't drink any alcohol, probably because alcohol seems to raise HDL (good) cholesterol. However, if you are a nondrinker, don't start! The benefit is not so clear that you should consider alcohol as something *good* for your heart. Remember, there are also a lot of calories in wine, and even more in other alcoholic beverages.

If you do drink, remember that moderation is the key. More than two drinks a day raises blood pressure; binge drinking can lead to stroke. What's acceptable? One glass of alcohol per day—one glass translates into 4 ounces of wine, 12 ounces of beer, or 1½ ounces of 80-proof spirits.

### Estrogen loss

The loss of estrogen precipitates an increase of coronary artery disease in women after menopause. (See Chapter 16 on menopause, for a discussion on the value of hormone replacement therapy in reducing heart disease.)

### Elevated homocysteine levels

Studies indicate that 25 to 50 percent of all heart attacks may occur in people without any currently known risk factors, which is one of the reasons why reducing the overall rate of heart attacks in the United States is such a challenge. However, in recent years, researchers have uncovered new predictors of heart disease risk that may one day lead to widespread screening tests. One of these tests focuses on measuring your blood level of the amino acid homocysteine.[12] High levels of this amino acid may play a role in damaging the arteries, which can lead to heart attack and strokes. To lower homocysteine levels and decrease your risk of heart disease, you need to increase your intake of folic acid and vitamin $B_6$. Women who regularly take B vitamin supplements have a 50 percent lower risk of heart disease than those not taking them. The suggested dose of folic acid is 400 mcg daily. Folic acid is found in beans, greens, broccoli, bananas, fish, and grains; cold cereals and some orange juices have been fortified with folic acid. It is found in multivitamin supplements as well. Also, increase your vitamin $B_6$ intake to 3 mg per day (the recommended daily allowance is 2 mg a day) and your intake of vitamin $B_{12}$ to 40 mcg.

### Infections

Scientists have theorized that infections such as those from the herpes virus, *Chlamydia pneumonia* (which causes respiratory illness), and a germ that causes gum disease may also be a factor in the development of fatty deposits and mineral deposits inside the coronary arteries. Harvard researchers reported in the *New England Journal of Medicine* in 1997 that elevated levels of C-reactive protein—a by-product of inflammation, which can be caused by infection—might act as a predictor of greater risk for having a heart attack. In 1998, similar results were found in participants in the Harvard's Women's Health Study, an evaluation of more than thirty-nine thousand healthy postmenopausal women. C-reactive protein levels were much higher in women who had heart attacks. In fact, women with the highest levels had more than a sevenfold increase in risk of heart attack and stroke than those women with the lowest levels. That's why simple good habits such as **flossing your teeth every day** are so important. Flossing, for instance, helps prevent or reduce inflammation in your gums, which in turn may decrease your risk for heart attack. And remember, **aspirin is an anti-inflammatory** agent, which is why doctors often recommend aspirin therapy for their heart patients.[13]

## IF YOU HAD EVERYTHING YOUR HEART DESIRES . . .

- *You would take life in stride.* Walking only thirty minutes a day can lead to a longer life.
- *You'd never let them make a monkey out of you.* Remember: Nicotine can be as addictive as cocaine.
- *You would be well read.* Every food label tells a story. Look for low-fat, low-cholesterol products, and take notice of how many calories come from fat in your foods. This will ensure a happy ending.
- *You wouldn't snap so easily.* Being quick to anger triples your risk of heart disease. Use your head to help your heart.
- *You wouldn't spend another lunch chewing the fat; instead, you'd spend more time in the garden.* Increasing your consumption of fruits and vegetables cuts your risk of heart attack in half.
- *You would make a lot more bread.* Soluble fiber in oat bran, fruits, and beans decreases blood cholesterol by 15 percent.
- *You would take a vacation every day.* The way we think affects the way we feel. Set aside time every day to listen to your self-talk (remember the self-talk exercises in Chapter 4?). Think optimistically; give yourself positive mental images. You will improve your health.
- *You would strike oil.* Polyunsaturated and monounsaturated fats— the good fats—decrease cholesterol.
- *You would let nothing go to waist.* Losing weight also decreases the fat around your stomach and waist, which is important in reducing your risk of a heart attack.

*Source:* Courtesy of ConAgra Foods.

## HIGH BLOOD PRESSURE (HYPERTENSION)

*A **primary risk factor for heart disease is hypertension.*** High blood pressure is so prevalent in the Black community, some physicians consider it the number one health problem for African Americans. One out of every three African Americans has high blood pressure, compared to one out of every four Americans in general. African Americans get hypertension earlier in life, which is also why high blood pressure is a much bigger problem in our community than among Caucasians.[14]

Hypertension is especially dangerous because there are no warning signs or symptoms for this condition, which is why it's often called the "silent killer." The statistics and research on high blood pressure are relentless:

- Fifty percent of all Americans over age 65 have high blood pressure.
- Women who are postmenopausal are more likely to have high blood pressure than men of the same age, beginning at age sixty in African American women and age seventy in Caucasian women.
- Older African American women who live in the Southeast are more likely to have high blood pressure than those in other regions of the United States.
- Women with high blood pressure have three to four times the risk of developing heart disease and seven times the risk of stroke as do those with normal blood pressure.
- Swedish research has shown that high blood pressure may cause subtle injury to blood vessels in the brain, which could lead to senility.
- Depression can be a symptom of high blood pressure.

### What Is Hypertension?

The traditional definition of hypertension is a blood pressure reading of 140/90 mm Hg or higher. A blood pressure reading of 130/80 is considered normal, but doctors recommend that you strive to achieve an optimal reading of 120/70. (See the table on the next page for a range of problematic blood pressure readings.)

# HYPERTENSION

| Stage | Systolic | Diastolic | Response |
|-------|----------|-----------|----------|
| STAGE 1 (MILD) | 140–159 | 90–99 | A second reading will be taken two months later. Health-care provider will encourage you to modify your lifestyle to reduce readings. *If lifestyle changes do not work, your doctor may consider treatment.* |
| STAGE 2 (MODERATE) | 160–179 | 100–109 | Health-care provider will recommend a medical evaluation and a modified lifestyle. *Your doctor will prescribe a treatment program. If lifestyle changes do not work, your doctor will prescribe treatment within 1 month.* |
| STAGE 3 (SEVERE) | >180 | >110 | Health-care provider will recommend a medical evaluation and a modified lifestyle. *Your doctor will begin a treatment program immediately.* |

# ARE YOU AT RISK FOR HIGH BLOOD PRESSURE?

Complete the following checklist to help assess your potential for developing this deadly disease and to help you see where you can change your lifestyle.

1. Do you have a family history of high blood pressure?
   YES     NO
2. Are you overweight for your height and age?
   YES     NO
3. Have you been diagnosed with high cholesterol?
   YES     NO
4. Do tests show you have high triglycerides?
   YES     NO
5. Do you have a sedentary lifestyle?
   YES     NO
6. Are you postmenopausal?
   YES     NO

7. Do you have a high-salt diet?

                           YES          NO

8. Do you have a high-fat diet?

                           YES          NO

9. Do you smoke?

                           YES          NO

10. Do you use medications that can raise blood pressure? (See p. 224.)

                           YES          NO

11. Have you been diagnosed with coronary artery disease?

                           YES          NO

12. Do you have kidney disease?

                           YES          NO

13. Have you ever had a stroke or small attacks of decreased blood flow to your brain (TIAs)?

                           YES          NO

If you circled yes for any of the questions, you should have your blood pressure tested at least once every six months by a health professional. You also need to pay close attention to the following Prime Time Prescription for hypertension.

*Source:* National Heart, Lung, and Blood Institute, National Institutes of Health.

 **PRIME TIME PRESCRIPTIONS FOR REDUCING HYPERTENSION**

You can prevent the onset of hypertension. If you already have it, you can reduce its severity. High blood pressure can be prevented and treated even if it can't be cured! By taking an active role in monitoring and controlling your blood pressure, you can improve the health of your heart and brain and reduce any complications that hypertension can cause when you have other illnesses. Here's how:

*Monitor your own blood pressure.* You can have high blood pressure and feel fine. That's why in midlife you need to track your own blood pressure between visits to the doctor. Before you start monitoring your blood pressure, though, talk with your doctor to make sure this is acceptable to him or her. If your doctor won't work with you, consider finding a health-care provider who will. Find one by visiting the Hypertension Network Web site at www.bloodpressure.com and searching its list of more than fifteen hundred doctors who specialize in treating hypertension.

A home blood pressure monitor will help you to keep a daily record of your blood pressure. If necessary, take readings throughout the day (such as when you're stressed, at rest, or after exercising). These machines are easy to use and only cost between $35 to $90. For many of us, that just means skipping a week of getting our hair and nails done. (See box for recommended units.)

After you purchase your monitor (the pharmacist can show you the basics of how to use it), consult your health-care provider for training on how to get the most accurate readings. Don't rely solely on the instructions that come with the unit. To make sure your home unit is accurate, check the readings against the professional unit used by your doctor or nurse.

Remember always to use the same arm, to keep your readings consistent, and check the cuff fit. (Refer to the monitor's instructions to make sure the cuff is the right size for your arm.) Also check the placement of the cuff, the lower edge of which should be one inch above the elbow on your upper arm.

If you have hypertension, discuss with your doctor when and how often you should take readings. We recommend that you start by taking your pressure twice a day (in the morning and evening) three days a week for about two weeks. Take it when you wake up in the morning or after a nap or short rest and in the evening after work or after you exercise. If you see a pattern of readings that are unusually high or low, call your doctor immediately. Otherwise, keep accurate records and share the results with your doctor at your next regular visit.

### KEEP A RECORD OF YOUR BLOOD PRESSURE

| DATE | TIME (A.M./P.M.) | YOUR STATE OF BEING (RESTED, STRESSED, JUST EXERCISED, ETC.) | READINGS |
|---|---|---|---|
| __/__/__ | | | __/__ |
| __/__/__ | | | __/__ |
| __/__/__ | | | __/__ |

*Commit yourself to the Prime Time Wellness Plan* (see Chapter 9). This plan offers a Prime Time Prescription for reducing or eliminating the leading five risk factors that contribute to hypertension—smoking, high blood cholesterol, obesity, inactivity, and stress.

## HOME BLOOD PRESSURE MONITORS

*Electronic blood pressure monitor (manual inflation).* This is a small battery-operated unit with an easy-to-read screen and an attached cuff that you inflate manually. This is simple to use by yourself because you don't need to use a stethoscope to listen for the beats to determine the pressure. To make record-keeping simple, consider a unit that will record your readings or allow you to print them out. Cost: $35 to $40.

*Electronic blood pressure monitor (automatic inflation).* This is a step up from the manual inflation model. You put on the cuff and push the button; the machine inflates the cuff and displays your numbers on a digital screen. This unit is very easy to use and wonderful if you have arthritis or are too weak to inflate the cuff. Cost: $70 to $90.

*Exercise more.* Increasing your exercise, even a little, will decrease your blood pressure 10 to 15 points. Thirty to forty-five minutes of daily walking, cycling, or swimming will work. If you don't have hypertension, these activities will help prevent your pressure from rising.

*Decrease your stress.* Meditate every day, Deep breathing and relaxation techniques will help reduce your stress and lower your blood pressure.[15] You will find instructions for these techniques in Chapter 13.

*Dramatically reduce the salt in your diet.* The amount of sodium in the average American diet is 3,500 to 5,000 mg per day, which far exceeds the amount needed by the body (about 200 mg). If your blood pressure is normal, you should consume no more than 2,400 mg of sodium a day (about one teaspoon of salt), which includes salt you add to foods as well as salt hidden in processed foods.

It's crucial to read food labels to determine how much salt you consume. Studies have shown that 75 percent to 80 percent of the salt we consume comes from processed food. Just one Big Mac or a serving of canned soup contains 1,000 mg of sodium—nearly half your daily requirement. Fresh foods are much more healthful. If you have high blood pressure, the goal is to consume only 1,200 to 2,400 mg of sodium each day. The best way to do this is not to add salt to your food, since there is likely to be 1,600 to 2,400 mg of sodium in the food you eat already.

Take the salt shaker off your table and away from your food preparation

# THE DASH DIET

| Food group | Daily servings | Serving sizes | Examples and notes | Significance of each food group to DASH's pattern |
|---|---|---|---|---|
| Grains and grain products | 7 to 8 | 1 slice bread, 1/2 cup dry cereal, 1/2 cup cooked rice, pasta, or cereals | Whole-wheat bread, English muffin, pita bread, bagel, cereals, grits, oatmeal | Major source of energy |
| Vegetables | 4 to 5 | 1 cup raw leafy vegetable, 1/2 cup cooked vegetable, 6 ounces vegetable juice | Tomatoes, potatoes, carrots, peas, squash, broccoli, turnip greens, collards, kale, spinach, artichokes, beans, sweet potatoes | Rich sources of potassium, magnesium, and fiber |
| Fruits | 4 to 5 | 6 ounces fruit juice, 1 medium fruit, 1/4 cup dried fruit, 1/2 cup fresh, frozen, or canned fruit | Apricots, bananas, dates, grapes, oranges, orange juice, grapefruit, grapefruit juice, mangoes, melons, peaches, pineapples, prunes, raisins, strawberries, tangerines | Important sources of potassium, magnesium, and fiber |
| Low-fat or nonfat dairy foods | 2 to 3 | 8 ounces milk, 1 cup yogurt, 1.5 ounces cheese | Skim or 1% milk, skim or low-fat buttermilk, nonfat or low-fat yogurt, part-skim mozzarella cheese, nonfat cheese | Major sources of calcium and protein |
| Meats, poultry, and fish | 2 or less | 3 ounces cooked meats, poultry, or fish | Select only lean; trim away visible fats; broil, roast, or boil instead of frying; remove skin from poultry | Rich sources of protein and magnesium |
| Nuts, seeds, and legumes | 4 to 5 per week | 1.5 ounces or 1/3 cup of nuts, 1/2 ounce or 2 tablespoons seeds, 1/2 cup cooked legumes | Almonds, filberts, mixed nuts, peanuts, walnuts, sunflower seeds, kidney beans, lentils | Rich sources of energy, magnesium, potassium, protein, and fiber |

area. Instead, use gourmet vinegars. Cook with herbs and spices instead of salt. For example, ginger, rosemary, thyme, curry powder, dill, cloves, oregano, tarragon, and sage add great flavor to your poultry dishes. Ginger, paprika, onion, marjoram, lemon juice, and curry powder are great on fish. (Added benefit: Curry powder also contains turmeric, which may help protect the walls of your arteries and balance your cholesterol levels.) Thyme, ginger, dill, garlic, onion, sage, cumin, tarragon, and rosemary work wonders on vegetables.

Garlic is a seasoning that almost works like a prescription drug to lower blood pressure and dilate blood vessels, thus protecting the heart. Taking 600 to 900 mg of allicin potential daily (which is equal to one or two cloves of fresh garlic) can lower blood pressure by 8 percent in one to three months. According to the Delaney sisters (authors of *Having Our Say*), garlic was one of the secret ingredients that kept both of them going well past their one hundredth birthdays.

*Load up on fruits and vegetables.* Numerous studies demonstrate that fruits and vegetables are anti-high-blood-pressure agents. They are important sources of potassium, magnesium, and fiber and the DASH (Dietary Approaches to Stop Hypertension) Diet recommends eight to ten servings. The most protective are apples, oranges, prunes, carrots, grapes, alfalfa, mushrooms, celery, and raw spinach.

The DASH Diet outlined in the box opposite is an example of how simple lifestyle modifications can effectively lower blood pressure.

A study in the *Archives of Internal Medicine*, February 8, 1999, found the diet was particularly effective in African Americans with hypertension and less effective in whites. In African Americans with hypertension the greatest decreases in blood pressure were observed (13–15 mm Hg lower).

The chart opposite outlines the number of servings to eat from each food group along with serving sizes and suggestions of what to eat.

*Eat more fiber.* High-fiber foods help keep your blood pressure down.

*Make sure your diet includes enough of the* **right fats.** As we have already pointed out, polyunsaturated and monounsaturated fats are most beneficial. Studies show that substituting olive oil for other fats lowers blood pressure. (Check out the box "Getting Bad Fat out of Your Diet" in Chapter 9.)

*Make sure you are getting enough of the right vitamins and minerals.* Your first step is to make sure you take plenty of vitamin C. According to research by Elaine B. Feldman of the Medical College of Georgia, people who take 500 mg of vitamin C daily tend to have lower blood pressure.

The big three antihypertensive minerals are calcium, magnesium, and potassium. Of the three, *potassium* seems to be the most potent in decreasing blood pressure, as it helps your body dispose of excess sodium. Since bananas are high in potassium, hypertension sufferers should start reciting the credo "A banana a day keeps the doctor away."

African Americans are especially sensitive to low potassium intake, so you must be extra sure that you get enough of this lifesaving mineral, about 3,000 to 4,000 mg of potassium a day. If you're taking a diuretic, you need 5,000 mg a day. This can lower your systolic pressure by about five points and your diastolic by about three points.

## PRIME TIME SMOOTHIE

*Start your day with a potassium boost (763 mg worth!)*
*2 bananas, sliced*
*2 cups nonfat vanilla yogurt*
*2 cups skim milk*
*½ cup pineapple juice*
*1 tbsp. honey*
*Process all ingredients in blender and serve immediately.*
*This recipe makes four servings.*
*Per serving: 763 mg potassium, 219 cal, 0.5 g fat, 134 mg sodium*

In addition to bananas, potassium is found in many other foods—apricots, dried fruits, oranges, milk, potatoes (with skin), dry peas, beans, poultry, yogurt, catfish, trout, plantains, and sweet potatoes. Therefore, you should be able to get enough potassium from eating a variety of foods. Just one banana contains 500 mg potassium; one potato with skin has 850 mg, and a half cup of spinach has 400 mg. *Don't take supplemental potassium unless your doctor prescribes it.*

On the other hand, you *should* supplement your diet with 350 to 400 mg of **magnesium** a day. In fact, magnesium is found in most multivitamins. Some research suggests that magnesium may also protect you from heart disease, irregular heart rhythm, and osteoporosis (the thinning of the bones that can happen after menopause). (See Chapter 16 for more information on menopause and osteoporosis.)

You'll also need to supplement your diet with at least 1,500 mg per day of **calcium**. Women with low calcium intake have higher rates of high blood pressure. Although there are many calcium-rich foods from which to choose, such as milk, dairy products, and leafy dark green vegetables (kale and collard greens, for example), midlife women should also be on supplemental calcium to prevent osteoporosis.

*Control your weight.* A major cause of increased blood pressure is being overweight. This is a major struggle for many African American women in midlife. Weight gain increases as we age and slow down. However, even a little weight loss has big rewards. Start by trying to lose 5 percent of your total weight at a time. Losing just six to nine pounds decreases the risk of hypertension by 50 percent! And if you have hypertension, losing weight may help you decrease your dosage of medication and perhaps even eliminate the need for medication.

*If making the lifestyle changes we recommend above doesn't bring down your blood pressure to the optimal level, you should discuss taking medication with your doctor.* If your blood pressure reaches the severe stages (see hypertension chart earlier in this chapter), you need medication immediately. You will also need to discuss the next steps with your doctor, including things you can do to help the medication work most effectively. Before you go off to the pharmacist with prescription in hand, ask your doctor the following questions:

- What is the medication and why did you choose it for me?
- Please explain the dosage instructions. (Ask for them in writing.)
- What are the side effects and how serious should they be before I call you?
- Are there any other medications or over-the-counter drugs that I should not take with this new prescription?

---

## INITIAL MEDICATIONS FOR HYPERTENSION

These are the most commonly prescribed medications for reducing high blood pressure and keeping it stable at optimal levels.

| | |
|---|---|
| DIURETICS OR "WATER PILLS," such as Maxide (triamterene) | Prescribed to promote water loss and decrease blood volume and blood pressure. Diuretics also help prevent abnormal blood clotting and therefore decrease the risk of coronary artery disease or stroke. |

| BETA BLOCKERS such as Tenormin (atenolol) | Prescribed to slow your heart and blood pressure. Solid research shows beta blockers prolong life and decrease complications from hypertension. *NOTE:* Taking beta blockers can increase your risk for diabetes. |
| --- | --- |

*An important reminder:* Certain chemicals, drugs, and medications can *increase* your blood pressure—even temporarily. You should avoid them and discuss them with your doctor if you have hypertension or several of the risk factors that lead to high blood pressure.

• Alcohol (two drinks), nicotine (two cigarettes), caffeine. Avoid all caffeine, including colas and decaffeinated coffee (which still has a small amount of caffeine).

• Decongestants (pseudoephedrine and phenylpropanolamine [PPA] which are found in over-the-counter cold, sinus, and allergy medications.

• Nasal decongestants such as Neo-synephrine (phenylephrine HCl)

• Diet pills such as Acutrim or Dexatrim

• Nonsteroidal anti-inflammatory drugs such as Indocin (in domethain).

• Popular pain relievers such as Motrin (ibuprofen), Aleve (naproxen), and Orudis (ketoprofen)

• Steroids (e.g., prednisone), antidepressants, and illicit drugs

• Popular herbal supplements (ginseng, ephedra or ma huang, kava, St. John's wort)

• Antidepressants such as Surmontil (trimipramine) and Effexor (venlafaxine)

• Monoamine oxidase (MAO) inhibitors such as Nardil (pheneiziine) and Parnate (tranylcypromine)

• Drugs that counteract antihypertensive medication such as Elavil (amitriptyline), an antidepressant

## DID YOU TAKE YOUR MEDICATION TODAY?

One of the biggest problems in controlling hypertension is that people don't take their medication regularly, if at all. Be sure to take any hypertension medication as prescribed. Here are some tips to help you remember:

- *Take your medication at the same time every day.* It must become a habit. Marilyn taped her medication to her toothpaste until she got in the habit of taking it every morning. You might want to tape yours to the refrigerator or mirror to remind you.
- *If the cost of medication is a problem, talk to your doctor.* See if your health insurance covers prescriptions. If not, your doctor may be able to replace the medication with a cheaper brand or a generic.
- *If you forget to take your medication, don't take an extra dose to make up for the lapse.* Instead, just take your next scheduled dose.
- *Take your medicine even though you feel great and don't feel sick.*

## STROKE OR BRAIN ATTACK

### MAKELA'S STORY

Makela was conducting her weekly staff meeting. She had been struggling with an unrelenting headache but was taking aspirin, which provided her some relief. As she talked, one of her staff members noticed that Makela was slurring her words. Fortunately, they all realized she was having a brain attack or stroke and took her right away to the closest hospital emergency room.

A stroke, sometimes also called a brain attack, is a medical emergency that requires immediate medical attention. Similar to heart attacks, strokes occur when the blood supply to the brain is severely restricted or cut off. Even though a stroke occurs every minute in America, very few victims realize they're having one, and way too many don't get help right away. That's not surprising, since the *Journal of the American Medical Association* reported that as many as 43 percent of Americans can't name one warning sign of stroke. Even more alarming, the University of Cincinnati stroke team found that nearly 40 percent of stroke victims couldn't identify any warning signs, either. Before you read further, take the following quiz to assess what you know about stroke.

---

## WHAT DO YOU KNOW ABOUT STROKE?

1. A stroke happens in the arms or legs.

                TRUE        FALSE

2. A slight temporary numbness on the left side of your face could be a stroke.

                TRUE        FALSE

3. Stroke is the leading cause of adult disability.

                TRUE        FALSE

4. Smoking, high blood pressure, and obesity are all risk factors for stroke.

                TRUE        FALSE

Answers: 1. F, 2. T, 3. T, 4. T

---

*Source:* American Heart Association and American Stroke Association.

---

Stroke treatment is literally a race against time, because rapid diagnosis and treatment (within three hours after the onset of a stroke) is the only way to minimize damage to brain tissue and possibly save the life of a stroke victim. *Every minute counts!*

As the chart opposite indicates, the mortality rates among African American women with stroke is twice that of American Indian/Alaska Native women, almost three times that of Hispanic women, and almost double that of White and Asian/Pacific Islander women.

The lack of understanding about the cause, prevention, and treatment of stroke may be why the statistics surrounding this disease are so brutal, especially for women and African Americans. Here are a few fast facts you should know:

- Four out of five American families will be affected by stroke.
- Stroke is the number one cause of long-term disability in adults. According to the Framingham Heart Study, 31 percent of stroke survivors need help

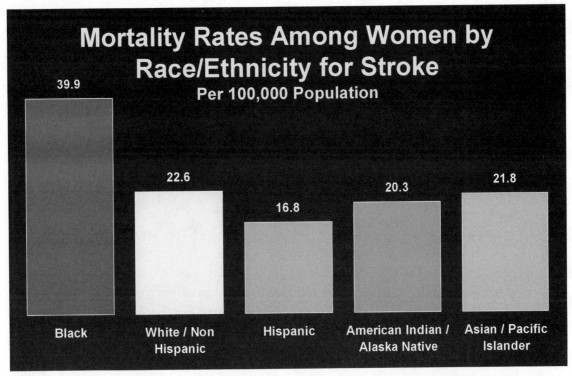

## Mortality Rates Among Women by Race/Ethnicity for Stroke
### Per 100,000 Population

- Black: 39.9
- White / Non Hispanic: 22.6
- Hispanic: 16.8
- American Indian / Alaska Native: 20.3
- Asian / Pacific Islander: 21.8

*Source:* National Center for Health Statistics, Health United States, U.S. Public Health Service, 1995.

caring for themselves, 20 percent need assistance to walk, and 71 percent have an impaired ability to work when examined an average of seven years later.

• African Americans have twice the risk of death and disability due to stroke than Whites.

• Ten times as many women die from stroke as they do from breast cancer.

• More women die from stroke than men.

• Stroke is the third most frequent cause of death for African American women in the middle years.

Prime Time African American women with high blood pressure are at the greatest risk for stroke. Our death rate from stroke is twice that of White women, mainly because we experience strokes at younger ages and have more risk factors that trigger an attack.

## What Is a Stroke?

What happens to the brain in a stroke is very similar to what happens to the heart during a heart attack. Eighty percent of strokes are due to a blocked artery leading to the brain. When the arteries in the neck or brain become so clogged with plaque (atherosclerosis) that the blood flow to the brain cells is restricted or cut off, the oxygen and nutrient supply to the brain is reduced and the brain cells die.

Blockage can also occur when a blood clot forms outside the brain (most typically in the heart) and travels up through the arteries into the neck or brain. A small clot in the brain cuts off the oxygen supply and triggers a buildup of toxins, which causes brain cells to die immediately. These strokes are common in people who've recently had heart surgery or who have defective heart valves or abnormal heart rhythms (atrial fibrillation).

Twenty percent of strokes are due to bleeding or hemorrhage in the brain, which decreases proper blood flow to the brain. This can occur in individuals who suffer from very high blood pressure. The high pressure causes a break in a weakened blood vessel or an aneurysm in the brain, resulting in blood leaking into the brain. (An aneurysm is an abnormal, balloonlike bulging of the wall of an artery.)

---

### THREE KEY STEPS TO LOWER YOUR RISK OF DEATH OR DISABILITY FROM STROKE

*Prevention of brain attack is the best medicine.*
- *Know the warning signs. (See the list opposite.)*
- *Act immediately if any signs occur.*
- *Control your risk factors for stroke.*

---

# Warning Signs of Stroke

One of the biggest problems with identifying the early warning signs of stroke is that they are painless. Too often, people don't take the symptoms of stroke seriously and therefore don't seek help right away. That's why it's crucial that you know the warning signs. In fact, if you have several risk factors for stroke (see page 230), you may even want to photocopy the warning signs, put the list on your refrigerator or near the phone, and give another copy to your family members and friends.

- Sudden weakness, numbness, or paralysis of the face, arm, or leg—especially on one side of the body
- Blurred or decreased vision
- Sudden difficulty speaking, slurred speech, or difficulty understanding speech
- Sudden confusion
- Sudden severe headache with no known cause, often described as "the worst headache of my life"
- Unexplained dizziness, unsteadiness, or sudden falls, especially with any of the other signs above

Transient ischemic attacks (TIAs), which are often called ministrokes, share the same warning signs or symptoms as a full-blown stroke, but TIAs only last for a short period of time; most subside within five to twenty minutes. But if you've had a TIA, your risk of having a full stroke is ten times higher than that of someone who hasn't had a TIA. So please report it to your doctor. The National Stroke Association estimates that more than a million people each year have a TIA but never tell their doctor.

If you are at risk for a stroke, if you have had a TIA, or if you have a carotid bruit, you should have an ultrasound, followed by magnetic resonance angiography (MRA), to evaluate the neck vessels. Fortunately, the narrowed blood vessels that cause TIAs are usually in the neck and can be surgically reopened. This procedure can really cut your risk of any future stroke. Discuss this procedure with your doctor to see if you are a good candidate for it. This is an important consideration if your carotid arteries are at least 70 percent blocked, as shown on an ultrasound. With this degree of blockage, surgery can reduce the risk of stroke by 65 percent over two years. If your carotid arteries are less than 50 percent blocked, discuss alternatives to surgery with your doctor. If surgery is not recommended, you should be treated to prevent a future stroke—simple aspirin (a baby aspirin, 81 mg/day) is effective.

Strokes and heart attacks are more likely to occur in the morning, between 6 A.M. and noon, and less likely to occur at night. Even though these warning signs and symptoms may last only a few moments and then disappear, *don't ignore them.* Call a doctor or 911 immediately! A brain attack is an emergency and as serious as a heart attack.

Stroke survivors are at substantial risk for a subsequent stroke. According to a 1999 Johns Hopkins White Paper, about 13 percent of stroke survivors will have another stroke within twelve months after the initial event, and 6 percent will have one each successive year after that.[16] (We will discuss more about the aftermath of a stroke later in this section.)

## Risk Factors for Stroke in Women

The following risk assessment quiz provides a pretty comprehensive assessment of risk factors that contribute to stroke.

---

### ARE YOU AT RISK FOR A STROKE?

Take this to see how you measure up.

1. Fill in your systolic blood pressure, which is the first (highest) number from a recent blood pressure reading. _____

2. Do you take medication to control your blood pressure?

                  YES      NO

3. Do you have a history of diabetes?

                  YES      NO

4. Do you smoke?

                  YES      NO

5. Have you ever had any of the following?

- *Coronary or cardiovascular disease*

                  YES      NO

- *Heart attack*

                  YES      NO

- *Chest pain*

                  YES      NO

---

- *Narrowed coronary blood vessels*
  YES        NO
- *Narrowed arteries in legs*
  YES        NO
- *Congestive heart failure*
  YES        NO

6. Do you have a history of rapid, irregular heartbeat (atrial fibrillation)?
   YES        NO

7. Do you live an inactive life? (Do you sit at work and/or spend leisure time watching TV or reading?)
   YES        NO

If you circled yes for any of these risk factors for stroke and your systolic pressure is 140 or higher, you need to pay close attention to the Prime Time Prescriptions for stroke listed on page 232.

*Source:* Adapted from a questionnaire by the American Heart Association.

As you can see, many of the risk factors for stroke are virtually the same as for heart disease, but high blood pressure is by far the most potent risk factor, playing a role in about 70 percent of all strokes. The risk of stroke in general increases about fourfold if your blood pressure is 160/95 or higher. Women with high blood pressure have seven times the risk of stroke as do those with normal blood pressure (130/80 mm Hg).

**African American women living in the southeastern states have some of the highest rates of hypertension and stroke.** Eleven states (Alabama, Arkansas, Georgia, Indiana, Kentucky, Louisiana, Mississippi, North Carolina, South Carolina, Tennessee, and Virginia) have such high stroke rates that they are called the "stroke belt states."

**Cigarette smokers have a 50 percent higher stroke risk** than nonsmokers. The greater the number of cigarettes smoked, the greater the risk. Even being around smokers can increase your risk of stroke because cigarette smoke decreases the blood flow and oxygen supply to brain cells.

As women age, our risk of stroke rises from being lower than men's to being higher. Once we turn fifty-five, the risk doubles. A new report revealed that the ability of blood vessels in the brain to maintain optimal blood flow falls significantly in women as we age, with the biggest drop occurring in our forties and fifties. The researchers speculate that the postmenopausal decline in estrogen levels may play a role in this drop, especially since women taking replacement estrogen did not have a similar decrease in blood flow.

Many of the risk factors for heart attacks—a sedentary lifestyle, high cholesterol, being overweight, alcohol and drug abuse, being diabetic—also contribute to increased risk of stroke. Heart disease and irregular heartbeat (atrial fibrillation) increase your risk because these conditions can result in blood clots in the heart that break loose and block vessels in the brain or in those leading to the brain.

The good news is that more than half of strokes can be prevented![17] And reducing your risk factors for stroke will also reduce your risk of heart disease.

**Rx | PRIME TIME PRESCRIPTIONS FOR REDUCING RISK FACTORS FOR STROKE**
*Get a thorough checkup, including the appropriate tests to screen for warning signs of stroke.* (See box on screening tests for stroke, below.)

---

### SCREENING TESTS FOR STROKE

1. *Make sure your blood pressure is normal.*

2. *Check for carotid narrowing.* One way is to have your doctor listen for *carotid bruit*. This is an abnormal sound made when blood rushes through a partially blocked artery. A doctor can hear this sound when the stethoscope is placed over the carotid arteries in the neck. Carotid bruit is a major warning sign for stroke. Also ask your doctor about using *ultrasound imaging* and *magnetic resonance angiography* to see if the arteries in your neck are narrowing.

3. *Find out if you have atrial fibrillation or an abnormal heart rhythm.* If you think your heartbeat is irregular, have your doctor check out your heart. In the meantime, Frederick Munschauer, M.D., at the State University of New York at Buffalo, School of Medicine, recommends doing self-checks using this technique: *Feel for the heart rhythm by putting your left hand on a flat surface, palm side up. Then place the first two fingers of your right hand on the area where your hand and wrist meet. Press until you feel your pulse. Then tap your foot each time you feel a beat. Do this for one minute. If your tapping is not consistent or regular, your heartbeat may be irregular. Check with your doctor immediately.*

---

*Commit yourself to the Prime Time Wellness Plan (see Chapter 9).* This plan will help you develop integrated Prime Time Prescriptions to reduce or eliminate the leading six risk factors that contribute to stroke—smoking, high blood pressure, high cholesterol, obesity, inactivity, and stress. Pay particular attention to any techniques, suggestions, or diet and exercise tips throughout this book that will help you keep your blood pressure at optimal levels. Remember that high blood pressure is found in 70 percent of stroke victims, so if you have high blood pressure, reread the section on hypertension earlier in this chapter.

*You must absolutely keep your hypertension controlled if you have it.*

*Reread the Prime Time Prescriptions for hypertension (earlier in this chapter), which also are appropriate for preventing strokes.*

---

### PRIME TIME TIP: POTASSIUM-RICH SNACK

*1 cup nonfat yogurt + 1 cup cubed cantaloupe
= 1,000 mg Potassium*

---

*Increase your consumption of vitamin B₆ and folic acid through supplements.*

*Check with your doctor about taking aspirin preventively every day.* If you are over fifty, you and your doctor should make a decision about aspirin therapy, because it is an effective blood thinner and decreases your chances of forming blood clots. (Tell your doctor if your stomach is sensitive to aspirin.)

Ask your doctor if you should consider taking estrogen to help prevent stroke, since this hormone can decrease LDL cholesterol and increase HDL cholesterol. It can also help improve your blood flow.

---

### REDUCE YOUR RISK FOR STROKE
### BY EXERCISING

Did you know that you can decrease your risk for stroke by 50 percent if you exercise enough to burn 2,000 calories a week? Here's how:

- *Walk one hour a day, five days a week*
- *Spend six hours a week gardening*
- *Swim five hours a week*
- *Play tennis four hours a week*
- *Bike five hours a week*

Note: Don't forget to discuss starting any type of exercise program with your doctor.

*Source:* Johns Hopkins White Paper, 1999.

## ANOTHER PRIME TIME TIP: DESK-DRAWER STRESS BUSTER

Keep some essential oils—try lavender, orange, or cedar—handy in your drawer. A deep whiff of these can soothe your stress.

## What to Do if a Stroke Happens

We repeat—with any of the signs of stroke, call 911 or your emergency medical services and get to a hospital right away. A new drug that breaks up blood clots requires that stroke victims get to the hospital, be evaluated, and be treated as quickly as possible. That's because the damage from a stroke can often be reversed if immediate care is provided within the first three hours of the stroke's occurrence. If the stroke was due to a blood clot, administering the new drug, t-PA, may increase the chance of surviving a stroke by 30 percent if given in the first three hours of the beginning of the attack. It will not work after three hours or if the stroke was due to a hemorrhage. Currently, less than 10 percent of stroke victims reach hospital emergency rooms within three hours of their first symptom. *Don't let this be you! When you first notice symptoms, get to a hospital.*

When a stroke patient arrives at the hospital, doctors must evaluate whether the patient has suffered a stroke from a brain clot or a hemorrhage. A radiologist will take a CT (computed tomography) scan or a more sophisticated MRI (magnetic resonance imaging) scan to determine the location and extent of brain injury.

Another important test is an angiography, in which special dyes are injected into the blood vessels and an X ray is taken. Angiography shows how the blood is flowing through the vessels. This test is important in diagnosing aneurysms (where a blood vessel balloons out and may burst) or where blood vessels are not formed correctly.

# Chapter 11

# COMBATING CANCER

## MARILYN'S STORY

In September 1998 Gayle and I had just returned from a wonderful three-week Mediterranean cruise with twelve other friends. We had had a ball. I was looking good and feeling even better. As I settled into my regular schedule, I realized that it was time for my annual mammogram. No problem. This was so routine, I didn't give it a second thought. Plus my monthly self-exams hadn't showed any change in the usual lumps, bumps, and cysts of the long-standing fibrocystic disease in my breasts. For the past ten years, the annual clinical examinations of my breasts performed by my doctor hadn't revealed a thing.

So you can imagine my surprise when I learned during a routine mammogram that I had multiple areas of tiny calcifications in my left breast and a suspicious mass in my right breast. An ultrasound was performed immediately on my right breast, which was fine. However, the biopsy of my left breast (performed one week after the mammogram) was positive for breast cancer. I couldn't believe it! I was living a preventive lifestyle—eating lots of fruits and veggies (broccoli, cabbage, collards) and hardly any meat, had increased my soy, was taking antioxidants (vitamins C and E, beta-carotene), had increased my daily exercise, was dealing with my stress—so why was this happening to me?

Initially I was terrified about being diagnosed with cancer, despite the fact that I'm a physician and I knew my chances of full recovery were quite good. Still, I was scared, and thoughts of my mother's death from cervical cancer when she was fifty-seven years old kept flashing through my mind. I knew I needed my personal support system right away, so my first two calls were to Gayle and my daughter. They immediately left work and showered me with flowers, love, and food.

I next called on my professional support system—my African American women doctor friends—who gave me both loving and medical advice.

Finally, armed with my mammograms and biopsy slides, I sought other expert opinions. I consulted Dr. LaSalle Leffall at Howard University, who is an expert on African American women with breast cancer; the Lombardi Cancer Center at Georgetown University; and Dr. Ruth Kirstein, the deputy director of the National Institutes of Health (NIH), who is a breast cancer survivor. Not only did she give me superb advice, but her husband, Dr. Al Rabson, the deputy director of the National Cancer Institute at NIH and a pathologist, reviewed my slides and referred me to other specialists. Quite a team, huh? The specialists agreed that only my left breast had to be removed, and I did not require radiation or chemotherapy. With this diagnosis in mind, I continued to consult other breast cancer survivors, who were wonderful to me.

The good news was that we had gotten to my cancer early—the disease was still confined to the ducts in my breast, with no invasion or spread outside the ducts. God is good! I will not be leaving too soon.

After many prayers, many opinions, and many tears, however, I decided to have both breasts removed (a bilateral mastectomy) so I wouldn't have to deal with every little lump, mass, and pain in my other breast for the rest of my life. I also opted for immediate reconstruction of my breasts using saline implants.

Two months later, after a successful bilateral mastectomy, I had the implants removed. They had caused me constant pain and discomfort, and the threat of leakage of the implants was more than I wanted to live with.

One of the best decisions I made during my healing process was to join an African American support group of breast cancer survivors, Rise Sister Rise, founded by Zora Brown, who is a survivor herself. Remember the ditty "Little Sally Walker" from those good ol' days?

*Little Sally Walker sitting in a saucer,*
*Rise Sally rise*
*Wipe your weeping eyes.*

*Put your hands on your hips,*
*Let your backbone slip.*
*Oh . . . shake it to the east.*
*And shake it to the west.*
*Shake it to the one that you love the best!*

This is the theme song of Rise Sister Rise.

Today I am doing well and my prognosis is excellent. My survival expectation is better than 90 percent. With so many unknowns about breast cancer, especially in African American women, I am living proof that the best defense continues to be early diagnosis and early treatment.

---

Although heart disease is the number one cause of death (cancer is number two) among the general population of all Americans (including African Americans), cancer is the leading cause of death of African American and Caucasian women between the ages of forty-five and sixty-four years. (See chart below.)

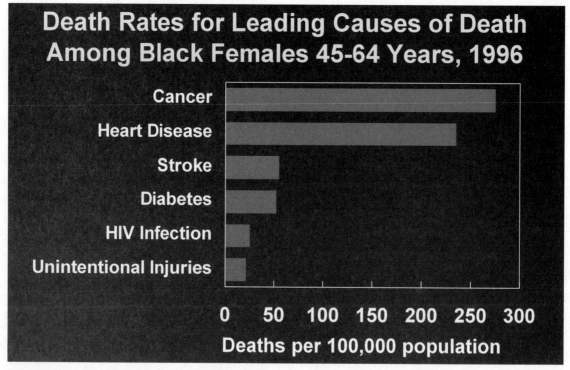

## Death Rates for Leading Causes of Death Among Black Females 45-64 Years, 1996

Cancer
Heart Disease
Stroke
Diabetes
HIV Infection
Unintentional Injuries

0    50   100  150  200  250  300
Deaths per 100,000 population

*Source:* National Center for Health Statistics.

The facts don't lie:

- Over the past thirty years, the cancer rate in African Americans has increased by 27 percent, whereas that number has risen only 12 percent among Caucasians.
- The chance of African Americans living five years or longer after diagnosis and treatment of cancer is only 42 percent; for White Americans, it is 58 percent.
- African American women and men are 30 percent more likely to die from cancer than any other racial or ethnic group.[1]

## WHAT IS CANCER?

According to the *Merck Manual of Medical Information*, cancer is "a cell that has lost its normal control mechanism and thus has unregulated growth." What does that mean in plain English? Cancer occurs when cells in your body that were previously normal go haywire and no longer respond to body signals that curtail cell growth and reproduction. Research indicates that the cause of uncontrolled cell growth can be a specific agent (called a carcinogen), such as a chemical, virus, radiation, or sunlight (or a combination of these factors). The agent causes the cell's genetic material to change. Some body cells have an inborn genetic flaw that can cause them to change. Even when a cell becomes cancerous, however, our immune system can often destroy it before it replicates. This is why cancer is more likely to develop when the immune system isn't functioning properly, such as in people with AIDS, or in people with poor nutrition and increased stress, which decreases the effectiveness of the immune system.

## HOW IS CANCER DIAGNOSED?

A recent study revealed that African American women over thirty-five years of age knew less about cancer and received Pap smears and mammograms less often than Caucasian women, even though we are at higher risk for breast cancer. The study demonstrated a connection between African American women's knowledge about cancer and how often they were screened. This is an important finding, especially since older women are at higher risk. Increased knowledge resulted in increased screening regardless of income level.

All cancer progresses from normal tissue to full-blown disease by stages:

*Stage one: dysplasia.* (You'll see this term on your Pap smear report. It means changed cell structure.) This is the very beginning of cancer, when changes start to occur at the cellular level but before the actual disease presents itself. At this stage, affected body cells may revert to normal or progress to the next stage.

*Stage 2: carcinoma in situ.* At this point, cancerous cells are present, but they have not invaded or spread beyond the surface of a tissue.

*Stage 3: full-blown tumors.* The cancerous cells keep multiplying and form a mass or tumor. These *malignant tumors* invade surrounding tissue, break loose, enter the bloodstream, and form tumors at other sites in the body. Once the disease has spread in this way, it is much more difficult to treat.

## TYPES OF CANCER

Since we are at greater risk in our age group, the more we know about the different types of cancer, the more we will be prepared to defeat cancer through early diagnosis and treatment. The table below list the six cancers that are the **most frequently diagnosed** among African American and Caucasian women.

### MOST FREQUENTLY DIAGNOSED CANCERS IN WOMEN

| AFRICAN AMERICAN WOMEN | RANK | CAUCASIAN WOMEN |
|:---:|:---:|:---:|
| Breast | 1 | Breast |
| Lung and Bronchus | 2 | Lung and Bronchus |
| Colon and Rectum | 3 | Colon and Rectum |
| Uterine | 4 | Uterine |
| Pancreas | 5 | Ovary |
| Cervix | 6 | Lymphoma (non-Hodgkin's) |

*Source:* National Cancer Institute, National Institutes of Health.

Compare this table with the next one, listing the cancers that are the **most common causes of death**. Note in particular the position of cancer of the cervix. The reality is that *there should not be any deaths from cervical cancer*, because this form of the disease can be diagnosed before the cells become cancerous.

Mortality rates for cervical cancer are higher in African American women than White women in this country. According to Dr. Harold Freeman, director of surgery at Harlem Hospital, at least half of the difference in survival is attributable to late detection of these cancers, especially in poor Black women.

Note also that while historically most of the cancer deaths in women have been due to breast cancer, with the dramatic increase in lung cancer, this pattern has changed, and now lung cancer is the number one cause of death from cancer for all women.

### MOST COMMON CAUSES OF DEATH FROM CANCER IN WOMEN

| AFRICAN AMERICAN WOMEN | RANK | CAUCASIAN WOMEN |
|---|---|---|
| Lung and Bronchus | 1 | Lung and Bronchus |
| Breast | 2 | Breast |
| Colon and Rectum | 3 | Colon and Rectum |
| Pancreas | 4 | Ovary |
| Ovary | 5 | Pancreas |
| Cervix | 6 | Leukemia |

*Source:* National Cancer Institute, National Institutes of Health.

Please note that even though breast cancer is the most commonly diagnosed cancer in women, it occurs much more frequently in Caucasian women than African American women. However, although African American women are diagnosed with breast cancer *less frequently*, we die *more often* from it. The chart below shows very clearly that our incidence or occurrence rate is lower but our death rate is higher.

Despite the grim reality of these research findings, the good news is that in the United States the number of new cases of all cancers is declining—around 1 percent a year from 1990 to 1996. These encouraging figures reflect healthful changes in lifestyle, particularly a drop in the number of Americans who smoke. The bad news is that these results are not as good for women and minorities—we have made fewer gains, and certain cancers, such as lung cancer, are on the rise in our population.

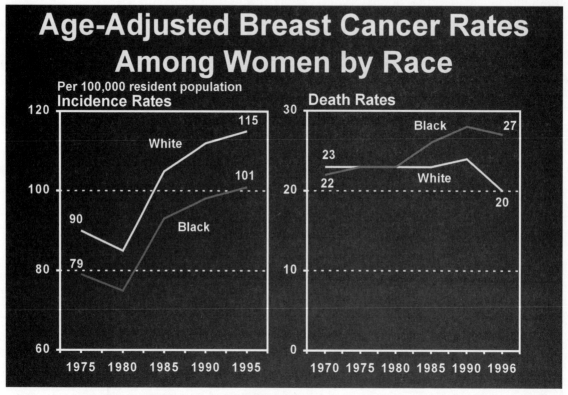

# Age-Adjusted Breast Cancer Rates Among Women by Race

*Source: U.S. Minority Health: A Chart Book, 1999.*

Nevertheless, this recent decline in cancer incidence underscores the fact that cancer is potentially preventable. By taking aggressive action to reduce risks by improving lifestyle habits, as well as by vigilant screening efforts, we can dramatically reduce our deaths from cancer.

**Remember: With all cancer, early detection and early treatment are key!** And, as in all of the Big Four diseases, understanding the risk factors and early warning signs for cancer can help save your life.

## RISK FACTORS FOR CANCER

- *Inherited changes in the genes*
- *Exposure to cancer-causing substances, such as arsenic, asbestos, and cigarette smoke*
- *Dietary factors, such as inadequate amounts of fruit and vegetables*
- *Ultraviolet light and other forms of irradiation*
- *Certain viral infections (HPV [human papilloma virus] which is linked to cervical cancer and HIV)*

## GENERAL WARNING SIGNS OF CANCER

The American Cancer Society has identified the known warning signs for cancer in general, of which you should be aware:

- *Change in bowel or bladder habits*
- *A sore that does not heal*
- *Unusual bleeding or discharge*
- *Thickening or lump in breast or elsewhere in the body*
- *Indigestion or problems with swallowing*
- *Obvious change in a wart or mole*
- *Nagging cough or hoarseness*

There are specific, routine examinations and tests you must do regularly in order to detect cancer early, even if you feel completely healthy. (See the following sections on specific types of cancers.) Thousands of African American lives could be saved with appropriate action. Yours could be one of them.

Let's examine in greater detail the main causes of cancer death, the risk factors, methods of diagnosis, and suggestions for prevention and treatment for the six major types of cancer found in women.

## Lung Cancer

*One week after her sixty-sixth birthday, jazz legend Sarah Vaughan died from lung cancer.*

Between 1973 and 1992, the incidence of lung cancer in African American women rose more than 100 percent, as did the death rate from this cruel disease. That makes lung cancer the leading cause of death due to cancer among Black women. **There are more deaths from lung cancer than from breast, colon, and pancreatic cancers combined.**

About 85 percent of the cases of lung cancer are attributable to smoking. This is why we continue to emphasize that *smoking is the number one preventable cause of all premature deaths and disability in the United States.*

Despite the strong antismoking warnings on packs of cigarettes and in public health messages, more women than ever are smoking, and women smokers are not quitting at the rate that men have over the past decade or two. (Could this be because we worry so much about gaining weight?) This is why women who smoke are more likely to get lung cancer than men who smoke; more men eventually quit.

Even though cigarette smoking causes more preventable deaths from cancer and heart disease than any other modifiable risk factor, a recent study reported that only 40 percent of current smokers perceived their risk of cancer as higher than that of nonsmokers of the same age and sex. Only 29 percent of the smokers thought that their risk for heart disease was higher than nonsmokers'.[2] Many smokers continue to deny their own personal risks for lung cancer, and many don't know about the association with heart disease.

### *Signs and Symptoms of Lung Cancer*

Lung cancer is devastating because symptoms usually don't appear until the disease is advanced and the cancer has started to spread. Early detection is very difficult, since chest X rays often don't reveal the early stages of the disease. Therefore, it's no surprise that the five-year survival rate is only 14 percent! When symptoms do appear, they include:

- Persistent cough
- Sputum streaked with blood
- Chest pain
- Recurring pneumonia or bronchitis

## Risk Factors for Lung Cancer

As we have stated before, smoking is an overwhelming risk factor for lung cancer. In fact, smoking is linked to more than four hundred thousand deaths in the United States annually. Women in general who smoke are more likely to get lung cancer than men who smoke because we have a harder time quitting than men. African American women have even more difficulty. According to a National Medical Association study, smokers may not fully comprehend the threat to health from smoking because of the powerful immediate stress reduction benefit from the nicotine.

Recent studies are showing that race is a factor in lung cancer. African Americans break down nicotine differently and perhaps more slowly than Caucasians do, and researchers have found that we absorb more nicotine than White or Hispanic smokers. There are also questions about our different physical reactions to mentholated cigarettes. On top of that, African Americans also find it more difficult to quit. Therefore, as women and as African Americans, we once again are at greater risk and suffer double jeopardy.

Secondhand smoke for nonsmokers is also dangerous. In fact, it's called "passive smoking"! If you don't smoke but live with a smoker, you are increasing your risk for problems. Each year about three thousand nonsmoking adults die of lung cancer as a result of breathing the smoke of someone else's cigarettes. It is estimated that as many as sixty thousand deaths occur from coronary artery disease related to passive smoke. If you do not smoke but are regularly exposed to secondhand smoke, you are also **doubling your risk of developing heart disease**. The ten-year Nurses' Study of 121,700 nurses (of whom 32,046 were smokers) found that the nonsmokers were twice as likely to have a heart attack if they were exposed regularly in bars or at home to secondhand smoke.

### PRIME TIME REMINDER

We know you don't want to hear this, but smoking speeds up the aging process in your entire body. It dries up and wrinkles your skin and yellows your teeth. It disturbs the balance of energy and blocks the normal flow of your life energy or *chi*. Women who smoke also lose bone mass more quickly after menopause than those who do not smoke.

Exposure to arsenic, radon, asbestos, and radiation from occupational, medical, and environmental sources also increases your risk for lung cancer.

### Diagnosing Lung Cancer

Because there are no adequate screening tests available at this time for lung cancer, early detection is very difficult. Chest X rays usually catch this disease only when it's in a later stage. The use of CT scans is being investigated, since they can find lung cancers earlier than chest X rays.

**Rx** | **PRIME TIME PRESCRIPTION TO STOP SMOKING**

*You can stop smoking!* But be patient, since it usually takes four, five, or six tries before you successfully quit. It is not easy, but it is one of the best things you can do for yourself. You are worth it. The health benefits are monumental and, as you can see in the table opposite, they occur almost immediately after stopping.

---

## MARILYN'S STORY

I finally quit smoking after four previous tries. It was one of the hardest things I ever did in my entire life. It ranks in difficulty with getting through medical school and having my children. Just knowing you shouldn't smoke is never enough motivation to help you successfully stop. I would see many smokers' lungs on the autopsy table—lungs black with tar, lungs eaten away and full of cancer, lungs swollen with emphysema. I would examine these lungs and then go right outside and take a smoke break!

Not until I got motivated to save my life and set a better example for my children, and then have a buddy really help me, encourage me, support me, be there for me, was I finally able to stop.

It's been seventeen years now, and I feel and look much better. And I sure am proud of myself! But above all, this was one of the most important gifts I have ever given to myself. Now my risk for heart disease and stroke is much, much lower—the same as any middle-aged African American nonsmoking woman.

---

Quitting can literally save your life—and it can also extend it. It's never too late to stop. Quitting at any time is important. The damage isn't all reversed overnight, but major damage reversal does occur. The following table shows the risk while you smoke and the decrease in risk after you quit.

## SMOKING IS A MAJOR RISK FACTOR FOR MANY DISEASES

| DISEASE | RISK IF YOU SMOKE (COMPARED TO NONSMOKERS) | RISK AFTER YOU QUIT |
|---|---|---|
| Heart Disease | Risk is 70% higher | Within 1 year, risk drops by 50% compared to nonsmokers. After 15 years, risk same as nonsmoker. |
| Stroke | Risk is 2 to 3 times higher | Risk drops steadily. After 15 years, same as nonsmoker. |
| Lung Cancer | Risk is 7 to 20 times higher | Within 10 years, risk drops by 50%. After 15 years, risk is 4 times that of nonsmokers. |
| Chronic Lung Disease | Risk is 9 time higher. | After 20 years, risk of death remains elevated 2 to 8 times compared to nonsmokers. |

Source: Harvard Health Letter, June 1998.

If you are thinking about quitting, try the Prime Time Eight-Step Smoking Cessation Program outlined in Chapter 9. It combines the medical, emotional, and spiritual recommendations you will need to make your effort successful.

## Breast Cancer

*Audre Lorde. Minnie Ripperton. Lorraine Hansberry. A poet. A singer. A playwright. All powerful sisters who died too soon from breast cancer.*

In recent years, deaths from breast cancer decreased by 5.5 percent for Caucasian women; however, African American women did not experience a similar decline. Our death rate **increased** by almost 3 percent during the same period. Between 1973 and 1992, both the incidence of breast cancer in African American women over the age of fifty and the death rate from the disease increased. Now breast cancer is the second leading cause of cancer deaths for Black women.

After skin cancer, breast cancer is the most common cancer among women in the United States. It is one of the diseases women fear the most. Breast cancer reports are constantly in the newspapers; television reporters do controversial stories on the topic, and most of us know someone who has faced it. You've seen the pink ribbons. Perhaps you wear one and know that *one in nine women will get breast cancer in her lifetime*. What's even more frightening is that only twenty-five years ago, this statistic was one in fifteen. This increase in breast cancer is of great concern to the health profession, partly because the rise in numbers can't be completely explained away by better early detection or the fact that this disease is being reported more often.

By the time most Black women get diagnosed for breast cancer, the disease has already advanced beyond the breast into other parts of the body. The National Cancer Institute's Black/White Cancer Survival Study found that the risk of dying was 2.2 times greater for African American women.[3] This was attributed mainly to the fact that when our cancer did get diagnosed, 30 percent of us had advanced disease compared to only 18 percent of the White women. Therefore, our five-year survival rate is lower than that of White or Hispanic women (see chart below).

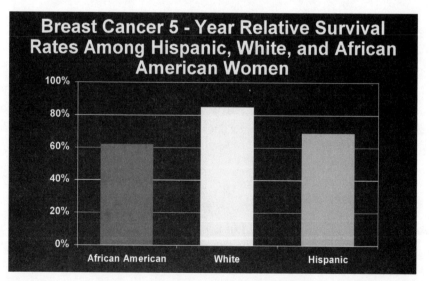

*Source:* National Cancer Institute Surveillance, Epidemiology, and End Results (SEER) Program, 1995.

There are a number of other reasons for this disparity in death rates.[4]

1. *Black women get breast cancer at earlier ages.* A 1998 four-state study by Dr. Edwin Johnson of the University of Alabama revealed that Black women at age thirty had the same incidence as White women at age forty. That is why more doctors are recommending that African American women start getting mammograms earlier than other women. By screening Black women at a younger age, we increase the chances of detecting our cancers early enough to treat them effectively.

2. *Black women's tumors may be far more aggressive and more dangerous than the cancers of White women.* Research is continuing in this area.

3. *Surveys indicate that African American women don't have sufficient knowledge about cancer and do not believe they need to be screened unless they already have a problem.*[5] We also have a great deal of fear surrounding cancer and cancer screening, such as the fear of radiation (even though it is harmless in this exam), fear of knowing we are ill, and fear of pain.[6] Whatever fear you may have, please, talk with your sisterfriend about it and face it so that you can take the steps necessary to save your life.

4. *Surveys reveal that many Black women rely solely on prayer and/or herbs to prevent and cure breast cancer.* Let us quickly emphasize that prayer is wonderful *in conjunction with* appropriate diagnostic procedures and follow-up treatment. Please do not rely on prayer alone. Use it to complement your health care.

5. *Cost may be a factor in why a number of poor African American women do not get annual mammograms.* Even though the number of free screening programs (as well as free follow-up treatments) is on the rise, the word is not getting out to many low-income women. One mammogram by itself is not enough. You must get them annually.

6. *Not all doctors recommend mammograms for their patients.* Whether or not your doctor says you need a mammogram, you need to take charge of your own health as a Prime Time woman. Keep track of when you're due for your annual screening.

### Risk Factors for Breast Cancer

We don't know the cause of breast cancer, but we do know there are several potential risk factors.

*Aging* is the single most important risk for breast cancer. Two-thirds of all breast cancer cases occur in women over the age of fifty. But you can counteract your risk with proper self-care and regular mammograms.

*A family history of breast cancer is also a strong indicator of risk.* If you have one first-degree relative (mother or sister), with breast cancer your risk increases up to threefold. With two or more first-degree relatives with breast cancer, your risk increases sixfold. If you inherit the genes of breast cancer—BRCA1 and BRCA2—your risk of breast cancer is up to thirtyfold that of women without this gene. You can find out if you carry these genes through genetic testing. If you have these genes, your risk of developing ovarian cancer also is increased. However, most breast cancer is not due to the BRCA genes. These genes cause breast cancer at an earlier age. BRCA1 is present in 30 percent of women diagnosed with breast cancer before age fifty, but less than 2 percent of those who develop it after age seventy.

*If you develop breast cancer in one breast, your risk increases fivefold for developing it in the other breast.*

*Studies indicate that having your first child later in life or not having children increases your risk of breast cancer.*

*Prolonged estrogen exposure* may be a risk factor for breast cancer. For instance, women who begin menstruating early (before age twelve) or enter menopause late (fifty-five or older) appear to have a higher incidence of this disease. Also, continued exposure of breast tissue to estrogen through hormone replacement therapy may increase risk. The controversy surrounding hormone replacement therapy (HRT) and breast cancer is a growing concern for many postmenopausal women. Approximately forty studies have looked at postmenopausal estrogen replacement and breast cancer. The findings vary considerably, but the higher incidence of breast cancer among women on estrogen seems to be correlated with the length of time on estrogen—five or more years.

Other risk factors to take note of:

- More than one drink or one ounce of alcohol daily
- Environmental factors such as air pollution, pesticides, or food additives
- Too much fat in your diet
- Being overweight (Since estrogen is stored in fat, having too much body fat increases your exposure to this hormone.)
- Lack of exercise
- Breast biopsies (Women who have had multiple breast biopsies have an increased risk.)

• Stress and depression (These suppress immune activity. More research is needed in this area, and more and more studies are documenting that people survive cancer longer when they use relaxation and imaging techniques.)

The National Cancer Institute has developed a computerized breast cancer risk assessment tool that can help you and your doctor look at your risk and determine what course of action you should take. The Breast Cancer Risk Assessment Tool comes on a standard computer disk and it calculates your estimated five-year and lifetime risk of breast cancer, and compares your risk with other women's. It is available free by going on-line to NCI's Web site at brca.nci.nih.gov/brc or by calling 800-4-CANCER (800-422-6237). This tool should only be used under the supervision of your health professional.

 **PRIME TIME PRESCRIPTION TO FIGHT BREAST CANCER:**

### Early Detection

Breast cancer *can be cured* if it is caught early. Experts say that when a breast tumor is found in the earliest stage, the five-year rate of survival goes up to 95 percent. That's good news! And the way to diagnose it early is by religiously practicing the three early-detection modalities:

1. *Once a month,* examine your own breasts.
2. *Once a year,* make sure that a health professional does a thorough exam of your breasts during your annual physical.
3. *Once a year,* get a mammogram. Have a baseline mammogram done when you turn thirty-five years old, and get annual mammograms starting when you're forty. (If there is a family history of breast cancer, consult your doctor about starting annual screenings at age thirty-five.)

*Remember, all three exams must be done regularly and consistently. You cannot stop after three years, five years, or ten years.* Breast care—examining yourself, getting examined by a health-care professional once a year, and having an annual mammogram—is critical for all Prime Time women. These three early-detection exams must become important routines in your life. Again, pick a convenient time to do your self-exams so you won't forget. If you're still menstruating, do it a few days after your period ends. If not, do the exam on the first or last day of the month, and mark the days on your calendar at the beginning of the year. Schedule your annual physical exam and mammogram on or near your birthday or during October, which is National Breast Cancer Awareness Month.

Why is consistency so important? Researchers estimate that the death rate from breast cancer for women age fifty and older could be reduced by more than 30 percent if we consistently obtained annual mammograms and clinical breast exams. The other piece of good news is that the effectiveness of these early-detection procedures increases as we get older because the density of our breast tissue diminishes with age, making it easier to detect a tumor.

Mammography is able to detect the tiniest of tumors before they become invasive and spread to other parts of the body and while they are still only a fraction of the size of lumps that can be felt during breast self-examination. That doesn't mean that breast self-examination is unnecessary, however. Women who practice breast self-examination regularly are able to recognize a lump that is three times smaller than ones found by women who are not trained in the technique.

### Breast Self-Examination

Remember, since cancer in Black women tends to occur earlier, it's important to obtain a baseline mammogram at age thirty-five. Remind your younger family members and friends. If you didn't get a mammogram at age thirty-five or forty, **get one now!**

Women discover more than 80 percent of their own breast lumps. Fortunately, most are benign. Self-examination takes no more than ten minutes. To examine your breast, you must *look* and *feel*:

1. In front of the mirror, *look*:

   • At the size and symmetry of your breasts
   • At the color and texture of your breasts
   • For changes in your breasts, such as skin dimpling, change in moles or nipples, or discharge

2. In the shower and lying down in bed, *feel* your breast. Press firmly using the flat surface of the middle three fingers, and check every part of the breast. Move your left hand over your right breast in a circle, vertically, or in a wedge pattern (see illustration below) going from top to bottom and

around, covering every part of the breast. Then use your right hand to check your left breast. Feel your breasts and armpits for:

• Lumps
• Hard knots
• Thick masses

By examining yourself every month, you will get to know your breasts very well and *you* will be the first to detect any change. Your mate or partner can also learn and assist with your exams. With any change, notify your doctor immediately. Also remember that 90 percent of lumps found are benign (not cancer) and nothing to worry about.

A physician, nurse-practitioner, or other trained health-care professional can instruct you in the proper way to do self-examinations. Local chapters of the American Cancer Society and other advocacy organizations can also assist. Call the ACS toll free at 800-ACS-2345 or go to its Web site at www.cancer.org.

## Below are some of the recommended SELF-EXAMINATION PATTERNS.

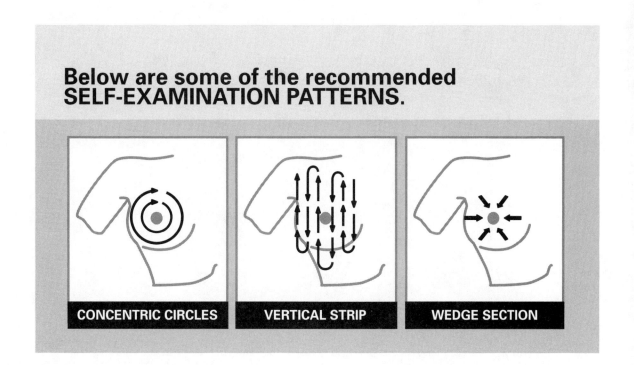

CONCENTRIC CIRCLES    VERTICAL STRIP    WEDGE SECTION

### Clinical Breast Examination

You should have an annual breast examination by your physician, even if your self-exams do not indicate that there is a problem. Either your primary care doctor (internal medicine specialist or family doctor) or gynecologist can perform a clinical breast exam during a routine office visit. Trained nurse-practitioners or other health professionals at cancer detection facilities can also perform the exam. Self-exams and clinical exams allow you and your health-care professional to check the sides of the breasts extending into the armpits, an important area that mammograms sometimes fail to screen.

## SMALLEST SIZE OF LUMPS DETECTED BY BREAST EXAMS

As illustrated below, mammography is able to detect tiny tumors that are not detectable by breast self-examination. That doesn't mean that breast self-exam is unnecessary, however. Women who practice BSE regularly are able to recognize a lump that is three time smaller, compared to women untrained in BSE.

1/8 inch
Found by a regular mammogram

1/4 inch
Found by a first mammogram

1/2 inch
Found by women who do regular BSE and by your health professional

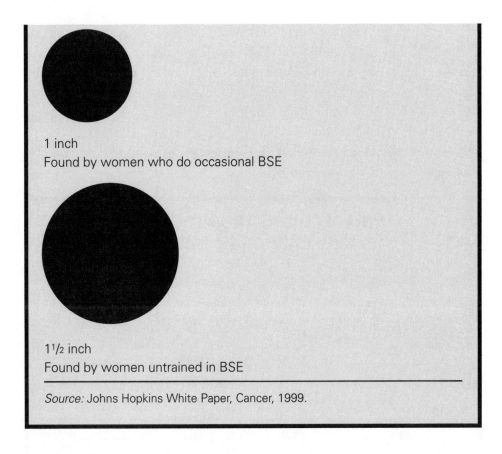

1 inch
Found by women who do occasional BSE

1¹/₂ inch
Found by women untrained in BSE

*Source:* Johns Hopkins White Paper, Cancer, 1999.

### How Well Are You Caring for Your Breasts?

If you are not following these three early-detection practices, ask yourself why. Think hard about what is preventing you from being serious about breast exams. We acknowledge that it can be very difficult emotionally for women to care properly for their breasts—maybe you're afraid of the tests, or perhaps you don't understand the disease. Or maybe you don't have enough money to pay for the exam. If you fit into any of these categories, you need to get support to address your concerns. As mentioned earlier, many communities now have mobile mammography units that are low- or no-cost. If you are sixty-five years of age or older, Medicare covers part of the cost, and you do not need a doctor's order to get a screening mammogram. Your local American Cancer Society has information about screenings and support groups in your area. To find out about mammography facilities certified by the Food and Drug Administration (FDA), call the National Cancer Institute's Cancer Information Service at 800-4-CANCER.

If you are afraid of finding out the diagnosis, as many women are, or are afraid of the mild discomfort and/or low-dose, harmless radiation associated with a mammogram, please use your Prime Time Sister and Prime Time Circle for support. They can remind you when it's time for your mammogram, and go with you for the exam. Your Prime Time Circle can also have discussions and explore the latest findings and recommendations regarding these health concerns.

You want to include the health of your breasts in your determination to keep self-care your foremost priority.

---

## WHAT KEEPS ME FROM PROPERLY TAKING CARE OF MY BREASTS?

What are your barriers from practicing preventive breast care and what would help you to stick to these preventive measures? Check some of the reasons we listed above and then write down your concerns and explore solutions for yourself.

1. _____
2. _____
3. _____
4. _____
5. _____
6. _____
7. _____

---

### Mammography

New methods of mammography currently under development might eventually lead to improved accuracy.

*Digital mammography* allows the image to be viewed from different angles on a computer and magnified or refocused. This helps identify smaller abnormalities. This will eventually replace regular mammography.

*High-definition imaging* (HDI) is an ultrasound technique that may reduce by 40 percent the number of biopsies done on suspicious lumps. It helps figure out the size of the mass and whether it is a tumor or a cyst (a benign noncancerous mass, frequently containing fluid).

We need to continue to advocate for better testing for breast cancer that is easier and has improved accuracy. For example, in 1999, *Nature* reported that X-ray analysis of hair may hold promise.

**PRIME TIME PRESCRIPTIONS FOR REDUCING RISK FACTORS FOR BREAST CANCER**

Remember, primary prevention of cancer means taking the necessary steps to prevent the occurrence of cancer in the first place. Secondary prevention (which focuses on the exams we discussed earlier) helps detect cancer as early as possible, preventing it from spreading or getting worse.

*Redesign your diet.* Our diet plays a major role in our rates of cancer occurrence and death from the disease, but we need more information on exactly what foods do help prevent cancer and the exact amounts we need to prevent the disease from developing.

*Limit your fat intake to 20 percent of your overall caloric intake.* A high-fat diet may increase your risk for breast cancer, but the type of fat you eat is also important. The omega-3 oils in tuna, salmon, mackerel, and sardines appear to be protective. North American Inuit women, who eat a diet extremely rich in omega-3 oils, have very low rates of breast cancer. Mono-unsaturated fats such as olive oil have been linked with lower rates of cancer. Animal fat, trans fat, and saturated fat all are linked to increases in cancer risk. (For more information on good fat versus bad fat, see the table "What You Should Know About Fats in Foods" in Chapter 9.)

*Buy organic.* Organic produce is free of pesticides such as DDT and other environmental toxins that have been linked to a higher risk of breast cancer.

*Eat mostly fruits and vegetables and limit meat intake.* A 1999 report from the American Institute for Cancer Research estimates that eating five to seven servings of vegetables and fruits each day may reduce the risk of cancer by up to 20 percent.[7] Not convinced? Well, think about this: When Asians move to the United States and change their diet from one that is rich in cabbage, sea vegetables, fish, soy products, and green tea—all foods that contain cancer-fighting substances—to the standard American diet, their cancer rates go up.

If you eat meat, definitely avoid meat that is heavily charred from barbecuing. These charred meats contain high levels of cancer-causing chemicals called heterocyclic aromatic amines. Also avoid cured and smoked meats such as sausage, bacon, and fatback, or other processed meats, because they contain nitrites and other potentially cancer-causing substances.

*Increase your intake of antioxidants and phytochemicals.* These build a powerful defense against cancer. Antioxidants are substances that protect against free radicals (which can damage cells and initiate cancer). Vitamins C and E and beta-carotene are important antioxidants. Phytochemicals, certain substances found in plants, stimulate the body's production of enzymes that detoxify cancer-causing substances. Antioxidants and phytochemicals are found in grains and a wide variety of fruits and vegetables, including cabbage, brussels sprouts, broccoli, tomatoes, collards, turnip and mustard greens, sweet potatoes, black-eyed peas, oranges, and watermelon. Here are some vegetables that you must absolutely include in your regular diet:

**Broccoli.** Broccoli is a potent cancer fighter loaded with natural chemicals called *indoles*, which help prevent tumors by blocking harmful cancer-causing chemicals before they do their dirty work. Indoles also help eliminate estrogen from the body and convert estrogen from cancer-promoting forms to forms that actually protect against breast cancer. One particular indole, *indole-3-carbinol*, inhibits the development of potentially cancerous cells in the breast. Cabbage, cauliflower, brussels sprouts, mustard, kale, and collard greens also offer great protection.

There is now a vegetable called *BroccoSprouts*, patented by Johns Hopkins University in Baltimore, that has twenty times more of the cancer-fighting compound *sulforaphane glucosinolate* (SGS). Sulforaphane increases the levels of protective substances inside cells that destroy cancer-causing chemicals and free radicals before they have a chance to cause cancer. As little as ¼ ounce of BroccoSprouts on a sandwich or salad each day reduces the odds of getting colon cancer by 50 percent. You would have to eat more than two pounds of broccoli every week to get the same result. BroccoSprouts are in supermarkets nationwide at a price of $2.99 for 4 ounces. Call 888-551-8989 for more information and a location near you.

**Tomatoes and garlic.** A study published in the *Journal of the National Cancer Institute* in August 1999 found evidence that people who eat lots of tomatoes and tomato products "are at substantially decreased risk of numerous cancers," including cancers of the stomach, lung, colon and rectum, esophagus, prostate, and cervix. The significant ingredient in tomatoes is lycopene, an antioxidant that gives them their red color. The cancer-fighting power of tomatoes increases when they are cooked; try tomato sauce with a dash of olive oil. And don't forget to add some garlic to the sauce, since garlic helps limit the production of cancer-causing chemicals. (Aged garlic extract is the most potent.) Other vegetables that are related to garlic and which also contain cancer-fighting substances are onions, leeks, and shallots. Compounds in these foods stimulate the production of enzymes that block the free radicals linked with cancer. Cut these vegetables up and let them sit for ten minutes to get the most effect. Eat vegetables raw, as cooking decreases their potency.

**Soy.** In one study, Seventh-Day Adventist women, vegetarians who eat a lot of soy, were found to have a lower-than-normal risk of breast cancer. If you have not introduced soy into your diet, please do! Soy does many things—it is a weak plant estrogen that binds to estrogen receptors in breast tissue, making it more difficult for stronger, cancer-causing forms of estrogen to connect with breast cells.

Soy contains a phytochemical known as *genistein*, an isoflavone, that has been proved in test-tube studies to stymie the growth of breast cancer cells. It also decreases the development of blood vessels that feed a tumor, increases cancer cell death, and contains enzymes that break down cancer-causing chemicals in the body.

Eat at least one serving a day of soy products, such as soybeans, tofu, miso, tempeh, and soy milk. That may decrease your risk of a number of cancers by 40 percent. Soy also has a cholesterol-lowering effect.

Highly refined soy products such as soy burgers and fake meats contain much less genistein than traditional Asian soy products and may contain artificial preservatives. Soybean oil and soy sauce are not good sources, either: soybean oil contains unhealthy fats, and soy sauce is high in sodium.

**Fiber.** High-fiber diets can decrease breast cancer risk by up to 54 percent.

**Green tea.** The Mayo Clinic has found that green tea has antioxidant components that can neutralize free radicals before they can damage the cell, a first step leading to cancer. These researchers suggest that drinking at least four cups of green tea daily could slow and/or prevent the growth of cancer cells. This may also explain the low rates of breast cancer among Japanese women. Make sure it's decaffeinated tea.

**Mushrooms.** Believe it or not, mushrooms—especially the Japanese varieties maitake and shiitake—appear to fight cancer by activating special immune cells. Immune system strength is key to conquering most forms of cancer.

*Take your supplements.* Vitamins C and E, grape seed extract, and selenium are antioxidants that reduce the damage done by free radicals. In 1996 the *Journal of the American Medical Association* reported that selenium (200 mcg daily) decreases the risk of colorectal cancer by 58 percent and the risk of lung cancer by 46 percent. Many doctors recommend coenzyme $Q_{10}$ to strengthen the immune system and zap free radicals, but the data on this are not clear yet.

*Investigate the pros and cons of drug therapy for preventing cancer if you are at high risk.* Studies of the so-called designer estrogens Nolvadex (tamoxifen) and Evista (raloxifene) seem to indicate that they are effective in the prevention of breast cancer.[8] They're synthetic hormones that look enough like estrogen to fool some parts of your body into thinking they are. They seem to act like your body's own estrogen and prevent your bones from thinning. Most important, these drugs don't encourage cancer cells to grow as our own estrogen can. Both drugs block the action of estrogen on breast tissue. Tamoxifen reduced the occurrence of breast cancer by 45 percent in a high-risk population, mainly women over sixty years of age with a strong family history. The bad news is that tamoxifen doubled the risk of uterine cancer over the placebo group and increased the occurrence of blood clots in the lungs and legs.

Raloxifene also reduced the occurrence of breast cancer by 60 percent. The good news is that it has fewer side effects than tamoxifen and does not produce cancer of the uterus in low-risk White women. This drug has been used to treat osteoporosis and is recommended to prevent and treat bone loss and decrease fractures.

The National Institutes of Health have started a major study evaluating the benefits and side effects of both tamoxifen and raloxifene. The results should be available in three to five years.

In the meantime, each woman must work with her doctor and make decisions based on her own particular situation, weighing the risks and benefits of drug treatment against her needs and medical history. It may be that the only women who should consider raloxifene are those at highest risk of osteoporosis, the group for whom it was originally designed. If that includes you, you should also consult your doctor about another drug, called Fosamax (alendronate), that may do a better job of preventing osteoporosis.

*Limit your alcohol intake.* Women who have two to four alcoholic drinks per week have a two to three times higher risk of developing breast cancer than those who don't.

*Engage in vigorous aerobic exercise.* Active women are 60 percent less likely to get cancer than couch potatoes. Breast cancer is linked to inactivity. The *New England Journal of Medicine* reported in 1997 that a huge study of twenty-five thousand women over a nine-year period found that women who exercised at least four hours a week had a 37 percent lower breast cancer risk compared to women who did no exercise at all. This may be because exercise enhances insulin use in the body, and there is a link between poor insulin utilization and increased risk of cancer.

Stay within ten pounds of your ideal body weight. Excess body fat stores estrogen and increases the risk of breast and uterine cancer.

*Sleep in total darkness.* Two studies suggest that light inhibits your body's production of the hormone melatonin, and lower levels of melatonin have been correlated with a higher risk of breast cancer.

**Get rid of your stress!** Stress inhibits your immune system and increases your risk for cancer.

### What Happens When a Lump Is Discovered?

If an abnormality is found on your mammogram, then ultrasound and magnetic resonance imaging (MRI) may be used to help with the diagnosis. However, since mammograms can't tell if a mass is just a benign lump or cyst or cancer, some tissue must be obtained and examined directly under a microscope. This can be done by one of three methods:

• Needle aspiration—a needle is inserted into the lump and fluid is withdrawn
   • Core biopsy—a larger needle is used to remove breast tissue
   • Removal of the lump (excisional biopsy)

Once again, remember that 90 percent of the lumps women discover are not cancerous. But if you do get a cancer diagnosis, always obtain more than one professional opinion.

Here are some of the other lessons that Marilyn learned from her experience with breast cancer:

1. Talk to breast cancer survivors to hear the many and varied scenarios they can share with you.

2. Use your personal support network for opinions, support, and love. This makes a real difference.

3. Remember, the final decision regarding your treatment is yours to make.

4. This human experience will change you in many ways spiritually. Take advantage of it. Remember the words of the great mystic Meister Eckhart: "We are not human beings here having spiritual experiences, but spiritual beings here having human experiences."

## Colon and Rectal Cancer

Colorectal cancer (cancer of the colon and/or rectum) is the third most common cause of death from cancer in middle-aged African American women. As with several other cancers, African Americans are more likely than Whites to be diagnosed with this disease. Men are more likely than women to have it. And for everyone, age is an important factor. In 1999 Supreme Court justice Ruth Bader Ginsburg, sixty-six, underwent surgery for colon cancer.

When colorectal cancer is detected before it has spread, the five-year survival rate is 92 percent. However, only about 40 percent of colorectal cancers are discovered at that stage. The five-year survival rate drops to 7 percent when it is diagnosed in an advanced stage, which is when the cancer has spread from the colon to other parts of the body such as the bones, liver, and/or brain.

Right now, the best way to prevent colorectal cancer is through a good diet low in fat, high in fruits and vegetables, and low in alcohol. Secondary prevention focuses on early detection and the removal of colonic polyps (growths) while they are in the precancerous state.[9]

**So again, the key is prevention, early diagnosis, and early treatment.** Beginning at age fifty, you should start having examinations of the colon and rectum. As we've said before, these are tests you must have done regularly, even if you feel great, nothing hurts you, and you are not sick!

### Signs and Symptoms of Colon and Rectal Cancer

A change in bowel habits is the first clue that something is wrong; constipation and diarrhea may be the first symptoms. Any bleeding, either in the stool or directly from the rectum, is a serious symptom, and you should seek medical attention right away. The most common cause of rectal bleeding is hemorrhoids, but they must be diagnosed first before you can relax. Don't assume that hemorrhoids are the cause of any rectal bleeding. Have your doctor check out the situation! Pencil-thin stools, bloating, fullness, stomach cramps, and unexplained weight loss are also symptoms that you need to have checked out. Frequently, colorectal cancer produces no symptoms and is found during a routine sigmoidoscopy or colonoscopy.

### Risk Factors for Colon Cancer

We are most susceptible to colon cancer in our middle years. The risk begins to increase after age forty, rises sharply between the ages of fifty and fifty-five, and continues to increase with age.

More than 20 percent of colon cancers are hereditary. The risk of getting colon cancer is doubled if a parent or sibling has the disorder. It is also linked to ovarian cancer and breast cancer. So if your mother had ovarian or breast cancer, you are at risk for three types of cancer: ovarian, breast, and colon.

Polyps increase your risk for developing colon cancer. Cancerous polyps and their precursors, benign polyps, may be present in the colon for years before invasive cancer develops. Reducing the number of deaths from this type of cancer depends on detecting and removing precancerous polyps at the earliest stages.

Lifestyle factors will increase your risk. Excess dietary fat, decreased fruits and vegetables, alcohol use, a sedentary lifestyle, and obesity are possible risk factors for colon or rectal cancer.

# Risk Factors for Colon Cancer

According to a recent report from the Harvard School of Public Health, about 50% of colon cancer cases could be prevented through simple lifestyle changes. For example, while a sedentary lifestyle raises your risk of colon cancer, getting just three or more hours of physical activity a week reduces your risk by about 40%, compared to getting no exercise at all. Moreover, current screening techniques, such as sigmoidoscopy, can identify early cancer, which is still treatable. And removing precancerous polyps during a sigmoidoscopy or colonoscopy can prevent the development of cancer.

The graph below illustrates the relative effects of a number of modifiable risk factors for colon cancer. For example, the risk of eating seven or more servings of red meat a week is compared to that of eating less than one serving a month, and eating five or more servings of vegetables and fruit a day is compared to eating less than three servings a day. By modifying the factors that raise the risk of colon cancer, increasing activities that offer a protective effect, and undergoing regular screening, you may lower your risk of colon cancer.

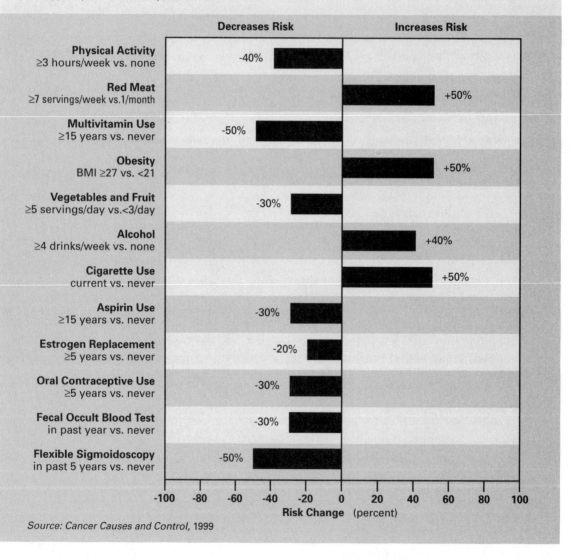

Source: Cancer Causes and Control, 1999

**℞ PRIME TIME PRESCRIPTION FOR DETECTING COLON CANCER**

Early detection and removal of colonic polyps can prevent the development of cancer in the first place. These procedures can be lifesaving, and they are not too painful and too uncomfortable to deal with. They have greatly improved from years ago. When you reach forty, you should start checking for any signs for colon cancer by taking the tests we explain in Chapter 8. You should begin these screenings earlier or have the screenings more often if you have:

- A personal history of colorectal cancer or polyps
- A personal history of chronic inflammatory bowel disease
- A personal history of breast, ovarian, or endometrial cancer
- A family history of colorectal cancer or polyps
- A family history of other inherited disorders of the colon or rectum

When colon cancer is diagnosed, survival depends on the stage of the disease at the time of diagnosis. If the tumor has spread to surrounding tissue, about 66 percent survive five years. Survival falls to about 7 percent if it has spread to distant organs, such as the liver.

Surgery is the initial treatment in all three stages. Often, chemotherapy is given afterward.

**℞ PRIME TIME PRESCRIPTIONS FOR PREVENTING COLON CANCER**

Diet, body weight, and physical activity all affect your risk for colorectal cancer. The National Cancer Institute and the American Cancer Society have issued the following guidelines for the prevention of colorectal cancer.

*Reduce fat in your diet.* A reduction of fat intake to less than 20 percent of calories has a big-time payoff. The death rate for colorectal cancer in different countries around the world is directly related to the availability of dietary fat and the consumption of high-fat diets. However, unlike heart disease, it is not clear whether specific types of fat, such as animal (saturated) or vegetable (monounsaturated and polyunsaturated) fats, influence the outcome differently.

*High-fiber diets can protect you against colon cancer.* Fiber speeds the passage of fecal material in the colon and reduces the concentration and time of exposure of the colon to carcinogens in the diet.

*Make sure you have an adequate intake of vitamins and minerals.* The

Nurses' Health Study, launched twenty-two years ago, found that women who took a daily multivitamin for at least fifteen years were 75 percent less likely to develop colon cancer than those who did not. Researchers reporting in a 1998 issue of the *Annals of Internal Medicine* suggested that the key ingredient appears to be folic acid and that the risk decreases more if this vitamin is taken in a daily supplement rather than only through food. The recommended dose is the same as for heart disease, 400 mcg daily, which is the amount in most multivitamins.

A recent study suggested that 1,500 mg of calcium per day can help prevent the development of precancerous polyps.[10] Calcium may also help prevent the development of additional polyps if you already have some. Antioxidants appear beneficial, but further study is necessary. Vitamin C, vitamin E, and selenium may protect the lining of the colon from cancer-causing damage.

*Hormone replacement therapy may significantly reduce the risk of colon cancer.* Some studies suggest that estrogen replacement in postmenopausal women reduces this cancer by 34 percent compared with women who have never had hormone therapy.

*Aspirin therapy may help.* A number of clinical and experimental studies have shown that aspirin protects against colorectal cancer by decreasing the formation of polyps. This is recommended for individuals at high risk for colon cancer, especially if this disease runs in your family.

*Regular exercise decreases the risk of colon cancer, possibly by helping to speed the stool through the colon.*

## Cervical Cancer

Although cervical cancer should have disappeared, it hasn't for Black women. Deaths of African American women from this preventable cancer still happen much too often. We are more than twice as likely to get cervical cancer, and three times more likely to die from it than White women. This is a tragedy because, when detected at an early stage, cervical cancer is one of the most successfully treatable cancers, with a five-year survival rate of 91 percent for cancers that have not spread.

Routine Pap smears detect abnormal cells even before they become cancerous. Since its discovery, the Pap smear has been responsible for a dramatic 70 percent decline in deaths from cervical cancer.

The Pap smear is a part of routine pelvic exams. It is simple and easy. (See Chapter 8 for more information on Pap smears.)

## JUDY'S STORY

Not too long ago, we buried our friend Judy. We all cried at the unnecessary loss of this smart, savvy businesswoman who was a good friend. Judy was financially solvent, practical, with sound common sense and a strong religious belief. She was loved by so many people. The people flocked to the front of the church to testify about how she had changed their lives with her wisdom, her insights into life, and her love. She had seemed totally in charge of her life.

But we buried Judy last week because of advanced cervical cancer, diagnosed only eight months before she died. Why? Why? Why? She had not had a Pap smear for *five years*. When Gayle asked her why, she sighed and simply said: "I just didn't get around to it." She was so busy taking care of her children, grandchildren, siblings, relatives, clients, and friends that there was no time or energy left for her to take care of herself.

And so we buried Judy.

## Signs and Symptoms of Cervical Cancer

Abnormal vaginal bleeding or spotting, bleeding after intercourse, and abnormal vaginal discharge are frequent symptoms. Pain and systemic symptoms are late manifestations of this disease.

## Risk Factors for Cervical Cancer

Cervical cancer risk is closely linked to sexual behavior and to sexually transmitted infections with certain types of human papilloma virus (HPV). Almost 90 percent of cervical cancer is due to HPV. It is thought that HPV produces cancer by releasing proteins that inactivate genes that suppress or keep tumors from growing. If your Pap smear is atypical or questionable, request a test for HPV. If you test positive for HPV, you should definitely have a biopsy to look for cancer. Herpes or genital warts also increase your risk for cancer. Women who began to have intercourse at an early age and have had multiple sexual partners are at increased risk. Another major risk factor is smoking.

**Rx** PRIME TIME PRESCRIPTION FOR PREVENTING CERVICAL CANCER

*Get an annual Pap smear.* Some women stop getting Pap smears after menopause despite the fact that the incidence of cervical cancer actually increases in older women. It's not safe to stop getting tested at any age. (Cost: $15 to $35.) Since one in five abnormalities are missed on standard Pap smears, some new methods that have been approved by the FDA have emerged to improve the accuracy of Pap smears. (See Chapter 8 for details.)

*Follow safe sexual practices and obtain early treatment for any venereal infections.* Safe sex consists of using condoms regularly and avoiding sexual activity with anyone who has a genital or anal sore, a visible rash, discharge, or any other sign of venereal disease.

*And as we keep saying, stop smoking.* Smokers have a higher risk of developing cervical as well as lung cancer.

## Uterine Cancer

Endometrial cancer (cancer of the lining of the uterus) is the most common cancer in the pelvic area. It is predominantly found in postmenopausal women between the ages of fifty and seventy.

### Signs of Uterine Cancer

Because it grows slowly, endometrial cancer is highly curable if detected and treated early. Symptoms are abnormal staining or bleeding (particularly in postmenopausal women). Late in the disease, patients may experience pain and weight loss.

### Risk Factors for Uterine Cancer

Your risk of developing uterine cancer is increased by diabetes, high blood pressure, and extreme obesity. Beginning menstruation before age twelve or ending menstruation after age fifty, having no pregnancies, and taking estrogen alone as hormone replacement after menopause also increase your risk, which is why hormone replacement therapy should include progestin. Nolvadex (tamoxifen), a synthetic estrogen-like hormone, also increases the risk.

**PRIME TIME PRESCRIPTION FOR DETECTING UTERINE CANCER**

The best defense is early detection through regular pelvic examinations and an immediate visit to a gynecologist if vaginal bleeding occurs after menopause. If this occurs, an endometrial biopsy should be performed. A new procedure for detecting cancer, endovaginal ultrasound (EVUS), is less invasive than a biopsy, but if that's positive, then biopsy of the lining of the uterus must be performed.

## Ovarian Cancer

Ovarian cancer is more common in White women than Black women—it is the fifth most common cancer in White women. It causes more deaths than any other cancer of the female reproductive system because it is a "silent" cancer, with no signs or symptoms until its late stages. This cancer is very difficult to diagnose early and in most cases it has spread when it is finally diagnosed.

### Symptoms of Ovarian Cancer

The symptoms of ovarian cancer are usually very vague:

- Loss of appetite, weight loss
- Fullness after even a small meal
- General discomfort in the lower abdomen

### Risk Factors for Ovarian Cancer

Postmenopausal women with a family history of ovarian cancer are at the highest risk for developing this disease. Other risk factors include:

- History of breast, uterine, or colon cancer
- Positive test for the gene BRCA1 or BRCA2
- Women who do not bear children or who have their first babies after age thirty

## Rx PRIME TIME PRESCRIPTION FOR DIAGNOSING OVARIAN CANCER

To diagnose ovarian cancer, multiple tests are usually performed:

- Ultrasound of the abdomen and transvaginal ultrasound
- CT scan
- Intravenous pyelogram (IVP) of the kidneys
- Lower gastrointestinal series (X rays of the lower abdomen)

A blood test is being developed that may help detect ovarian cancer at its earliest and most treatable stage. CA-125 levels in the blood are elevated in ovarian cancer patients; however, CA-125 can be elevated in people who do not have ovarian cancer. Lysophosphatidic acid (LPA) levels were significantly higher in patients with ovarian cancer than in healthy women, in a study reported in the *Journal of the American Medical Association* in August 1998. Ninety percent of the women in the earliest stages of ovarian cancer had elevated LPA. This test appears to be more specific than CA-125 for ovarian cancer.

## WHERE ARE WE HEADED IN THE TREATMENT OF CANCER?

Medical experts are predicting that cancer will be the number one cause of death in this century, surpassing heart disease. Clearly, we need to be more committed than ever to prevention and early detection and treatment. Now that you know about the different risks and how to lower yours, you can save your own life and help your sisters save theirs. Here's how:

1. Help disseminate information about cancer. We all need to be better informed and eliminate as many fears, misconceptions, and inaccurate bits of information as possible. So it's important that you initiate discussions about cancer whenever you have the opportunity to clear up misperceptions—in church, at the beauty parlor, at sorority meetings, at club events, and wherever else you can. Encourage others to do the same.

2. Advocate for quality care for everyone.

3. Advocate for improved and better testing methods, especially since mammography is less accurate for women under forty.

4. Demand that African American women be included in new cancer studies. Call your local chapter of the American Cancer Society or the National Institutes of Health to express your concern. See Resources for contact information.

# Chapter 12

# DEALING WITH DIABETES

*My mother lived with diabetes for many years. It took her sight. But for her, and our family, education was the key to her living successfully with this disease. And because she had all the available facts about this disease, she was able to live a long, and productive life.*

— Gladys Knight, quoted in *Heart and Soul*, December 1997

Gladys Knight lost her mother, Elizabeth Knight, from the complications of diabetes. She also has a brother and cousin (one of her legendary backup singers in the Pips) who have been diagnosed with diabetes. So to support research and awareness programs in communities across the country, Gladys established the American Diabetes Association Elizabeth Knight Fund in memory of her mother.

We wanted to begin this section on diabetes by thanking Gladys Knight for this gift. Diabetes affects African American women so disproportionately that it has become the number one disease causing blindness, kidney ailments, and amputations of feet and legs in Black women. It is now the fourth leading cause of death among African American women and the sixth among Black men.[1] Here are the facts:

• The National Center for Health Statistics reports that diagnosed diabetes in African Americans has increased fourfold in two decades.[2] This is twice the rate of increase among White Americans.

• Diabetes has increased in the United States as obesity has increased.

• Of African American women in our age group, one in every four has diabetes—which is double the rate of White women. At this level, diabetes is reaching epidemic rates among Black women.

- Only 19 percent of Black men in this age range are diabetic.
- Black women are twice as likely as all other women to develop the complications associated with diabetes: heart disease, stroke, kidney failure, blindness, and amputation of our legs and feet.
- Compared to White women, Black women are three times more likely to be blind and four times more likely to have kidney failure.
- Black diabetics undergo twice as many amputations as do Whites.
- Depression occurs three times more often in diabetic women than in diabetic men.

It doesn't have to be this way for African American women. We can do something about diabetes. We can reduce our risk for it and reduce its severity if we do develop it.

As critical as the statistics above is the fact that half of the women who have diabetes don't know it! Could you be one of them? When you factor in the undiagnosed cases, our diabetes rates start becoming stratospheric.

Why are so many women unaware they have this disease? According to Dr. James Gavin, chairman of the American Diabetes Association's African American Program, many people with diabetes don't exhibit any symptoms until a life-threatening complication such as a heart attack, stroke, and/or kidney failure occurs. That's why having a "touch of sugar" is nothing to shrug off lightly.

---

## COULD YOU HAVE DIABETES AND NOT KNOW IT?
### Take the test. Know the score.

To find out if you are at risk, write in the points (in parentheses) next to each statement that is true for you. If a statement is not true, put a zero. Add your total score.

| | | | |
|---|---|---|---|
| 1. | My weight is equal to or above that listed in the chart below. | Yes (5) | ___ |
| 2. | I am under sixty-five years of age and I get little or no exercise during a usual day. | Yes (5) | ___ |
| 3. | I am between forty-five and sixty-four years of age. | Yes (5) | ___ |
| 4. | I am sixty-five years old or older. | Yes (9) | ___ |
| 5. | I had a baby weighing more than nine pounds at birth. | Yes (1) | ___ |

| 6. | I have a sister or a brother with diabetes. | Yes (1) ___ |
|---|---|---|
| 7. | I have a parent with diabetes. | Yes (1) ___ |
| | | TOTAL ___ |

SCORING

3 to 9 points: You are probably at low risk for having diabetes now. New guidelines recommend that everyone age forty-five and over should consider being tested for the disease every three years.

10 or more points: You are at high risk for having diabetes. Only a doctor can determine if you have diabetes. See a doctor soon and find out for sure.

*Source:* Developed by the American Diabetes Association.

# At-risk Weight Chart

**HEIGHT (without shoes)**

| 4'10" | 4'11" | 5'0" | 5'1" | 5'2" | 5'3" | 5'4" | 5'5" | 5'6" | 5'7" | 5'8" | 5'9" | 5'10" | 5'11" | 6'0" | 6'1" | 6'2" | 6'3" | 6'4" |
|---|---|---|---|---|---|---|---|---|---|---|---|---|---|---|---|---|---|---|
| 129 | 133 | 138 | 143 | 147 | 152 | 157 | 162 | 167 | 172 | 177 | 182 | 188 | 193 | 199 | 204 | 210 | 216 | 221 |

**BODY WEIGHT IN POUNDS (without clothes)**

## WHAT IS DIABETES?

Diabetes is a disorder in which your levels of blood sugar (glucose) are abnormally high. People develop diabetes when either their bodies don't produce enough insulin (which is made by the pancreas) or the insulin they make doesn't do its job. Insulin is a hormone that allows blood sugar to enter our cells and generate energy that fuels our body. When there isn't enough insulin or the insulin is malfunctioning, the simple sugar glucose cannot get into the cells to produce the fuel we need.

There are two major types of diabetes. *Type 1 diabetes* occurs when the pancreas doesn't produce enough insulin. This form of the disease usually begins in childhood, and sufferers must take daily shots of insulin to survive. *Type 2 diabetes* occurs in individuals who usually make enough insulin, but whose body is having problems using it correctly. Type 2 accounts for 95 percent of all diabetes cases and is more common in African Americans, Hispanics, Native Americans, and Native Hawaiians than Caucasians. The onset of Type 2 diabetes usually occurs in adults over forty-five years old, which is why we must pay close attention to this disease in our Prime Time years.

## WARNING SIGNS OF DIABETES

The symptoms of diabetes may begin gradually and are hard to identify at first. Warning signs include:
- *Excessive thirst*
- *Frequent urination, especially at night*
- *Extreme hunger*
- *Unexplained weight loss*
- *Fatigue or unusual tiredness (We know you're thinking: "Oh, my God, I'm always tired! Could I have diabetes?" We're all tired—all the time. But this fatigue is more pronounced and severe and does not let up with rest.)*
- *Nausea and vomiting*
- *Tingling in fingers*
- *Urinary tract infections*
- *Vaginal itching, perhaps an increase in vaginal infections*
- *Sores that are slow to heal*

These symptoms do not mean you have diabetes, but if you have any of these problems, you must see your doctor for an appropriate workup.

## WHAT DO YOU KNOW ABOUT DIABETES?

1. Eating too much sugar causes diabetes.
TRUE          FALSE
2. Sugary foods are off-limits for people with diabetes.
TRUE          FALSE

Both are false. But don't feel bad if you got either of them wrong. According to experts, many doctors do, too.

Myth 1: Eating too much sugar causes diabetes.

Fact: *Sugar per se has nothing to do with it. Excess calories and inactivity are the problem. At least 80 percent of those with Type 2 diabetes are overweight.*

> Myth 2: Sugar and sugary foods are off-limits for people with diabetes.
> Fact: *Carbohydrates in general raise blood sugar, and sugar is only one type of carbohydrate. With diabetes you must count how many grams of carbohydrate you eat, not how many grams of sugar. Carbohydrates are in milk, fruits, desserts, rice, cereal, and so on.*

## RISK FACTORS FOR DIABETES

**Age, sex, weight, physical activity, diet, and family health history** all affect our chances of developing diabetes. While we can't change family history, age, sex, or race, we can do a lot to control our weight, diet, and physical fitness.

**Being overweight, not exercising, and having high blood pressure** are three primary risk factors for diabetes. Unfortunately, 50 percent of Black women are considered overweight, compared to only 33 percent of our White counterparts, and 67 percent of Black women report that they do very little physical activity, according to a study published in the *Archives of Internal Medicine* in 1998. The location of the excess weight is also a factor for Type 2 diabetes; excess weight carried above the waist is a stronger risk factor than excess weight carried below the waist.

**Taking antihypertension medicine** (particularly beta blockers) can increase your risk for diabetes.[3]

Your doctor will also want more information about your pregnancies if he or she is concerned that you have diabetes. Two particular risk factors are having given birth to a baby weighing more than nine pounds and a history of high sugar levels in your blood during one of your pregnancies, even though it returned to normal after delivery.

**Rx** PRIME TIME PRESCRIPTION FOR PREVENTING DIABETES

*Find out if your family has a history of diabetes,* since this disease truly runs in families.

*Get tested for diabetes.* All adults forty-five years and older should be tested for diabetes every three years. For higher-risk African American women—those who are overweight and have a family history—testing should begin at a younger age and be done more frequently.

A doctor will diagnose diabetes by looking for four kinds of evidence:

• *Risk factors such as excess weight and a family history of diabetes*

• *Symptoms such as the ones we listed on page 275, especially thirst and frequent urination*

• *Complications such as heart disease*

• *Signs of excess sugar in your blood and urine*

**Control your weight and reduce fat in your diet.** Not only should you limit the total number of calories you take in, but you must diligently reduce the fat calories you consume. That's because the more fat there is in the diet, the harder time insulin has in getting sugar into the cell. Minimizing your intake of fat helps insulin do its job better.

**Increase the amount of grains and vegetables you eat.** Developing better eating habits will be easier if you know how to prepare tasty foods without the life-threatening fat and sugar that are found in so many of our favorite recipes. That's why the American Diabetes Association published the *New Soul Food Cookbook for People with Diabetes.* To order, call 800-ADA-ORDER (800-232-6733).

**Get up and move around.** Regular physical activity is also a protective factor against Type 2 diabetes. Thirty minutes of aerobic exercise daily helps weight control, helps the sugar to enter the cells, lowers your blood pressure, and builds a healthy heart.

---

## TESTS FOR DIABETES

**Test for sugar in your urine:** This is performed during a routine test of your urine. However, the results of this test alone are not enough to make the diagnosis of diabetes.

**Fasting blood sugar:** A test for the sugar level in your blood in the morning after ten to twelve hours of fasting.

Normally, the sugar in a person's blood rises quickly after eating something with sugar in it (often called a *sugar load*) and then falls gradually again as insulin signals the body to metabolize the sugar. In someone with diabetes, the blood sugar rises and remains high after consumption of the sugar load because of a lack of insulin from the pancreas or an inability to use a normal amount of insulin appropriately.

The following two tests detect diabetes even when a simple blood test for sugar does not. In these tests, blood sugar is measured before and at specific times after a person has consumed a certain amount of sugar.

---

> **Two-hour postprandial blood test.** This test may be performed two hours after eating or after consuming a special sugar solution. A diagnosis is made if the value at two hours is 200 mg/dL or more. Glucose levels below 140 mg/dL are normal. Between 140 and 200 mg/dL, you should be watched carefully.
>
> **Oral glucose tolerance test.** This measures multiple blood sugars at specific times over a six-hour period after the sugar load has been given. Fasting blood glucose is normally less than 110 mg/dL. If it is above 125 mg/dL on at least two tests, a diagnosis of diabetes is made. If values are between 110 mg/dL and 125 mg/dL, your condition should be followed closely.

## R̽ PRIME TIME PRESCRIPTION IF YOU HAVE DIABETES

Implementing all of the above prescriptions will minimize complications and improve control of your illness. For example, regular exercise can frequently reduce the need for insulin injections and oral medications.

*Keep your medical appointments faithfully.* A critical part of controlling diabetes is regular checkups and examinations. Annual eye exams (even if you're not having any problems) are absolutely crucial to prevent blindness. Also, having your feet and legs examined regularly for sores, infection, and sensation is essential to help prevent future problems. Because diabetics suffer from circulatory problems (especially in their feet and legs), they can lose sensation in these extremities. This is why diabetics sometimes don't notice sores until they become infected. Even when treated, sores on diabetics are more difficult to heal, which also promotes infection.

You should receive special training on how to care for your feet to prevent sores that don't heal properly, become infected, or develop gangrene. Infections and gangrene are two reasons why some diabetics get their toes, feet, or lower legs amputated. If you take care of your feet (remember the power of self-care we discussed earlier?) and are examined regularly, you can reduce the risk of amputation by 70 percent. Some doctors recommend special shoes to prevent sores, and don't worry about how you look in "those shoes."

*Monitor your blood sugar and understand what it means to have your diabetes under control.* Consult your doctor about the variety of tests used to monitor blood sugar, and learn how to take and read the test he or she recommends. Controlling your blood sugar and hemoglobin A1c will decrease the chance of complications.[4]

# DIABETES EXAMINATION SCHEDULE AND CHECKLISTS

*During every visit you must:*
- *Have your weight and blood pressure taken*
- *Have your feet examined*
- *Review your self-monitoring blood glucose record*
- *Review self-management skills, dietary needs, and physical activity*
- *Discuss recommendations to help you lose weight, exercise, and give up smoking*
- *Review the medications you are taking*

*Twice a year you must:*
- *Get your hemoglobin A1c checked. HbA1c or glycohemoglobin measures the amount of glucose attached to hemoglobin in the red blood cells. The amount of glucose attached to hemoglobin increases as the blood glucose level rises. This test helps determine how well your diabetes is being controlled.*

*Once a year you must:*
- *Schedule the following annual tests: fasting lipid profile, serum creatinine, urinalysis for protein and microalbumin*
- *Monitor any damage to the kidneys (if you have kidney abnormalities, you should see a kidney specialist). Twenty percent of people with Type 2 diabetes develop kidney damage. The first sign is small amounts of the protein albumin in the urine.*
- *Have your eyes examined by an ophthalmologist (your eyes must be dilated so that the entire retina can be examined). Diabetic retinopathy is damage to the retina (back of the eye that transmits visual images to the brain) and is the leading cause of blindness among adults in the United States. Keeping your blood sugar low significantly reduces your risk of developing retinopathy. As reported in the August 1999 issue of* Diabetes Care, *high doses of vitamin E (over 1,000 IU) may prevent blindness and kidney damage due to diabetes.*
- *Schedule your dental and foot exams*
- *Get your Influenza (flu) vaccine*

## CONTROL GOALS

| LEVEL OF CONTROL | Hemoglobin A1c |
|---|---|
| Excellent | <7% |
| Good | <8% |
| Take action | >8% |
| SELF-MONITORING BLOOD GLUCOSE | |
| Preprandial glucose goal: | 80–120 mg/dL |
| Bedtime goal: | 100–140 mg/dL |

*Learn about all aspects of your disease and diligently follow your prescribed treatment plan.* Be a complete partner with your physician in the management of your disease. The more you know and do, the better you will be able to control your diabetes.[5] Self-management is critical if you want to control this disease. That means exercising, monitoring your diet, monitoring your blood sugar, and keeping up with your scheduled checkups and self-exams.[6]

*Join a support group.* Remember the 1998 movie *Soul Food?* It highlighted how for us, soul food is truly "food for our soul." However, as we know, much of what we eat as soul food is not good for our bodies, especially if we have diabetes. The matriarch character in this movie had diabetes, and there was no evidence that she was trying to take charge of her illness; certainly her family, by encouraging weekly food orgies disguised as Sunday dinner, was not helping her control it.

Many families are like the one in the movie, loving each other to death. That's why getting support from others who are successfully controlling their diabetes can be very helpful in your struggle.[7] Fortunately, Elizabeth Knight had Gladys and the rest of her family to help her manage her disease. Whom do you have?

Diabetic support groups share information, advice, experience, and tough love. This is the type of support and motivation you'll need to keep your diabetes in check. Will your family or Prime Time Circle be knowledgeable or objective enough to keep you on track? Even if they will be, call the local chapter of the American Diabetes Association or a local hospital to find a diabetic support group near you.

# PART V

# Staying Sane in a World that Can Seem Insane

# Chapter 13

# STRESS CAN BE MANAGED

*Did you ever wonder why so many sisters look so angry? Why we walk like we've bricks in our bags and will slash and curse you at the drop of a hat? It's because stress is hemmed into our dresses, pressed into our hair, mixed into our perfume and painted on our fingers. Stress from deferred dreams, the dreams not voiced; stress from the broken promises, the blatant lies; stress from always being at the bottom, from never being thought beautiful, from always being taken for granted, taken advantage of; stress from being a black woman in white America.*

—Opal Palmer Adisa, quoted in Evelyn White, ed., *The Black Woman's Health Book*

Unfortunately for many Black women, all of the points writer Opal Palmer Adisa makes ring true. But we could also add one more: Maybe we're stressed because we can't even imagine not being chronically stressed. Consider these poignant words from Iyanla Vanzant's *The Value in the Valley*: "Many black women have become so accustomed to hard times and bad situations, we think that is all life has to offer."

Far too many African American women seem to believe consciously or unconsciously that our lives must be filled with a variety of difficult, traumatic, or burdensome events over which we have no control. While it's true that we can't control major stress-inducing events such as the death of our spouse or partner or whether our employer is moving to Mexico, we can learn to make better decisions about our everyday lives. We can choose what we eat, how we manage our time and money, how much we indulge our adult children, and how often we exercise or pamper ourselves with a relaxing bath or a good book. We can choose how much we use our Prime Time Sister and Prime Time Circle for support.

In fact, the situations that are most apt to spike our blood pressure or drive us crazy are those over which we do have some degree of control—but we deny, minimize, or fail to appreciate the impact of these circumstances on the quality and length of our lives.

The passage though the middle years can be particularly challenging and stressful for African American women. To gauge just how stressful this time period is for you, please take a few minutes to fill out the test that follows. We developed and administered the Black Women's Midlife Stress Test questionnaire to more than two hundred African American women between the ages of forty and seventy.

## BLACK WOMEN'S MIDLIFE STRESS TEST

Below is a list of thirty-one different typical life events that midlife women have identified as potentially stressful. Please read each one carefully and consider how each one makes you feel. After reading each item on the list, check the most appropriate answer with respect to how that event has affected your life over the past twenty-four months. This isn't a test to be scored. It will help you identify the areas in your life that you find most stressful. This information will help you develop a stress management program.

| EVENT | DOES NOT APPLY | NOT STRESSFUL | SOMEWHAT STRESSFUL | VERY STRESSFUL |
|---|---|---|---|---|
| 1. DEATH OF A SPOUSE/PARTNER | | | | |
| 2. DEATH OF A CHILD | | | | |
| 3. DIVORCE | | | | |
| 4. DEATH OF A FAMILY MEMBER | | | | |
| 5. PERSONAL ILLNESS/INJURY | | | | |
| 6. DEATH OF A CLOSE FRIEND | | | | |
| 7. INJURY/ILLNESS OF A FAMILY MEMBER | | | | |
| 8. SUBSTANCE ABUSE BY AN ADULT CHILD | | | | |
| 9. ARREST OR INCARCERATION OF AN ADULT CHILD | | | | |
| 10. BEING A SINGLE PARENT | | | | |
| 11. PRIMARY CARE RESPONSIBILITIES | | | | |
| 12. CARETAKING OF PARENTS OR OLDER RELATIVES | | | | |
| 13. RELATIONSHIP WITH SPOUSE OR PARTNER | | | | |

| EVENT | DOES NOT APPLY | NOT STRESSFUL | SOMEWHAT STRESSFUL | VERY STRESSFUL |
|---|---|---|---|---|
| 14. LACK OF A ROMANTIC RELATIONSHIP | | | | |
| 15. RELATIONSHIP WITH CHILDREN | | | | |
| 16. RELATIONSHIP WITH OTHER FAMILY MEMBERS | | | | |
| 17. RELATIONSHIP WITH FRIEND(S) | | | | |
| 18. DIFFICULTY FINDING SUITABLE EMPLOYMENT | | | | |
| 19. RACIAL/SEXUAL DISCRIMINATION AT WORK | | | | |
| 20. ONLY BLACK FEMALE ADMINISTRATOR | | | | |
| 21. DIFFICULTY WITH COWORKERS | | | | |
| 22. DIFFICULTY WITH BOSS | | | | |
| 23. RETIREMENT | | | | |
| 24. FINANCIAL DIFFICULTIES | | | | |
| 25. RETURNING TO SCHOOL | | | | |
| 26. CHANGING JOBS | | | | |
| 27. COMMUNITY ORGANIZATION/ RELIGIOUS OBLIGATIONS | | | | |
| 28. ADULT CHILD RETURNS TO LIVE IN HOUSE | | | | |
| 29. CHANGES IN PHYSICAL APPEARANCE | | | | |
| 30. NONIMMEDIATE FAMILY OR FRIENDS LIVING IN HOUSE | | | | |
| 31. COMMUNITY VIOLENCE | | | | |

The results of the discussions with the women who took the stress test confirmed what Gayle and her colleagues are hearing in their private practices: African American women in midlife identify stress as their number one emotional health concern. When asked what stresses them, Black women's answers are surprisingly consistent:

1. *We are concerned about what our adult children are doing or not doing*—such as abusing drugs, staying in relationships that we think are harmful to them, not taking care of their physical and spiritual needs, not being financially responsible, or not providing consistent and adequate care for their own children.

2. *We often have financial difficulties that are related to how much money we lend to, give to, or spend on our adult children.*

3. *We want to be in a positive, nurturing romantic relationship or we're currently in a difficult relationship.*

4. *We are concerned about our relationships with our coworkers and our boss. We are apprehensive about sex, race, and age discrimination at work.*

5. *We are worried that changes in our physical appearance as we age will make us less attractive and desirable.*

6. *We are concerned about our physical and emotional health and that of our family and friends.*

Another stress point for Black women is how conflicted we feel after interacting with our loved ones—feelings that often center around guilt, anger, and anxiety that stem from our difficulty in putting our needs first, even when our needs (such as a pressing health concern or a problem at work) are more critical than our family's or friends' difficulties.

---

## BARBARA'S STORY

Barbara is a fifty-seven-year-old divorcee. She has three adult children in their thirties—Renee, John, and Robert. All three have their own children. Over the years, Barbara has been very emotionally and financially supportive of her children and grandchildren.

Unfortunately, Barbara has hypertension and within the last two years has started suffering from headaches and lower back pain. Too tired to think about dieting or starting an exercise program, Barbara has gained more than forty unwanted pounds in the last year.

Barbara works as a supervisor in a very demanding post office station and frequently works overtime by both choice and necessity. Her physician thinks most of her physical complaints are stress-related and has recommended that she lose weight, exercise, reduce her hours at work, and learn to relax. The doctor has warned Barbara that if she does not take these steps, she will increase her risk of having a stroke or a heart attack. Although Barbara is anxious about not heeding her doctor's suggestions, she's worried about the impact on her cash flow if she stops working overtime. Barbara earns a decent salary, but her savings are meager—primarily because of her loans to her kids. Barbara does not share her health information with her family because she doesn't want to worry them.

Barbara's oldest daughter, Renee, is thirty-eight, is single, and has two children, a sixteen-year-old son and a thirteen-year-old daughter. Renee dropped out of school when she became pregnant with her son, and she recently informed her mother that she wants to go back to college. She wants to move in with Barbara, who lives in a small, three-bedroom house, so that she can save money. Renee also wants Barbara to watch the kids while she attends night school. Barbara feels very stressed and conflicted about the request. She was disappointed when Renee became pregnant and dropped out of college and was quite upset when Renee had a second child. Nonetheless, Barbara loves her daughter and grandchildren very much and has prayed that Renee would go back to college, so she wants to be supportive.

Barbara thinks fleetingly about her own health and the difficulty of relaxing with two teenagers living in the house. She realizes that she's too old and too tired to baby-sit her grandchildren, but she keeps asking herself: Isn't that what mothers and grandmothers are supposed to do? Barbara starts to feel guilty even thinking about saying no and quickly hugs her daughter and agrees to let her move in.

---

How often does a scenario similar to Barbara's play out across Black America? Many African American women like Barbara continue to accept additional responsibilities and burdens long after they are emotionally or physically unable to manage them effectively. Although we know many of our sisters would vehemently deny this, we believe that Black women often choose to bring additional stress into our lives. As Iyanla Vanzant writes in *The Value in the Valley*, we must "be honest enough to say what [we] will do, won't do, can do, cannot do."

Whatever your reasons for continuing to live with stress and not deal with it, you have to open your mind and reevaluate these reasons, because as good, noble, unselfish, and loving as those reasons may be, they are killing you. The negative, cumulative effect of stress on your emotional and physical well-being is undeniable and devastating, from increasing your risk of feeling depressed or anxious to decreasing your immune system's ability to fight off physical ailments ranging from colds to cancer.

## WHAT IS STRESS?

Stress is our inner mental, physical, and emotional response to external demands or pressures. We can feel stress from both positive and negative events. In fact, some degree of stress is a normal part of living. Many life events, though stressful, can be wonderful, such as getting a college degree at fifty, starting your own business, or retiring from your job. However, Dr. Hans Selye, often called the father of stress research, distinguished between favorable stressful events, which he called *eustress*, and adverse ones, *distress*.

Dr. Selye found that prolonged or recurrent exposure to distressing experiences—such as caring for a terminally ill parent, the boss repeatedly insisting that you work overtime, ongoing serious arguments with your spouse/partner—can be detrimental to your emotional and physical health and well-being. When we use the term *stressors* throughout this chapter, we are referring to these types of negative, traumatic, overwhelming situations.

The signs of stress can be very subtle. You might notice only a slight headache, but the internal physiological reactions, depending on the stressor, can be dramatic.

---

### THE MOST COMMON EMOTIONAL SIGNS OF STRESS

- *Tension/anxiety*
- *Anger*
- *Reclusiveness*
- *Pessimism/cynicism*
- *Boredom*
- *Irritability*
- *Resentment*
- *Inattentiveness*

---

### FREQUENT PHYSICAL SYMPTOMS OF STRESS

- *Recurrent headaches*
- *Fatigue*
- *Insomnia*

---

- *Digestive problems*
- *Skin problems*
- *Neck/back pain*
- *Loss of appetite*
- *Overeating/obesity*

When you perceive you are in danger (whether emotional or physical) your usual reaction is a fight-or-flight response, which has three stages.

## Phase 1: Alarm

To prepare the body for action, the adrenal glands produce hormones (adrenaline and noradrenaline) that cause your blood pressure and heart rate to increase and your muscles to tighten, which leaves you feeling excited or frightened. Dr. Christiane Northrup, author of *Women's Bodies, Women's Wisdom,* refers to the adrenal glands as our "shock absorbers." Some women respond quickly to a situation by producing a lot of stress hormones quickly, while others tend to respond much more slowly. Dr. Northrup explains that when we are exposed to several negative stressors at once, for extended periods of time, the glands' ability to secrete and monitor appropriate hormonal levels can become compromised. When this happens, it's very difficult for your body to calm down between stressful events— even when the stressor is no longer threatening.

Following the story of our friend Barbara after her daughter's family moved in can shed some light on just how ongoing multiple stressors ready the body for action and eventually trigger uncomfortable physical reactions. You've probably had days when you felt just like Barbara. We certainly have had our share.

### BARBARA'S STORY (CONTINUED)

As Barbara got out of her car, she could hear the music blaring. Teenagers! She had asked them repeatedly to keep the music down. But after a long, difficult day at work filled with arguing staff and complaining customers, Barbara didn't have the energy to ask them once more. Reacting to the noise, she could feel her muscles tensing up as she opened the door. She was starting to get a headache, and her heart felt as if it was racing.

---

## Phase 2: Resistance

During the second phase of stress, your body attempts to recover from a state of alarm and repair any damage caused by the stress. The brain tries to understand the stressor and figure out how to avoid it in the future. However, if the stressful situation continues, your body won't have time to rest, recover, and replenish itself. The immune system starts reducing its activity in an attempt to increase your energy flow.

Unfortunately for our friend Barbara, the ongoing confrontations with her grandchildren and long hours at work were beginning to take their toll.

---

### BARBARA'S STORY (CONTINUED)

When Barbara opened the door, the house was a mess. Dishes and teenagers were everywhere. She had asked her grandchildren not to bring anyone to the house when there was no adult at home, but the kids always had a reason why Omar, LaShonda, Amir, and Shaneequa had to be at their house.

Barbara hated to start fussing as soon as she walked through the door, but she was angry that her grandchildren had broken the rules. Even though Barbara insisted that the visitors leave, her grandchildren begged her to let their friends stay until their favorite television program was over, and they promised to clean up once everyone had gone. Barbara argued with them for a few minutes, then finally gave in and went to her bedroom.

---

## Phase 3: Exhaustion

The final stage of unrelenting stress is when our internal resources are depleted and more obvious and sometimes damaging emotional and physical symptoms start to appear. It is at this stage when stressed-out women often try to alleviate their emotional and physical discomfort by adopting inappropriate behavior, such as

- Smoking
- Substance abuse—alcohol and other drugs
- Excessive gambling
- Overspending

Feeling overwhelmed by her out-of-control home situation, Barbara could no longer find appropriate ways to relieve her never-ending tension. Instead of heeding her doctor's advice, Barbara tried to find comfort in unhealthy habits and thought about smoking to calm her nerves.

## BARBARA'S STORY (CONTINUED)

After closing her bedroom door, Barbara started craving a cigarette for the first time in ten years. Her head was pounding and she felt totally drained. As she drank a soda to wash down a handful of potato chips that she had grabbed on the way to her room, Barbara realized that she was too exhausted, frustrated, and angry even to fix herself a decent meal. Despite her overwhelming sense of fatigue, Barbara was unable to fall asleep.

### Rx QUICK PRIME TIME PRESCRIPTION FOR BARBARA

Barbara didn't realize until a few months after her daughter's family moved in what a serious mistake she had made. After getting dizzy at work, Barbara went to see her doctor. He was concerned that her blood pressure was so high and that she had gained ten more pounds. That's when Barbara realized she needed to reclaim her home and start taking better care of herself.

Our first recommendation for Barbara was to start thinking of herself as a miracle of God who has the right and responsibility to take care of her own emotional, physical, and spiritual needs. To help her reframe her thinking, she began each day reading one of the meditations in Iyanla Vanzant's *Acts of Faith: Meditations for People of Color* or reviewing some of the tenets in Debrena Jackson Gandy's book *Sacred Pampering Principles: An*

*African-American Woman's Guide to Self-Care and Inner Renewal.* Both books help Barbara stay appropriately focused on herself.

Barbara also identified a Prime Time Sister and developed a Prime Time Circle of Sisterfriends. One of their main purposes is to remind her that one of the most important parental responsibilities is helping children develop into self-reliant, responsible adults. Barbara will need their moral support and common sense to develop and implement a plan to reclaim her home from her daughter and grandchildren. (To get started, Barbara will give her daughter a deadline to move out as soon as her classes end for the semester.)

Barbara also plans to use her company's employee assistance program to find free or low-cost financial counseling, stress management and assertiveness training/workshops, and weight and exercise support groups. You can find this information, too, in the Resources section in *Prime Time.*

Barbara's decision to ignore her health needs increased her feelings of anger and sadness, which made her even more vulnerable to stress and major health complications.

Everyday stressors, from traffic jams to washing the dishes, take a cumulative toll on our health. The stressors that seem to evoke the most intense, destructive responses are events that are life-threatening to ourselves or our family members, intentionally violent (especially acts of sexual violence), or unexpected, uncontrollable, and multiple (such as the death of a spouse soon after you have been diagnosed with cancer).

A number of studies have documented that significant life changes—death of a spouse or family member, divorce, major work difficulties, involuntary decrease in financial status—increase the prevalence of illness or sudden death. Racial minorities are more apt to be exposed to violence, unexpected illness or death, work difficulties, and financial concerns.

## RISK FACTORS THAT MAKE MIDLIFE PARTICULARLY STRESSFUL FOR AFRICAN AMERICAN WOMEN

Sex, age, race, personality, socioeconomic status, and childhood conditioning are probably the most potent determinants of what stresses us and how we cope with life events, good and bad. For instance, Black women who experience sexual harassment from a Black male colleague or supervisor are more reluctant to report it to a White supervisor than to a Black female supervisor.

Let's explore some of the factors that influence our ability to handle everyday stress.

## Personality

There is increasing evidence that your behavioral and emotional characteristics influence how you respond to stress. After surveying numerous post-heart-attack patients, San Francisco cardiologists Drs. Meyer Friedman and Ray Rosenman studied patients who appeared to be more vulnerable to coronary disease. The most vulnerable patients were folks who tended to respond to any stressor with anger, competitiveness, impatience, increased blood pressure, and a rapid heart rate. The doctors referred to these individuals as *type A personalities*. Type A's struggle incessantly to achieve more and more in less and less time. On the other hand, patients who seemed more relaxed, more cooperative, more optimistic, more even-tempered, less aggressive, and less competitive were not as susceptible to cardiovascular disease. People with these characteristics were described as having *type B personalities*.[1]

Although type A characteristics are usually associated with men, many women also exhibit them. Type A men usually expend most of their energy on their profession, while type A women attempt to give their personal and professional lives the same amount of time and attention. The stereotypical strong Black woman would certainly be described as a type A personality— she would expect and be expected to do it all. These women are often considered to have an attitude (which often seems to be hostile). Some wear this hostile attitude as if it were a badge of honor. Does this sound like anyone you know? (For advice on how to reduce or eliminate your anger and attitude problems, see Chapter 6.)

## Childhood Experiences

Individuals raised in homes where there was a high degree of chaos, tension, anger, parental conflict, domestic violence, or parental substance abuse are often very vulnerable to stress-related physical and psychological difficulties. According to Dr. Frank Treiber of the Medical College of Georgia, people whose blood pressure rises as a result of stress are likely to have been raised by parents who were often irritable, tense, argumentative, or unstable.[2]

Children who experienced a high degree of fear, neglect, physical or sexual abuse, death of a parent, or divorce can find it difficult to feel comfortable as adults without a high degree of stress. Dr. Jay Gidd of the National Institutes of Health believes the young child's brain is very responsive to the environment, and his writings stress that the brain can "become hardwired to deal with high fear states . . . As adults, these children feel empty or bored if they're not on edge."[3]

## Racism

Most midlife African American women grew up experiencing some degree of racism, which sometimes intensifies our reactions to even routine stressors such as a rude salesperson in a store. Sensitive about how we are treated by others, especially Caucasians, many Black women automatically interpret a salesperson's rudeness as racism, which triggers an internal fight-or-flight physical reaction. That's because those of us who experienced daily or recurrent acts of discrimination as children learned to suppress our anger even when we are boiling over inside. For instance, Marilyn and her African American classmates could only swim in her high-school pool on Friday afternoons. The pool was drained and cleaned on Friday evenings, and thus the Caucasian students who swam daily didn't have to swim in water used by Blacks. Every summer as a young girl, Gayle visited relatives who lived in the South. She was forced to sit in the back of the bus no matter how empty the bus was.

Women our age also remember being extremely frightened and angry when we heard about or witnessed acts of race-engendered assaults (verbal and physical) on African American leaders and Freedom Fighters. The murder of fourteen-year-old Emmett Till and the bombing deaths in an Alabama church of four young girls—Addie Mae Collins, Denise McNair, Cheryl Robinson, and Cynthia Wellsberg—shattered any myth about the safety of Black children and childhood. Some of us believed that Whites in general or at least segregationists would kill us simply because we were Black.

The chronic, suppressed race-related anger and anxiety experienced by many African American women and men in childhood often continue into adulthood. Contemporary acts of prejudice and discrimination—from cab drivers refusing to pick us up to never being invited to the Super Bowl party given by colleagues at work—can be insidious and damaging, but more difficult to identify or legislate. However, the destructive impacts on our emotional, physical, and social health are all too obvious. These impacts include our rage or attitude, which sometimes seems disproportionate to the precipitating event; our dramatic rates of adult hypertension; and a tendency by many of us to attribute most, if not all, of our individual and collective stress to racism.[4]

## Socioeconomic Status

While it's probably true that money can't buy happiness, it certainly influences the quantity and types of stressors to which we are exposed. Poverty increases the likelihood that we will have inadequate health care, poor housing and schools, violence in our neighborhoods, and meager community resources. Poverty also decreases the likelihood that we will have access to social and institutional networks that can truly change our level of vulnerability to chronic stressors. Women with lower incomes and poor education often have multiple stressors and higher rates of disease and death. Since minority women constitute the poorest adult segment of our population, it is understandable why their high level of stress is related to their economic condition.

## THE BIG SIX STRESSORS FOR BLACK WOMEN

Earlier in this chapter, we listed six major concerns that African American women identified when they took our Black Women's Midlife Stress Test. Exploring each of these concerns plus some others we've identified over the years provides some insight into the kinds of issues that are most problematic for us. To help explore these concerns, we divided our stress triggers into six areas: relationships, personal illness/injury, loss, work, financial issues, and physical appearance.

## Relationships

At some time, every relationship goes through stressful periods. Even happily married women, like several of our friends who've been married for more than forty years and who have successful, happy, and well-adjusted adult children, would readily agree with the title of Langston Hughes' poem "Life Ain't Been No Crystal Stair."

The historical legacy that has pressured many African American women to assume the role of the "Black matriarch" or "universal mother"—mothering our nuclear and extended families, friends, and members of our church and community—can have a profound and very stressful effect on all our relationships. The expectations to provide financial assistance and information often intensify if we have a college education or are single and without children, because then everyone assumes we have the money, time, and energy to tackle these responsibilities.

Also, many of us are part of the "sandwich generation," expected to care for elderly, perhaps sick parents while we're dealing with the continuous demands of our children and grandchildren. For time-squeezed women like this, even sleep is considered a luxury.

---

## MARY'S STORY

Mary is forty-five years old and has been married to John, fifty-two, for more than twenty years. They have three children—a nineteen-year-old son who is a sophomore in college, a seventeen-year-old daughter who is a high-school senior, and a fourteen-year-old daughter who is a freshman in high school and involved in sports and other extracurricular activities.

Mary is a sales manager and John is an attorney. She is the youngest child and the only daughter of her parents, who are both in their mid-seventies. Her husband is the oldest of six children of his widowed seventy-two-year-old mother.

Mary and her father, who is recovering from a stroke, are concerned about her mother's forgetfulness and mood swings. Mary has noticed that her mother is starting to repeat herself and that her house isn't as clean or neat as it always had been. Initially she attributed the changes in her mother's behavior to the normal aging process, but now she's worried that something more serious might be the cause.

John brags about his wife's cooking and the way she manages the house and the kids. When her husband compares her favorably to her sisters-in-law, who all have help with their household chores, Mary is pleased and starts believing that her ever-growing sense of fatigue is worth it.

When Mary called her mother's doctor and told him about her concerns, the doctor suggested that Mary should help out a little more. At first Mary felt sad and hurt by the doctor's implication that she wasn't doing enough for her parents—not only does she help them around the house and run errands for them, but she takes her mom shopping, first stopping by John's mother's house to see if she needs something—but then she started to question whether she really was a dutiful daughter.

So even though Mary was already exhausted, she started going to her parents' house every day, often cooking for them. She would then rush home, cook, straighten up her own house, tend to her kids' needs, and finish any paperwork from her job. As a result, Mary was rarely in bed before midnight, only to be up by 6 A.M. to cook breakfast.

These days Mary is an exhausted working mom and caring daughter who needs at least three or four cups of coffee a day just to stay alert. When she tried to cut back, her head felt as if it would burst. Always a picky eater, lately Mary has been having trouble digesting most of her food and has started suffering from heartburn. Even her skin has been breaking out. After several months of this marathon existence, Mary told her best friend, Rita, "I feel like an old, tired teenager."

---

Mary's inability to put herself and her own health first, before competing needs, was making her too exhausted to take care of anything appropriately. She needs to reframe her perceptions of what absolutely needs to be done by her and where she can turn to get help to survive this demanding period of her life.

### Rx QUICK PRIME TIME PRESCRIPTION FOR MARY

Mary needs to rethink her approach to life and why she is so determined to be the stoic, stereotypical strong Black woman, despite the toll her overburdened agenda is taking on her health and well-being. A Prime Time Sister or Prime Time Circle of Sisterfriends could help her explore why she refuses to ask other members of her family to help take care of her parents and mother-in-law or pitch in at her home. A caring support network also will give her the encouragement to cry out for help.

Mary will benefit from reading bell hooks' *Sisters of the Yam* daily, until she finds her own voice. She will also learn how to identify and speak up about her needs in *Prime Time*'s Chapter 14, on anxiety, and Chapter 6, on assertiveness. Finally, Mary must make time so that she can relax and pamper herself.

Our relationship with our adult children is one of the biggest stresses for African American women. Many women are expected to be ATM machines for their children or to become the surrogate parent or primary baby-sitter for their grandchildren. After years of never-ending demands from her children, our friend Jean decided to take back her life.

---

## JEAN'S STORY

At sixty Jean decided to move into her own apartment. She had shared an apartment with her daughter and grandchildren for almost twenty years. Several of her friends expressed their concern that she might be lonely. Jean's response: "I might be lonely, but I won't be so tired."

---

Renegotiating, ending, or starting relationships with spouses, partners, or lovers can be more difficult for us because of inter- and intraracial stereotypical depictions of African American women. As middle-aged women, we are usually portrayed as asexual, caretaking mammies or as domineering, sarcastic Sapphires. The media rarely depict our need for intimate, mutually satisfying emotional and sexual relationships. Thus it can be very difficult and stressful for us to recognize and ask for what we want and need.

## Personal Illness/Injury

As we revealed earlier, a major stressor for many African American women during this period is our health and that of our families and friends. The Big Four chronic illnesses, which often run in families, start to manifest themselves in midlife. African American women are two to three times more likely to suffer from these major health concerns than our Caucasian counterparts but only half as likely to have adequate health care and the information and financial resources to combat them.

Unfortunately, many of our risk factors for these diseases—overeating, overworking, and overgiving—are heightened by how we respond to other stressors in our lives.

## Loss

One of life's most stressful experiences is separation from someone whom you care about, especially if that person has provided you with love and support. In fact, the death of a spouse or partner is often rated as life's most stressful event. *In Stress, Diet, and Your Heart*, Dr. Dean Ornish notes that there is a 40 percent increase in the death rate of widows and widowers within the first six months of their spouses' deaths.

Divorce and the death of spouses, partners, family members, and friends often occur when we are at midlife. When you combine the high rate of divorce in our community with the higher incidence of life-threatening diseases among older African Americans, it's no wonder that we're apt to experience multiple losses at this time in our lives. The resulting emotional, social, and financial toll can be devastating.

Appropriately grieving these losses can be more difficult for us because many strong Black women believe we're supposed to hide our tears, to minimize, ignore, or deny our sad feelings, and to focus our energy on supporting family and friends as they grieve. How many times have you heard someone—maybe even you—say, "Oh, Mary will be all right, she's a strong sister"? But how does anyone know how Mary really is coping? No one has bothered to ask her how *she* feels or what *she* needs to work through her grief. What's really scary is that Mary might not know how to answer either question because she never bothered to focus on her own feelings or ask herself what she needs.

## Work

The workplace is rated by many people as their number one source of stress. According to Mitchell Marks, author of *From Turmoil to Triumph: New Life After Merger and Downsizing*, people today equate work with stress.

According to the *Columbia University College of Physicians and Surgeons Complete Home Medical Guide*, a work-stress study conducted by Dr. Robert A. Karasek of Columbia University determined that the incidence of coronary disease was higher among workers whose jobs entailed high psychological demands (multiple tasks that had to be performed in a short period of time) and low decision control (little to no input in working conditions).[5] Many women, especially poor and minority women, are often concentrated in occupations that Dr. Karasek labels as high-stress jobs.

These include assembly line workers, clerks, cashiers, or nurses' aides—all low-paying positions with little job security.

African American women often attribute their low-status work positions and lack of job advancement to race-related prejudice and sex discrimination. They cite inadequate institutional support and information related to career opportunities as prime examples of racism, report University of Michigan researchers.[6] This type of work-related stress results in a greater sense of burnout, irritability, fatigue, impatience, and lower work productivity.

Race and class issues can also affect the availability of an adequate support network for college-educated African American women in supervisory roles. Many middle-aged African American women were the first among a small handful of college graduates in our families. Thus, it can be difficult for us to discuss our salary or work concerns with family members, spouses, or friends who have lower-paying and lower-status jobs. Dr. Mary Snapp documented that it can also be more difficult for us to get support from our colleagues because we are frequently the only African American or female supervisor at our workplace.[7] The stress associated with feeling anxious because of our isolation often heats up when we're in a supervisory role in a setting with different racial and ethnic groups.

---

## SHIRLEY'S STORY

At forty-four years old, Shirley was thrilled to become the assistant principal at a high school that serves primarily students from upper-middle-class families. The school is located in a changing neighborhood—the families had been predominantly Caucasian, but now a significant number are African American, Korean, and Cuban.

Shirley was assigned to the school after a group of minority parents demanded that a minority person be assigned to the administrative office. They believed that their children were being discriminated against because of their race or ethnicity. Shirley believes that her principal, a well-respected, older Caucasian male, would have preferred a male or a Caucasian woman. Plus, most of the administrative staff is Caucasian.

Shirley has felt an increasing amount of stress because of her conflicted feelings, anger, and anxiety toward her colleagues, the parents, and the students. She agrees with the minority parents that a few of the Caucasian teachers have low academic expectations of the minority students, especially the African Americans, and will also more quickly give them a disciplinary referral. She is also aware that some of the African American staff and students expect her to allow them to bend or break the rules without sanction, because of the unwritten rule of "us against them."

Shirley wants to be fair but feels anxious and caught in the middle. Even though she believes that the principal is in her corner, Shirley experienced too much racism in professional and social settings to really trust him.

Being organized was never Shirley's real strength, but in the last few months her office has become a disaster area. She's having difficulty sleeping, so she's always tired. She's also having difficulty completing her routine tasks.

---

Shirley was so accustomed to "handling" every situation that it was difficult for her to prepare for a new professional experience or even to realize how stressed she was feeling.

### $R_X$ QUICK PRIME TIME PRESCRIPTION FOR SHIRLEY

Shirley had never felt comfortable asking other people for help. As the eldest daughter, she was the person everyone went to for answers. Thus, accepting her principal's idea of discussing her management problems with other African American supervisors was, initially, very difficult.

Shirley eventually called the principal she used to work for, a Black woman, who talked with her and supplied the names of several other administrators. Shirley was relieved to discover that they had common experiences. Their recommendations were extremely helpful.

Shirley decided to join a Prime Time Circle so that she could learn how to give and receive information and support. Her circle strongly recommended that she read Debrena Jackson Gandy's *Sacred Pampering Principles*, which focuses on women accepting their right to nurture themselves.

## Financial Issues

The middle years often present complex financial problems for everyone, as more money is required to cover children's college tuition, care for family members, and pay increased medical bills. Sexism and ageism compound these problems for all women, for the following three reasons: (1) women earn 70 percent of what men earn even though they have equal years of education and similar jobs; (2) 60 percent of all women are in lower-paying, traditionally female jobs, and (3) 15 percent of older women are poor, compared with fewer then 8 percent of older men.

Even though African American women who work rarely have the same self-imposed breaks (such as extended maternity leaves) as Caucasian women, Black women are more likely to be poor and have less discretionary money. That's because we earn only 82 percent of Caucasian women's income, are three times more likely to work in service occupations than Caucasian women, and are more apt to be single or widowed and have raised our children alone. We are also more likely to be financially responsible for our grandchildren, our elderly relatives, and sometimes our friends. Although older African American women with college degrees tend to have an annual income that surpasses that of their Caucasian counterparts, the financial assets of this small group of Black women are often quite meager because of their single status, spending patterns, and family demands.

Some Black women undeniably worship at the altar of consumerism (using our Kmart salary to purchase Lord and Taylor clothes) and have a crisis-management approach to handling money. We also spend more of our income—no matter how much we earn—on products that help us look good, including makeup, hair products (you know the ones we mean), nails, and clothes. Don't get us wrong—we want you to take care of and pamper yourselves, but not in a way that leaves you financially stretched and stressed. Far too many of us are full of professional potential and promise but lack the financial skills to properly manage our growing income.

## REGINA'S STORY

Regina is a forty-two-year-old single mother with a nineteen-year-old daughter, Kim. She's an extremely hardworking secretary who has just been hired for a new position. Regina's job offers her tremendous potential for growth, but the beginning salary is slightly less than she was making at her old office. She was already struggling to make ends meet on her previous income.

Despite her financial difficulties, Regina is very generous—she's always willing to lend money to a friend (even if she's not sure it will be repaid) or contribute to the office pool for weddings or baby showers. Regina and her daughter are also impulsive shoppers. However, spending more than she earns has left Regina dodging creditors (who are now calling her at her job) and feeling anxious whenever she sees an envelope that she thinks might contain a bill. She's having difficulty sleeping and is so tired in the mornings that she has been getting to work later and later.

---

How often have you, unknowingly, tried to "buy" love and friendship or acceptance at the expense (no pun intended) of implementing a realistic budget?

### ℞ QUICK PRIME TIME PRESCRIPTION FOR REGINA

Regina's daughter Kim was extremely worried and angry when Regina finally told her the truth about the seriousness of their financial problems. Kim reminded Regina that when asked, she had repeatedly denied having any financial problems. However, when Kim threatened to quit school and get a job to help pay the bills, Regina promised that she would get some financial counseling.

Regina can use her employee assistance program to obtain information about two organizations, the National Association of Credit Counselors (NACC) and Debtors Anonymous, which work with people who are "balanced-budget-challenged." They can help her to negotiate with her creditors and develop long-term strategies to stay out of debt. After joining Debtors Anonymous, Regina should read *Talking Dollars and Making Sense: A Wealth Building Guide for African-Americans*, by Brooke Stephens. She might be amazed at how many of the money myths described in the book she actually believes—from "high income equals great wealth" to "White people won't let us." Two other books she should check out: *Wealth Happens One Day at a Time*, also by Brooke Stephens, and *It's About the Money*, by Jesse L. Jackson Sr. and Jesse L. Jackson Jr.

Regina would also benefit from some short-term cognitive-behavioral counseling. The focus of the counseling would be to help Regina change her unspoken belief that to secure love you have to give or spend money on people or buy them gifts. Practicing relaxation and deep breathing techniques could also make a tremendous difference in Regina's ability to talk with her creditors and develop a realistic budget. Whenever she starts feeling anxious about her debts, she could relax and start visualizing a zero balance on her credit cards. After changing her spending pattern, Regina should think about getting into a long-term therapy group. She needs to find out what other silent beliefs are negatively affecting her life.

Regina would also benefit from having a Prime Time Circle of Sister-friends. They could meet on a regular basis and read the biographies of African American women who overcame tremendous difficulties to become financially solvent—Madame C. J. Walker, Mary McLeod Bethune, Sarah Spencer Washington, Oseola McCarty, Cathy Hughes, Oprah Winfrey. Her circle would also help her to realize how much of her time, money, and energy were focused on others. They could encourage her to schedule time in the morning and at night to meditate and read books focused on spirituality, some of which we mention throughout this book.

## Physical Appearance

Americans' cultural obsession with thinness and youth makes it more difficult for middle-aged women in general and African American women in particular to accept and love our bodies. As part of our African cultural legacy, Black Americans tend to have positive feelings about obesity and age. These feelings are in conflict with contemporary American standards of beauty, which extol thinness, white skin, straight hair, blue eyes, and youth. Many of us have been unable to resolve this conflict appropriately—especially those of us who grew up in households where our color wasn't light enough, our hair wasn't straight enough, our body wasn't thin enough, or our features weren't aquiline enough to satisfy our mothers, grandmothers, or fathers. That's a large part of why Black women are major consumers of cosmetics—we're constantly trying to stave off feelings of stress or depression when we believe that we are inadequate or ugly because we are too fat, too dark, or too old.

---

### JOAN'S STORY

Joan is a fifty-seven-year-old widow. Five years ago her husband, Phil, died unexpectedly of a heart attack. They had been married for almost thirty years and have two adult, married children. Joan's beauty shop keeps her busy during the day, but she is often very lonely at night and on the weekends. She would love to remarry but is afraid that she will not find another spouse because of her age and appearance. Joan is short, dark, and almost plump, and she has never really believed that she is attractive. Her family even told her that she was lucky to catch a husband such as Phil, who was tall and light-skinned and had good hair.

Joan often feels very tense and angry but hides her feelings by making funny, usually sarcastic remarks. Joan only shops at stores such as Saks and Nordstrom, hoping her expensive clothes will compensate for, as she puts it, her "fat, black body." Joan has many associates but only one or two women whom she considers close friends, and both of them are married. For a while, Joan's main way of relaxing was to drink four or five glasses of wine a night.

---

Joan's story shows how we can compromise our own self-esteem—no matter what our achievements—if we judge ourselves by other people's standards.

 **QUICK PRIME TIME PRESCRIPTION FOR JOAN**

After Joan's children expressed their concern about her drinking, she decided to join a local meeting of Alcoholics Anonymous (AA) and also see a certified addiction counselor to help her stop drinking. We also recommend that she study Chapters 5 and 6 and Part V in *Prime Time*, which focus on emotional health. Joan and her therapist must develop strategies to help her cope appropriately with her feelings of sadness, anger, and fear.

Joan also needs a Prime Time Circle to explore and share their feelings and concerns about their appearance. The group should read books such as *Skin Color*, edited by Elena Featherston, which can help Joan and her sister-friends to redefine beauty in a nonracist, nonsexist manner.

Finding a church that meets her spiritual needs and reading the *Daily Word* or her Bible will help Joan to claim and nourish her spiritual self. Developing her spirituality will enable Joan to find the strength and inner peace to continue on her journey toward taking charge of her emotional, physical, and spiritual health. Reliance on alcohol or other substances often stems from a spiritual thirst.

 **PRIME TIME PRESCRIPTIONS TO HELP YOU REDUCE STRESS**

*Ugi ni kihoota.*
*Knowledge is power.*

—Kikuyu proverb

Knowing what stresses you are subject to and how your mind and body register the effects of stress are the first steps to managing your stress level. The second step is doing something about it without becoming a lot more stressed in the process. Responding to a specific stressful event is much easier if we have developed some effective coping strategies when life becomes overwhelming. Barbara, Mary, Shirley, Regina, and Joan all had to learn some positive, effective stress management techniques.

Building, maintaining, and nurturing a network of friends who have varied interests and strengths is critical to managing stress. Friends can provide invaluable physical, emotional, and moral support and good practical advice during stressful periods. Having more than one good friend or circle of friends (men and women) can offset the sense of isolation and fear of being alone that often occurs with the loss of an important relationship.

Your Prime Time Sister or Prime Time Circle of Sisterfriends can help you cope with your stressors and can also prolong your life. In fact, a team of researchers found that having a supportive network of friends calms us down, reduces our pulse rate, and lowers our blood pressure.

## Destress Your Mind

Your ability to have an open mind about your social and professional interactions can help you to avoid or at least minimize potentially stressful situations. Writing in your health journal can help you explore how you feel when faced with a new situation or meeting new people.

There's a popular maxim almost chanted by many Blacks: "Just because I'm paranoid, that doesn't mean that somebody isn't out to get me." This statement vividly describes the contradictory but concurrent feelings many of us experience in professional and social settings. Thus, being able to evaluate an experience from diverse perspectives is critical if we are to function appropriately in various situations.

---

### DO YOU INVITE STRESS INTO YOUR LIFE?

Following are three sets of responses to the statement "My boss, who is White, never compliments me on my work."
Each set represents a different frame of reference.

---

SET A

1. He's a racist.
2. He's a sexist.
3. He's a poor administrator.
4. He's uncomfortable making positive statements.
5. He's a jerk.
6. All of the above.

SET B

7. My work is no good.
8. I never do anything right.
9. I'm going to be fired.

SET C

10. I don't know why he doesn't, but I can compliment myself about my work because I know it's good.
11. I will ask my coworkers about his behavior.
12. I will have a meeting with him to discuss my feelings.
13. I will ask for a midyear evaluation.

If you would typically select a response from Set A or B, you are probably adding stress to your life. Set A responses assume the worst about the other person. Set B responses assume the worst about yourself. The other problem with Sets A and B is that none of the responses acknowledges our power to have a positive impact on situations. Selecting a response from Set C indicates that you have a positive attitude about your ability to effect change.

You can increase your ability to see situations from different points of view and perspectives by opening yourself daily to new experiences and by interacting with people whose race, sex, life experiences, insights, and frames of reference are different from yours. Reading self-help books, biographies, and autobiographies about people who have successfully worked through stressful situations also exposes you to alternative ways to interpret and respond to different situations. Taking classes on multicultural issues can expose you to other cultural mores and traditions. If your paranoia about race hinders you from developing comfortable relationships—social or professional—with non-Blacks, try joining a support group or seeing an individual or group therapist to work through your prejudices, fears, or discomfort. If you open your mind to alternative points of view, you can lessen the stress on your mind and body.

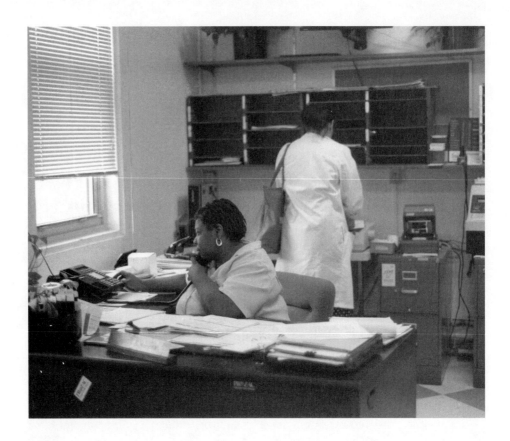

Here are some other ways to destress your mind:

***Learn how to become more assertive.*** Decide to express your wants and needs consistently in an open, honest, direct, courteous manner. Listen with the same manner to others communicating theirs.

Assertiveness means being comfortable putting your own needs first and saying yes or no without reservation, guilt, anger, or resentment. You have a right and responsibility to express what you are thinking and feeling, but you don't have to do it in a hostile or aggressive manner. You really are less stressed when you're not feeling angry and upset. Learning to be assertive or becoming more consistently assertive is a skill you can acquire. Classes in assertiveness training are frequently offered through universities, women's organizations, and church groups. More information about assertiveness is in Chapter 6, "Confronting the Two A's: Attitude and Anger."

***Become more resilient.*** The ability to translate lessons learned from adversity into opportunities for growth (a process that Iyanla Vanzant refers to as seeing the "value in the valley") is one of the major reasons why some individuals, such as Oprah Winfrey, bounce back from difficulties while others, such as the late actress Dorothy Dandridge, become overwhelmed. Resilient people have strong personal convictions and are honest with themselves about how they react to stressful situations. They know how to gather and use information that will help them learn to cope with stress. They are also confident that friends and family will support them during difficult times.

*Embrace the power of positive self-talk.* In Chapter 4, we asked you to think about the self-talk in your head that motivates you or makes you question your abilities. Many of us grew up in homes where we were more apt to be teased or criticized for making a mistake than verbally praised for an accomplishment. Concern about a child becoming big-headed, uppity, or a braggart often discouraged friends and relatives from offering too many compliments or positive, congratulatory remarks. Even though many of us decided to interact differently with our children or grandchildren, we continue to find it difficult to affirm our own accomplishments verbally. Making positive statements about ourselves can prevent and reduce stress and increase feelings of happiness. Look in the mirror and say at least these three positive things about yourself:

- I can set and accomplish my goals.
- I am an effective professional.
- I am a beautiful Black woman! *(We all are!)*

## Destress Your Body

Because prolonged stress can have a devastating effect on your physical health, developing healthy living habits is critical.

*Don't skimp on sleep.* Your mother was absolutely right when she said, "You need your rest." Developing and maintaining good sleep habits is a staple of good health and a sound mind. Sleep is not a luxury. Just remember: There is nothing on Leno, Letterman, or *Nightline* worth losing sleep over. If you must see a late-night program, tape it or have a friend tape it for you.

Too many of us have good intentions of getting to bed early, but then the phone rings and our friend, our sister, our colleague just must have our ear for a few minutes. How can you cut off these late-night calls? Turn off your phone! Voice mail or an answering machine will allow your friends and relatives to keep in touch with you if they must hear your voice in the middle of the night. (For many of us, that's anytime after 9:30 P.M.)

If you're experiencing insomnia, try establishing a regular bedtime routine.

You may want to exercise a few hours before sleep (but not too close to bedtime), meditate, practice deep breathing exercises, take a hot bath, or have a glass of warm (soy) milk and honey. You should also stop trying to fall asleep with the lights and television on.

*Eat something from each of the food groups every day.* Eating well-balanced meals (especially for breakfast) nourishes and calms your mind, body, and spirit. So forget the jelly doughnut and Kentucky Fried Chicken on the run. Fresh fruits and vegetables, whole-grain breads and cereals, fish, and poultry are particularly helpful in reducing stress levels. (To find out more about eating balanced meals, see Chapter 9, "Developing Your Prime Time Wellness Plan.")

Caffeinated foods (I'm afraid that does include chocolate-chip cookies—yes, chocolate actually contains some caffeine) and drinks (such as coffee, tea, and colas) can actually worsen your physical and emotional responses to stress. Caffeine stimulates the production of noradrenaline and increases your heart rate. This artificial energy booster only sets your body up for a big letdown.

*Learn more about herbs.* Chamomile, lavender, lemon balm, valerian, and other herbs have been used in various cultures for thousands of years for stress relief. The remedies are often given in the form of salves, teas, ointments, tablets and inhalants. To find out more about stress-reducing herbs, check out these books: *A Path to Healing* by Dr. Andrea Sullivan or *The Green Pharmacy* by Dr. James Duke.

*Exercise, exercise, exercise.* Regular physical activity can generate a sense of calmness and relaxation. Exercise reduces the level of stress hormones (adrenaline and noradrenaline) and stimulates the production of endorphins, which are brain chemicals that produce a sense of well-being. Walking (up and down steps if you can't go outside), jogging, and dancing are activities that most of us can do without any training or expensive equipment. Start off slow, just five minutes the first day, and build up your stamina over a few weeks until you can easily work out thirty minutes or longer. (For more information on starting an exercise program, see Chapter 9.)

*Take up yoga or tai chi.* The oldest, most widely practiced holistic approaches to health and healing, yoga and tai chi unite and balance the mind, body, and spirit. Controlled breathing, various postures, and a meditative focus help to relax the body, calm the mind, and nourish the spirit. There are many yoga and tai chi videotapes available at your local video store or sports store. Some local cable television stations air yoga exercise programs early in the morning. To find out more about the benefits of yoga and tai chi and how to get started, read *Stress, Anxiety and Depression* by the Natural Medicine Collection.

*Practice stress-relieving breathing.* Most of us think about breathing only when we're having trouble doing it. Breathing correctly involves more than forcing air in and out of your body, and it can decrease your stress level by lowering your heart and blood pressure rates.

When practicing deep breathing, also known in yoga as "belly breathing," you slow down your breathing rate to seven to eight cycles (inhaling and exhaling) per minute instead of the usual fifteen to sixteen cycles. To practice deep breathing, lie on your back and place a book on your belly. When you breathe from your abdomen, the book will rise and fall.

---

## DEEP BREATHING

Stress-Buster Breathing #1

To increase the amount of oxygen you receive, do this exercise at least once a day for three weeks. This will help you learn the basic approach to switching from shallow to deep breathing. The more often you do it, the better the results.

1. Sit in a chair without armrests, feet flat on the floor and thighs parallel to the floor. Hold your back straight. Place your hands in your lap.

2. Inhale through your nose and breathe deeply, without forcing. Let your abdomen expand. Imagine air filling your abdomen.

3. In one continuous breath, imagine filling your chest and lungs with air. Feel your chest expand fully and your shoulders rise slightly (keep your shoulders relaxed). Imagine the air expanding your abdomen and chest in all directions.

4. Exhale slowly through your nose. Breathing out should take longer than breathing in.

5. Do this breathing for at least a minute. Stay in a comfortable rhythm and don't strain yourself. Focus on keeping your breathing deep and full and your body relaxed.

Stress-Buster Breathing #2

1. As you inhale, count very slowly from one to four.

2. As you exhale, count slowly back down.

3. Do this for several breaths or as long as you need to.

---

Stress-Buster Breathing #3

1. As you inhale, begin to count down from ten, saying "ten" aloud.

2. Exhale.

3. As you inhale again, say "nine."

4. Keep counting down with each inhalation. If you start to feel light-headed, slow down.

5. When you get to zero, you should be feeling much calmer! If not, start over at ten and keep going.

*Try muscle relaxation.* Learning how to relax your muscles can reduce your overall feelings of tenseness. Progressive muscular relaxation (PMR) and deep muscular relaxation (DMR) are the two most popular types of muscle relaxation. However, it's important to use them with caution if you have muscular weakness or injuries. Also, since blood pressure is elevated when the muscles are tensed, anyone with hypertension should use DMR instead of PMR because it does not require tensing of the muscles.

## PROCEDURE FOR PROGRESSIVE MUSCULAR RELAXATION (PMR)

Warning: Do not overtense or overstretch your muscles. Stop if you feel uncomfortable or experience any pain. Those with high blood pressure are advised to practice deep muscular relaxation instead of using PMR. Allow fifteen minutes to complete this procedure. You will need a biodot, a small handheld instrument that changes colors based on your body temperature, which is an indication of how relaxed you are. You can buy one at most health-food stores.

1. Place a biodot on your hand and note the color. Sit comfortably well back in the chair so your back is supported and both feet rest flat on the floor a little way apart. Rest your arms in your lap. Keep your head straight, with your chin parallel to the floor. Your breathing should be abdominal and relaxed—gentle, slow, and unforced.

2. Close your eyes and direct your attention to each part of the body in turn. Tense each set of muscles and hold the position for five seconds or so. Concentrate on the tenseness and tightness. Then relax the muscles and concentrate on the sensation of relaxation. Notice how the tenseness disappears and the muscles feel at ease, warm, and heavy. Stay in this position for about ten seconds.

3. Pull your shoulders up toward your ears as far as you can. Feel the tenseness in your shoulders and neck. Hold for five seconds. Now relax; feel the muscles relax. Relax for ten seconds.

4. Now pull your shoulders down toward the floor. Concentrate on the tenseness. Hold for five seconds and relax for ten seconds.

5. Bend your right arm and make your biceps muscle stand out as much as you can; hold the tenseness for five seconds. Now lower the arm and relax for ten seconds. Turn the palm of your right hand upward. Clench your fist as firmly as you can. Concentrate on the tenseness for five seconds and then relax, unfolding your fist, for ten seconds. Now stretch your fingers out as far as they will go; feel your fingers stiffen and the thumb pushing away from the fingers. Hold it, feeling the tenseness; then relax, feeling the fingers curl gently inward. Always hold the tenseness for about five seconds and the relaxation for about ten seconds.

6. Bend your left arm and make your biceps muscle stand out; tense the muscle. Then lower the arm and relax. Turn the palm of your left hand upward. Clench your fist as firmly as you can and concentrate on the tenseness. Hold it. Now unfold your fist and relax. Stretch your fingers as far as they will go. Feel the fingers stiffen, the thumb pushing away from the fingers. Hold it. Now relax and notice the fingers curl gently inward.

7. Concentrate on your legs. Straighten your right leg and push your foot away from you. Feel the tenseness of the muscles on the front of your thigh. Point your toes as far away as you can; now bend your foot back at the ankle. Feel the muscles tense in your right calf. Hold it, and then relax. Tighten the muscles in your right foot. Curl your toes, and when your foot feels as tense as you can make it, relax.

8. Straighten your left leg and push your foot away from you. Feel the tightness of the muscles at the front of your thigh. Point your toes as far away as you can; now bend your foot back at the ankle. Feel the muscles tense in your left calf. Hold it, and then relax. Tighten the muscles in your foot. Curl your toes, and when your foot feels as tense as you can make it, relax.

9. Now lift yourself up by tensing your buttock muscles. Lift higher and higher; hold it. Now let the muscles relax.

10. Contract your abdominal wall muscles—make your waist as small as you can. Feel the tenseness. Hold it and then relax.

11. Now turn your attention to your head. Move your head gently forward until you feel the muscles in your neck and back tighten. Hold it and then return your head to the center and relax. Tilt your head to the right, feel the tenseness in your muscles, and then return your head to the

center and relax. Now tilt your head to the left, feel the tenseness, and return your head to the center and relax.

12. Now clench your teeth tightly—feel the pressure and tenseness of your jaw muscles. Allow your jaw to sag slightly; feel the muscles ease. Let your mouth drop open and feel the tenseness ease further. Now close your mouth and push your tongue against the roof of your mouth; feel the tenseness and pressure. Now relax the tongue behind the lower teeth.

13. Smile broadly and feel the change in muscle tenseness. Hold it and then relax. Screw up your eyes, tighter and tighter. Hold it, and then relax them back into the sockets. Now first pull your eyebrows down, and then raise them as high as you can. Hold it and relax.

14. Concentrate on your breathing. Feel your abdominal muscles move slowly out and up as you breathe in, and then down and inward as you breathe out. Your breathing should be slow, gentle, and shallow.

15. Now quiet your mind. Allow your thoughts to drift through your head without trying to pursue them. As easily as thoughts come into your mind, they leave, and as easily as they leave, more thoughts effortlessly come in. Recall happy memories. Picture a walk along the seashore, the waves, warm water lapping around your feet as they sink in the sand, sun glistening on the water, a deep blue cloudless sky, and the cries of the seagulls.

16. Sit quietly for five minutes and enjoy the state of relaxation you have created throughout your body. Your body should feel warm and heavy—totally relaxed.

17. After five minutes, open your eyes slowly and look at your biodot. If you are more relaxed than when you started, its color should be more toward the blue end of the scale.

18. Before you stand up, gently stretch your body and take two or three deep breaths.

## PROCEDURE FOR DEEP MUSCULAR RELAXATION (DMR)

Allow fifteen minutes to complete this procedure.

1. Place a biodot on your hand and note the color. Sit comfortably well back in a chair so your back is supported and both feet rest flat on

the floor a little way apart. Rest your arms in your lap. Keep your head straight, with your chin parallel to the floor. Your breathing should be abdominal and relaxed—gentle, slow, and unforced.

2. Close your eyes. Direct your attention to each part of your body in turn. Each time, relax the muscles and concentrate on the sensation of relaxation. Notice how tenseness disappears and muscles feel at ease, warm and heavy (stay in this position for about ten seconds).

3. Concentrate first on your left leg. Focus your attention on each part of your leg in turn, starting at your toes and working toward your hip. As you relax each set of muscles, feel the tension drain away and notice the sensation of limpness, heaviness, and warmth. Relax your toes. Concentrate for about five seconds on the feeling of relaxation (do this between relaxing each part). Now relax the instep, then the heel, and then the ankle. Now relax your calf muscles. Feel them become limp, heavy, and warm. Now relax your knee, then your thigh, and then your hip. Concentrate on the relaxation of your left leg, heavy, limp, and warm.

4. Now focus your attention on your right leg. Concentrate on each part of your leg in turn, starting at your toes and working toward your hip. As you relax each set of muscles, feel the tension drain away and notice the sensation of limpness, heaviness, and warmth. Relax your toes. Concentrate for about five seconds on the feeling of relaxation. Now relax the instep, then the heel, and then the ankle. Now relax your calf muscles. Feel them become limp, heavy, and warm. Now relax your knee, your thigh, and your hip. Concentrate on the relaxation of your right leg, heavy, limp and warm.

5. Now concentrate on your left arm. Focus your attention on each part of your arm in turn, starting with the fingers and working toward your shoulder. Relax your fingers and thumb. Feel them curl inwards. Relax your palm, now your wrist, your forearm, your elbow, upper arm, and lastly your shoulder. Concentrate on the limp, heavy, and warm sensation.

6. Now concentrate on your stomach muscles. Let them relax, limp, heavy, and warm.

7. Relax your neck muscles but keep your head straight, your chin parallel to the floor. Your head should now be balanced on your spine. Now focus your attention on your head. Relax your jaw, let it drop, and feel your mouth slightly open. Relax your tongue and feel it drop behind your lower teeth. Relax the muscles around your eyes; feel them become limp, heavy, and warm. Relax your forehead and scalp. Your head should feel totally relaxed, heavy, and warm.

8. Concentrate on your breathing. Feel your abdominal muscles move

slowly out and up as you breathe in, and then down and inward as you breathe out. Your breathing should be slow and gentle.

9. Now quiet your mind. Allow your thoughts to drift through your head, without trying to pursue them. As easily as thoughts come into your mind, they leave, and as easily as they leave, more thoughts effortlessly come in. Recall happy memories. Picture a walk along the seashore, the waves, warm water lapping around your feet as they sink in the sand, sun glistening on the water, deep blue cloudless sky, the cries of the seagulls.

10. Sit quietly for five minutes and enjoy the state of relaxation you have created throughout your body. Your body should feel warm and heavy—totally relaxed.

11. After five minutes, open your eyes slowly and look at your biodot. If you are more relaxed than when you started, its color should be more toward the blue end of the scale.

If you have not worked on relaxation techniques before this, you might find that you have to practice these exercises to learn to relax. Try not to expect instant success. With the aid of biodots, you will be able to monitor your progress and the effects of the techniques. Eventually you should be able to do a short meditation or muscular relaxation anytime, anywhere.

*Get a massage.* Massage can stimulate circulation, lower blood pressure, and soothe muscle tension and headaches. Toxins and lactic acid buildup in the lymphatic system (the lymph nodes throughout the body that fight infections) are broken up through the stroking and pressure techniques used in massage, and then leave the body through the lymph system and blood circulation.

There are various types of massage, but Japanese shiatsu, Swedish massage, and reflexology are the most widely practiced in the United States. *Shiatsu* uses principles similar to those in acupuncture and helps stimulate and facilitate the movement of energy around the body. In *Swedish massage*, the hands touch the body with various degrees of pressure. *Reflexology* involves rubbing and pressing various parts of the foot, which reflexologists believe correspond to various organs and body parts.

## Destress Your Spirit

The more severe and uncontrollable the stressor, the more critical it is that you have an inner space from which you can draw strength and comfort. Here are ways to soothe your spirit.

*Nourish your inner spiritual life.* Prayer is the coping mechanism most widely used by African American women of all ages. Numerous studies have documented the positive impact of prayer and meditation on our sense of well-being and our recovery rates from illness and surgeries. Starting the day with the *Serenity Prayer*, reading a daily meditation from *One Day My Soul Just Opened Up* (Iyanla Vanzant), *Soul Quest: A Healing Journey for Women of the African Diaspora* (Deneser Shervington), or *Daily Cornbread: 365 Secrets for a Healthy Mind, Body, and Spirit* (Stephnie Stokes Oliver) is an effective way to help you get in touch with and stay in touch with your spiritual self. Other good books to read include *Acts of Faith: Meditations for People of Color* (Iyanla Vanzant) and *Sisters of the Yam: Black Women and Self-Recovery* (bell hooks).

Finally, if you have stopped allocating specific time for focusing on God, your spirit, Allah, The Buddha, or the orishas, give that back to yourself. Going to a church, temple, synagogue, or mosque or any other place of worship on a regular basis affirms your commitment to keeping healthy this essential part of yourself.

*Learn how to meditate.* This ancient Eastern method of reducing stress actually helps you relax your mind. There are different forms of meditation, so it's important that you find the one that works best for you.

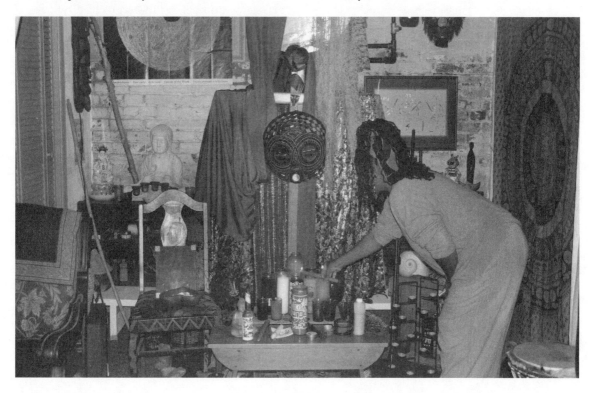

A widely practiced variation involves the repetition of a single word: *om*, *peace*, or *one*. Numerous studies of meditation have documented that an increase in brain-wave alpha rhythms is associated with a relaxed state. One explanation for this is that while the left side of the brain (the thinking side) is occupied with repeating the word or sound, the right side (the creative, intuitive lobe) becomes dominant.

Check with your physician before starting to meditate, because certain types of meditation practices may not be good for you if you have epilepsy or an emotional disorder.

## PROCEDURE FOR MEDITATION

(Allow twenty minutes)

1. Find a quiet, warm place where you will not be disturbed. Sit in a comfortable upright position, place a biodot on your hand, and note the color. Make a note of the time. Breathing should be slow, gentle, and abdominal. Close your eyes, then repeat aloud the word *om* or *one*. Do this several times, then repeat the word more quietly and then quieter still until you are not moving your lips but merely thinking the word over and over in your mind. Do not concentrate on keeping the word in the forefront of your mind—it should not be like counting sheep. You will find that your mind begins to wander.

2. Let thoughts wander into your mind and then let them leave by simply thinking the sound over and over again. (The sound of the word is purely a means of helping you clear your mind.) Continue in this manner for twenty minutes, then stop and sit quietly for a minute or so. Gradually and slowly open your eyes. Note the color of the biodot. You are looking for the color of your biodot to change toward the turquoise/blue range, to show that you have achieved a state of calm and relaxation and reduced level of stress. Look for signs of relaxation such as warm hands and feet and salivation.

3. End your relaxation by gently stretching your arms and legs and taking two or three slow deep breaths.

Do not use an alarm to tell you when the twenty minutes is up—open your eyes slowly and look at a clock when you feel that the time has passed. With practice you will find it easy to judge twenty minutes. The time will pass very quickly. Sometimes you will find it hard to believe you have sat and relaxed for twenty minutes. After practicing meditation regularly, twice a day for about two to three months, you may experience periods of deep mental relaxation.

Try to meditate regularly each morning and evening at a time when your home or office is reasonably quiet. Take precautions so you will not be disturbed. While you are learning the technique, you may find it helpful to use earplugs (available from drugstores). Unplug the telephone. Avoid eating for about two hours beforehand. Late evening meditation may affect your sleep, since meditation usually increases alertness.

We recommend you practice PMR, DMR, and meditation in the sitting position without supporting the head. If you are lying down with your head supported, it is easy to fall asleep. The aim of practicing a relaxation technique is to achieve a state of physical and mental calmness different from sleep.

*Check out the healing powers of aromatherapy.* In aromatherapy, aromatic essences (essential oils) extracted from plants are either inhaled directly, inhaled from a burning candle, or used in a bath or massage. Just as smelling certain aromas (such as perfumes and baking bread, for instance) can evoke physical and emotional reactions, aromatherapists believe certain scents can be used to relieve various physical and emotional health concerns. The most commonly used oils for stress relief are bergamot, chamomile, clary sage, geranium, lavender, rose, rosemary, verbena, spearmint, and ylang ylang.

If you have allergies or respiratory problems such as asthma or emphysema, it's extremely important that you talk to your physician or a qualified aromatherapist before you begin using this treatment.

*Laugh more.* Smiling, laughing, and having a good sense of humor will not only reduce your stress level, but can actually improve your emotional and physical well-being. During stressful periods, harmful hormones are released and toxins are stored in the body. Laughter and tears facilitate their excretion through the eyes and the nose.

In *Anatomy of an Illness*, Dr. Norman Cousins described his remarkable recovery from a major illness through "laugh therapy." He believes that spending several days laughing at old movies and television comedies saved his life. Humor is an integral part of Black life, but often it takes the form of teasing. When we're stressed, we might find it more difficult to handle a certain type of teasing, so it can be more useful to talk with a nonteasing but amusing and supportive friend, read a humorous book, or see a funny movie.

*Practice visualization.* Using your imagination in conjunction with muscle relaxation and positive affirmations can be a powerful method for combating stress. Most of us have a memory of a time or place in which we felt calm and relaxed. Recalling or fantasizing about that time or place can reduce your physical and emotional tension.

## TAMING A MAJOR STRESSOR—TIME

Time management skills are critical components of any stress management program. Our multiple roles and responsibilities as wife, partner, mama, grandmama, daughter, sister, niece, aunt, friend, supervisor, supervisee, church sister, sorority sister, and so on (it's stressful just thinking about all these relationships) require that we learn to balance and prioritize our various activities or lose our minds, our physical health, our jobs, or our loved ones.

The first step to effective time management is to accept that our time is truly our own. Every day we decide—either actively or passively—how we will spend the next twenty-four hours. Just as financial planners tell us we should pay ourselves before we pay anyone else, we're suggesting that you include taking care of your emotional, physical, and spiritual needs when you plan your day. Allot time for talking with at least one positive, affirming person, eating properly, exercising and praying, meditating, or reading something inspirational. (Notice we didn't mention sitting in front of the TV.)

Every day you should make a to-do list—what you *must do, should do, want to do*. Prioritize the to-do list and assign a date or time to complete each item on it. Don't try to do them concurrently or in an unrealistic time frame.

Ask your family or assistant for help or delegate some tasks to others. If you don't have a secretary, use your voice mail to screen your calls. Time how long you spend off the task you aim to get done. You might be shocked at how much time you spend "chatting" on the phone, spot-checking the television, or visiting with a coworker even while feeling anxious about how little time you have left to meet your deadline.

Unless you have an infant or a toddler, close the door at home and at work when you need time to take care of yourself or complete a task.

*Take time off to rejuvenate.* Plan vacations that will allow you to relax and focus on replenishing your mind, body, and spirit. Consider frequent short, inexpensive trips. For instance, two nights at a bed-and-breakfast or small inn can cost less than $150. Use the Internet or a travel agent to plan longer trips that won't leave you stressed out about the costs.

Time with your children and grandchildren can be wonderful, exciting, educational, and loving, but you will probably assume some sort of caretaking role during your stay, so don't think of these visits as vacations. Some married or partnered couples take separate vacations or go with friends to destress and rediscover themselves as individuals. Single people also need to take some time alone in a different setting to reassess their priorities. Remember that vacations with folks who require you to entertain them, plan for them, worry about them, or provide for their good time, including your spouse or partner, aren't really vacations—they're just more work.

*Pace important life events.* We have no control over many life events, such as unexpected deaths or Christmas, but many others, such as retirement, reunions, or marriage, can be scheduled, delayed, or canceled altogether. Research conducted on thousands of patients demonstrated that planning the timing of major life events could reduce stress levels and the risk of developing a stress-related illness. Using the Life Change Index, a forty-three-item scale in which events were scored from a high of 100 to a low of 11, the researchers determined that people with a score of 150 or higher dramatically increased their chances of developing a serious illness within two years.[8] Trying to negotiate a divorce and move into a new home while grieving the recent death of a parent, for example, dramatically increases our risk of becoming ill. Deciding to delay the divorce proceedings or the move could save your life.

| Life Event | Average Stress Score |
|---|---|
| Death of spouse | 100 |
| Divorce | 73 |
| Marital separation | 65 |
| Jail term | 63 |
| Death of close family member | 63 |
| Personal injury or illness | 53 |
| Marriage | 50 |
| Being fired from work | 47 |
| Marital problems | 45 |
| Retirement | 45 |
| Change in health of family member | 44 |

| Life Event | Average Stress Score |
|---|---|
| Pregnancy | 40 |
| Sexual difficulties | 39 |
| Gain of new family member | 39 |
| Business readjustment | 39 |
| Change in finances | 38 |
| Death of close friend | 37 |
| Change to different line of work | 36 |
| Change in number of arguments with spouse | 35 |
| Mortgage or loan for major purchase (such as a home) | 31 |
| Foreclosure of mortgage or loan | 30 |
| Change in responsibilities at work | 29 |
| Son or daughter leaving home | 29 |
| Trouble with in-laws | 29 |
| Outstanding personal achievement | 28 |
| Spouse begins or stops work | 26 |
| Beginning or finishing school | 26 |
| Change in living conditions | 25 |
| Revision of personal habits | 24 |
| Trouble with boss | 23 |
| Change in work hours or conditions | 20 |
| Change in residence | 20 |
| Change in school | 20 |
| Change in recreation | 19 |
| Change in church activities | 19 |
| Change in social activities | 18 |
| Mortgage or loan for lesser purchase (such as a car or television) | 17 |

| Life Event | Average Stress Score |
|---|---|
| Change in sleeping habits | 16 |
| Change in number of family get-togethers | 15 |
| Change in eating habits | 15 |
| Vacation | 13 |
| Christmas | 12 |
| Minor violations of the law | 11 |

Determine which life events have occurred in your life over the past two years and add up your total stress score. For example, if you got married, changed to a different line of work, changed residence, and took two vacations, your total stress score would be 50 + 36 + 20 + 13 + 13 = 132. If your total stress score is under 150, you are less likely to be suffering the effects of cumulative stress. If it is between 150 and 300, you *may* be suffering from chronic stress, depending on how you perceived and coped with the particular life events that occurred. If your score is over 300, it is likely you are experiencing some detrimental effects of cumulative stress. Please note that the stress scores on the above survey are averaged over many people. The degree to which any particular event is stressful to you will depend on how you perceive it.

*Source:* Reprinted from "The Sacral Readjustment Scale," by T. H. Holmes and R. H. Rahe, *Journal of Psychosomatic Research*, 11(2), August 1967.

Review your Life Change Index score. How many things are happening in your life? How many stressors on the Black Women's Midlife Stress Test did you rate as very stressful? When we look at the multitude of changes that occur during this critical stage in our lives, it is not surprising that so many of us feel stressed out. Even if many of the transitions are positive, it can be less stressful to spread them out. If we are experiencing traumatic events, it is critical that we try to prevent or minimize nonrandom stressors.

***Schedule personal time-outs.*** In *Sacred Pampering Principles*, Debrena Jackson Gandy encourages us not only to pamper ourselves, but also to differentiate the time we spend on "grooming" versus "pampering." Grooming, she contends, consists of activities that keep our external selves looking our best, such as getting our hair or nails done. *Pampering* involves nurturing and giving joy and peace to our inner selves. Taking a warm bath, getting a massage, listening to music, reading, and sitting quietly are daily rituals that can help prevent or reduce our stress.

## USING STRESS MANAGEMENT IN OUR DAILY LIVES

Stress prevention does work, but we have to learn the strategies and practice them on a daily basis. Preventing and reducing stress makes life easier, but remember that you're human, so allow yourself some time to adapt to new behaviors. You also need to get comfortable with the fact that sometimes (many times, in fact), we must learn from our mistakes as well as from the advice and actions of family members, friends, colleagues, teachers and books like this one. Accepting that you're not perfect and that you don't have to be perfect to be a good person allows you to acknowledge your mistakes and to rectify them. Writing about these feelings in your health journal or notebook is a great way to come to grips with your own shortcomings.

Being flexible and open to changing life events gives us the opportunity to, as Marilyn's daughter, Ami, says, "change our plate size." As Black women, we often act as if we are "serving platters" who can carry all of our own needs and those of everyone around us. We can't and never could, but trying to do it all now, when our midlife emotional, physical, and sometimes financial resources are more limited or strained, can be extremely stressful. By developing effective coping strategies, we can reduce our platters to plates or maybe even saucers. You can use many of the techniques described above on a daily basis, but they are particularly effective during acute periods of stress.

Although the Quick Prime Time Prescriptions we recommended earlier in the chapter to help our friends Barbara, Mary, Shirley, Regina, and Joan may not fit your needs exactly, feel free to borrow from these prescriptions and the Prime Time Prescriptions we offer elsewhere and modify them to work for you. Taking charge of your stress will be challenging. You must realize that taking responsibility for managing the stressors that you can control will give you opportunities to increase your sense of power and your growth and development.

# Chapter 14

# OVERCOMING WORRY, FEAR, AND ANXIETY

*There are only two emotions in life, love and fear. Either we are acting out of love or we're acting out of fear.*

—Iyanla Vanzant, *The Value in the Valley*

How many times have you had trouble getting to sleep or woken up in the middle of the night because you're so worried about anything like the following?

• Your grandson, who just dropped out of college
• Your daughter, whose rent you've just paid for the third time in the last six months
• Your spouse, who just won't quit smoking even though his cough is getting worse
• Your work relationship with a new young Caucasian administrator, who seems only to hear and certainly only to acknowledge comments made by younger management or staff
• The results of your Pap smear

How many times have you tossed and turned through the night, unable to calm down enough to fall asleep? For many Black women, the answer would be too many times to keep count.

We all worry about our personal safety and that of our families and friends—and with good reason: African American women of all ages are victims of physical assault, rape, and homicide at a rate greater than that of any other group of women. We're always worried about money—and with good reason: More of us are in debt than Caucasians, and fewer of us have adequate savings. We worry about our health—and with good reason: More of us die from major diseases than any other group of women. We worry about our relationships or lack of them—and with good reason: African American women are more likely to be single compared to other ethnic groups. We also have the highest rate of divorce and the lowest rate of remarriage of any group of women. Many of us are lonely and want to be in permanent relationships—and so we worry that we'll grow old without a partner or a spouse.

We worry about the impact of racism and sexism on our personal and professional lives—and with good reason: Anecdotal stories have been supported by studies indicating that our health-care coverage is inferior and our job promotion rates are lower than those of Caucasians and African American men. Some of us worry about groups of people whom we don't know but to whom we feel connected—poor people, the homeless, political prisoners.

At this age, many of us don't give a second thought to how our fears have limited our lives, because we've been afraid or worried for so much of our lives that we take these emotions for granted. We assume that they just come with the package of being a Black woman. We may feel sad but often are resigned that we can't fulfill our dreams. Do any of the following stories sound familiar?

• You're unable to give your only sibling, who's also your best friend, a public tribute at her birthday party because you're afraid to speak in front of people.
• You don't take your dream trip to Egypt because you can't get there by driving and you're certainly not going to fly.
• You're tired all the time because worrying keeps you from getting a good night's sleep.
• You didn't go to the historic Million-Woman March with your daughters and granddaughters because whenever you're in a crowd, your heart pounds, you start to sweat, you get dizzy, you gasp for breath, and you feel as if something awful is going to happen to you.

When you stop and think about it, just how much of your life is controlled by worry, anxiety, and fear? Probably more than you want to admit. It can be difficult to differentiate between the acute worries, anxieties, and fears that are a function of being alive and the feelings of panic, terror, or distress that are associated with anxiety disorders.

This chapter will enable you to identify the thoughts, feelings, and behaviors that often accompany an anxiety disorder and prevent you from doing things you want to do or should do to live as fully and productively as you can. We also offer a variety of suggestions for handling your everyday worries and fears more appropriately, and explanations of effective treatments for anxiety disorders.

## WHAT IS AN ANXIETY DISORDER?

Feeling anxious or frightened is not unique to African American women. Most people (if they live long enough, and probably just making it through the birth process is long enough) will experience instances of anxiety and fear. These are normal, recurrent emotions that are not only useful, but can be lifesaving (for instance, worrying about AIDS motivates us to practice safe sex). Although the terms *fear* and *anxiety* are often used interchangeably, they're related but not synonymous.

**Fear** is a reaction to a specific, identifiable, *present* threat to your well-being. **Anxiety** is a mental and physical response to what you believe is a *future* threat to your psychological or physical well-being. (*Anxiety* is Latin for "twisted rope"—that's how you often feel when you're anxious.) When you feel anxious or afraid, your mind believes that you're going to be emotionally or physically harmed, and your body prepares to fight or flee: your heart rate quickens, your muscles tense, and you become more aware of your surroundings.

---

## JENNIFER'S AND ROBERTA'S STORIES

Jennifer, fifty-six, and her sister Roberta, fifty, were going to visit their mother. When the sisters got out of Jennifer's car, a pit bull ran toward them, growling and baring its teeth. They were frightened and their hearts started beating faster as they started running—Jennifer back to the car, Roberta to their mother's house.

While driving to their mother's house the following week, the sisters discussed how frightened they had felt when they saw the dog. Even though she was anxious, Jennifer laughed and said she would look both ways when she got out of the car. But Roberta started to feel really frightened. She was breathing hard, her heart was pounding, and she started to perspire. Even though the dog had stopped before he was really close to either one of them, Roberta started thinking of stories of pit bulls attacking and seriously harming their victims. As they approached their mother's house, Roberta began feeling really tense.

When they finally arrived, Jennifer slowly got out of the car and looked both ways. She then laughed and gave a loud sigh of relief in celebration of the "wonderful quiet." However, Roberta was unable to move, and sat huddled in her seat. She started to cry when Jennifer opened her door. Her heart was pounding and she felt faint. Within a few minutes, she became convinced that she was having a heart attack. Jennifer drove her to the emergency room, where the doctors diagnosed her as having a panic attack.

---

Jennifer and Roberta experienced the same stressful event and shared some of the same mental, emotional, and physical responses. They were both initially frightened, and both felt anxious returning to their mother's house. There was a qualitative difference, however, in the severity of their reactions. Jennifer's anxiety left her slightly nervous, somewhat agitated, and a little more cautious—a normal reaction. Roberta's feelings of terror and impending doom were so intense and overwhelming that she met the medical criteria for an anxiety disorder known as a *panic attack*.

*Anxiety disorders* are the most common of all mental disorders. Approximately 16 percent of adults between the ages of eighteen and thirty-four experience chronic anxiety. However, a 1999 Surgeon General's report on mental health revealed that 21 percent of women over fifty-five suffer from anxiety disorders. *Disorders* are medical illnesses that have both mental/emotional and physical/behavioral components.

An anxiety disorder occurs when anxious feelings are constant, overwhelming, and uncontrollable and interfere with our ability to function effectively in our personal or professional lives.

## PHYSICAL SYMPTOMS OF ANXIETY DISORDERS

- *Trembling, twitching, or shaking*
- *Restlessness*
- *Fatigue*
- *Breathlessness*
- *Pounding heart*
- *Sweating*
- *Cold, clammy hands*
- *Dry mouth*
- *Dizziness or light-headedness*
- *Frequent urination or diarrhea*
- *Nausea*
- *Difficulty swallowing*
- *Backache or headache*

## PSYCHOLOGICAL (EMOTIONAL) SYMPTOMS OF ANXIETY DISORDERS

- *Apprehension or feelings of dread*
- *Difficulty concentrating*
- *Irritability*
- *Insomnia*
- *Excessive worrying*
- *Excessive caution*
- *Feeling of a lump in the throat*
- *Butterflies in the stomach*
- *Reduced sex drive*

*Source:* American Psychiatric Association, *Diagnostic and Statistical Manual*, 4th ed., 1994.

Anxiety and stress share many of the same symptoms because both emotions activate a fight-or-flight response—an almost immediate arousal state that causes tensed muscles and increased heart rate and breathing. This response is triggered whenever we think we're in an actual or potentially dangerous situation that makes us fearful and anxious. It also occurs whenever we're confronted by internal or external demands that threaten our sense of physical or emotional well-being. This is stress.

Our earliest ancestors were frequently confronted by life-threatening environmental dangers—human, animal, and natural. Almost instantly and sometimes intuitively, their brains assessed the situation and mobilized the action section of the nervous system, called the sympathetic nervous system. Blood flow to the heart, leg, and arm muscles increased. All five senses became more alert. The lungs expanded. Internal temperature rose slightly, which triggered sweating and flushing.

However, according to the 1999 Surgeon General's report, anxiety reactions differ from stress states in a number of significant ways:

> First, with anxiety, the concern about the stressor is out of proportion to the real threat. Second, anxiety is often associated with elaborate mental and behavioral activities designed to avoid the unpleasant symptoms of a full-blown anxiety or panic attack (such as avoiding air travel, public speaking or leaving home). Third, anxiety is usually longer-lived than stress. Fourth, anxiety can occur without exposure to an external stressor.

You are probably thinking that as crazy and fearful as the world can still sometimes seem—random shootings and hate crimes, for instance—we need to stay hyperalert for our own survival. Even when we don't feel physically threatened, many African Americans believe that our anxiety is justified as a realistic reaction to racist, sexist, and ageist acts and attitudes against us. Reading this next passage from Delia Garlic, reproduced in *Remembering Slavery*, might put this anxiety into perspective:

> I was growed up when de war [Civil War] come . . . an' I was a mother befo' it closed. Babies was snatched from dere mother's breas' an' sold to speculators [slave auctioneers]. Chilluns was separated from sisters an' brothers an' never saw each other ag'in. Course dey cry; you think dey not cry when dey was sold lak cattle? I could tell you bout it all day, but even den you couldn't guess de awfulness of it. It's bad to belong to folks dat own you soul an' body; dat can tie you up to a tree, wid yo' face to de tree an' yo' arms fastened tight aroun' it. Who take a long curlin' whip an' cut de blood ever' lick.

The words of our foremother document the fear and anxiety that are part of our legacy as granddaughters and great-granddaughters. Our forebears' abduction and subsequent enslavement robbed them—and to some extent us—not only of physical freedom, but also of a sense of cultural and emotional security. During slavery, our foremothers worried that they or a loved one would be beaten or killed over an imagined or real "rule" violation. They worried that they or their children, partners, parents, other relatives, or friends would be sold to a different owner. They worried that they or their daughters or granddaughters or mothers would be raped by their owners, overseers, or other slaves. They worried that they would not have enough food or adequate clothing for themselves or their families.

Their worries and fears continue to resonate with us because most of us have had direct experience with the residual impact of slavery. Just think about it—"Jim Crow laws," which gave legal sanction to discriminatory practices against Blacks, were still in effect when midlife African American women were teenagers or young adults. Thus we worried ourselves, and felt the concern of our parents and grandparents, about our ability to obey the "law" to the satisfaction of Caucasian observers. Many of us had to sit in the back of buses or trains. Some of us were beaten, bitten by dogs, or jailed as we marched for the right to vote or desegregate restaurants. All of us were sad and fearful at seeing our leaders shot or bombed or burned as they tried to secure our civil rights.

The passage of the Civil Rights Act of 1964 did not eliminate racism. Contemporary studies indicate that almost 98 percent of Blacks report some degree of racial discrimination on an annual basis—from job discrimination to verbal or physical assaults—which negatively affects our quality of education, health, life circumstances, and financial status. Racism also has a substantial effect on our mental health.[1]

Gayle and her colleagues find that their clients often attribute their general feelings of fear, anxiety, anger, and helplessness to living with racism. The prejudice and discrimination they experience in the workplace causes particular pain. Their anecdotal stories of their development of these negative emotions have been further validated by studies that indicate that the development of certain psychiatric disorders, in particular anxiety and depression, is significantly influenced by racial discrimination.

Anxiety disorders, however, are inappropriate responses to present-day challenges, for they drain energy and often immobilize us. For some people, these experiences are occasional, but for others, feeling anxious, worried, or afraid is a chronic, disabling way of experiencing the world. Their worries and fears can make it difficult for them to make good decisions about their personal or professional life and can keep them from normal interaction with families, friends, and the world at large. In extreme cases, some women are too anxious even to leave their homes.

There are several types of anxiety disorders: *phobic disorder*; *generalized anxiety disorder* (GAD); *panic disorder* (PD), which is often associated with *agoraphobia* (a fear of open places, of being outside alone, or of being in a crowd); *post-traumatic stress disorder* (PTSD); and *obsessive-compulsive disorder* (OCD).

Each of these disorders is characterized by worry and physical and emotional symptoms, but each also has its own distinctive characteristics and its own incidence rate among the general population. Anxiety disorders are the most frequent diagnosis given to African American women who seek mental health treatment. According to recent research on phobias and African Americans, generalized anxiety disorder, post-traumatic stress disorder, and panic disorder with agoraphobia are two to three times more common in Black women than Black men.[2]

There are conflicting data about the incidence of generalized anxiety disorder, phobia, and agoraphobia in African Americans compared to Caucasians. Some studies indicate that African Americans have higher rates of these disorders than their Caucasian counterparts, but others indicate that there are no differences.[3]

## PANIC DISORDER (PD)

Panic disorder is characterized by unexpected episodes of intense fear and thoughts of approaching death. Panic attacks are often accompanied by physical symptoms that mimic signs of a heart attack or other life-threatening illnesses. Because these attacks resemble physical illnesses (such as in the case of Roberta, which we discussed earlier in the chapter), victims and their families, friends, and physicians often misdiagnose panic disorder. For instance, a panic attack is often misdiagnosed as hypoglycemia (an abnormal decrease of sugar in the blood that can be a separate condition but is often a medical complication of diabetes) because they have the same symptoms—sweating, rapid heartbeat, and trembling. In many cases, health professionals prescribe numerous costly medical procedures to rule out any physical basis for their patient's disability before diagnosing a panic attack.

People who suffer from panic disorder may make several trips to the emergency room before being properly diagnosed, which may be why many individuals who suffer from this form of anxiety fear they are losing their minds. Not surprisingly, friends and family often accuse PD sufferers of being *hypochondriacs* (imagining they are ill).

## SYMPTOMS OF PANIC DISORDER

To be diagnosed with panic disorder, you must exhibit at least four of the following symptoms:
- *Racing, palpitating, pounding heart (tachycardia)*
- *Chest pain*
- *Shortness of breath or smothering sensation (dyspnea)*
- *Tingling or numbness in the hands*
- *Flushes or chills*
- *Feeling of unreality or a sense of losing control*
- *Fear of impending doom or dying*
- *Fear of going crazy or doing something uncontrolled*
- *Choking*
- *Rapid breathing (hyperventilation)*

**In general, African Americans are two to three times more likely than Caucasians to report the following symptoms:**
- *Numbness/tingling in extremities (toes and hands)*
- *Strong fear of dying*
- *Worry about going crazy*

*Sources:* American Psychiatric Association, *Diagnostic and Statistical Manual*, 4th ed., 1994; Lisa C. Smith, Steven Friedman, and Jeffrey Nevid, "Clinical and Social Differences in African American and European American Patients with Panic Disorder and Agoraphobia," *Journal of Nervous and Mental Disease* 187(9) (1999): 550–61.

Panic disorder affects between two million and six million people each year. Women are two to three times more likely to be diagnosed with this disorder than men are, and we are also more apt to have recurring episodes of panic disorder. Many people with PD associate their panic attacks with the place or situation in which the attack occurred—elevators, supermarkets, and crowded stores—and develop a phobic reaction to that place.

As these attacks increase, PD sufferers may restrict their activities to places they know and feel safe in, and so they may eventually become agoraphobic. This behavior is memorably depicted as a response to a traumatic experience by Miss Havisham in Charles Dickens' *Great Expectations*, who did not leave her home after her fiancé stood her up at the altar, and Eva Pearce, the main character's grandmother in Toni Morrison's *Sula*, who permanently retreated to her bedroom after a meeting with her husband, who had deserted the family years before. These characters' devastations and self-imprisonment are extreme, but their stories help make the point that many women need to become more resilient and find more productive ways of dealing with life's setbacks.

**Several noted African American researchers report that panic disorder is significantly correlated with hypertension in African Americans, although this connection often goes undetected and misdiagnosed.** One reason may be that a majority of African American women diagnosed with hypertension and panic disorder do not report their panic symptoms to their primary-care physicians. The women themselves believe that the PD symptoms they experienced are caused by high blood pressure. Black women who have both hypertension and PD also report more instances of *isolated sleep paralysis* (ISP). This experience is a condition that occurs just as an individual is going to sleep or waking up. "During this period the individual is unable to move the body and may experience vivid hallucinations and feelings of acute danger. When the paralysis ends, the individual sits up and experiences panic-like symptoms, including tachycardia, hyperventilation, and fear [like a] 'witch is riding you.' "[4]

Blacks who have panic disorder and agoraphobia are also more likely to have had multiple medical emergency-room visits; deaths and separations from parents during childhood; physical and sexual abuse; paternal and sibling abuse of alcohol and other drugs; psychiatric hospitalizations and post-traumatic stress disorder.[5]

Panic disorder is associated with other physical and mental illnesses such as irritable bowel syndrome, mitral valve prolapse (damaged heart valve), and increased rates of major depression (approximately 75 to 80 percent of all panic disorder patients have a history of depression) and dependence on alcohol or illegal drugs. Panic disorder and agoraphobia are also associated with increased suicide attempts.[6]

## Effective Treatment Plans for Panic Disorder

If you have PD, a cognitive-behavioral therapist will help you examine negative or irrational thoughts you might have during an attack, such as "I'm having a heart attack" or "I'm going to die," and replace them with more realistic, reassuring thoughts, such as "I'm feeling anxious, but I'll feel better in a few minutes." They will also teach you relaxation and deep breathing techniques, which will help you relax during an attack and avoid hyperventilation. You will probably be given "homework" assignments to practice these techniques and to reinforce other things you've discussed in the office.

A process called *interceptive exposure* or *conditioning* is often done in the therapist's office. During this procedure, the therapist assesses your internal sensations and thoughts by having you simulate a panic attack. Sometimes they have you exercise to increase your heart rate or breathe rapidly to induce light-headedness, or spin around to trigger dizziness. The therapist can then assess your thoughts and feelings and have you replace "I'm dying" with "I'm dizzy."

If your panic attacks are severe, are frequent, and prevent you from functioning, medication might be recommended. The most commonly prescribed medications are benzodiazepines (BZDs), selective serotonin reuptake inhibitors (SSRIs), monoamine oxidase inhibitors (MAOIs), and tricyclic antidepressants.

## GENERAL ANXIETY DISORDER (GAD)

GAD is characterized by chronic, excessive worry that is usually unfounded and possibly irrational. It affects approximately four million to six million people and is twice as common in women as in men. At least six of the general systems of anxiety must be present for at least six months for someone to be diagnosed with generalized anxiety disorder.

## GENERAL ANXIETY DISORDER SYMPTOMS

- Feeling keyed up or on edge
- Impatience
- Difficulty concentrating or mind going blank
- Inability to relax
- Trembling, twitching, or feeling shaky
- Irritability
- Sleep disturbances, insomnia, or difficulty staying asleep
- Fatigue

*Source:* American Psychiatric Association, *Diagnostic and Statistical Manual,* 4th ed., 1994.

Patients suffering from generalized anxiety disorder not only focus on family, interpersonal relationships, money, work, and physical illness, but also worry excessively about their appearance, being late for appointments, and other daily matters such as commuting, getting meals, or the weather. African American women are even more worried than other people about violence, relationships, their children, money, and physical illness.

## ESTELLE'S STORY

Estelle, a sixty-two-year-old retired social worker, was known in the family as the worrywart. None of her siblings was as anxious as the "baby of the family." She was born prematurely, and her mother had been afraid that she was going to die because of the lack of adequate medical care in their segregated community. Estelle's mother, however, worried about Estelle's health long after her baby grew up to become a healthy adult.

Estelle worried about everything—her adult children, grandchildren, husband, siblings, friends, and clients. She was always on edge and very impatient. Even after she retired, she was always tired and rarely felt relaxed. She listened to the news and always focused on the most horrifying and unusual news stories. And then she discussed these incidents as if they were everyday events.

When Estelle's husband retired, he discovered that she was a closet smoker.

After a few months, he told Estelle that she was driving him crazy with her nervousness and smoking.

---

**R̲x̲ QUICK PRIME TIME PRESCRIPTION FOR ESTELLE**

Estelle joined a Black women's support group when her husband threatened to leave her if she didn't get some help. Her support group recommended that she take a class on complementary therapies, which included relaxation techniques, meditation, and yoga.

Estelle's lifelong habit of worry, her preoccupation with others, and her lack of knowledge about anxiety disorders initially prevented her from seeing her need for help. Research shows that people who are diagnosed with generalized anxiety disorder often suffer from depression, panic disorder, and substance abuse as well.

## Effective Treatment Plans for Generalized Anxiety Disorder

Generalized anxiety disorder is one of the most common anxiety disorders and is quite responsive to cognitive-behavioral therapy, which helps you examine the thoughts that cause you to assume the worst about any potential situation. Relaxation training, deep breathing, and visualization (picturing a calm, peaceful scene) are three techniques taught for generalized anxiety disorder.

Preferred medications for treating GAD are BuSpar (buspirone), Valium (diazepam), or the antidepressant Tofranil (imipramine). If Valium is prescribed, care should be taken to keep its course of treatment short (five to seven days) to avoid potential side effects.

## PHOBIC DISORDER

Phobias are persistent, unrealistic fears of certain objects or situations. Simple phobias are specific and focus on a particular object—snakes, rodents, birds, dogs, cats, insects, closed spaces, heights, driving, flying, water, blood, or injections. Social phobias include a fear of performing or speaking in a public setting.

Phobic disorder is the most common of the anxiety disorders. Approximately 10 percent of Americans, or 25 million people, have one or more clinically significant phobias.

---

## SYMPTOMS OF PHOBIC DISORDER

Simple and social phobias share many of the same symptoms:
- *Persistent fear*
- *Exposure to object or situation evokes intense anxiety*
- *The object or situation is avoided or endured with intense anxiety*
- *The fear or avoidance behavior interferes with occupational function, usual social situations, relationships with others or there is marked distress about having the fear*
- *The person recognizes the fear is excessive or unreasonable*

*Source:* American Psychiatric Association, *Diagnostic and Statistical Manual*, 4th ed., 1994.

---

African Americans report rates of simple phobias that are two to three times greater than Caucasians'. People with simple phobias are often terrified that they will be unable to escape from the situation or object they fear. **Black women are more phobic than Black men.** Phobias related to snakes, bats, cats, dogs, insects, mice, storms, confined spaces, heights, and being in water **are far more likely to be reported by African Americans than Caucasians**. This difference is constant, regardless of education, socioeconomic level, or birthplace.[7]

Fear of humiliation or embarrassment in front of others is the key feature of social phobia. People with this disorder are often afraid of choking on their food, saying something stupid or crazy, or having their minds go blank.

---

### KAREN'S STORY

Karen, fifty-four, is a radiology technician for a medium-sized hospital in Philadelphia. She is an excellent employee and very knowledgeable about her job. On several occasions, her boss has asked her to represent the hospital at various high schools on career days. He wanted her to give a short speech about her field, but she has always found a reason to refuse.

Karen's family and friends know that she is shy, but she has always been ashamed to tell anyone how she actually feels about public speaking. Even when she's asked to give a speech, her heart starts to pound, her skin flushes, and she feels faint. She has convinced herself that she will start to stutter or forget everything.

She also never told anyone about the hurt and pain she experienced when she was teased as a child by her sibling and classmates because she stuttered. Speech therapy was quite effective, so no one would guess that she had ever had any concerns about the way she talks. Still, Karen continues to feel overwhelmingly anxious whenever she thinks about speaking in public.

Her job evaluations have suffered and she has not been promoted because she seems so passive and unwilling to express her opinions in staff meetings or to participate in meetings outside of the office. Karen has become increasingly anxious and depressed as she watches her career stall.

---

### Rx QUICK PRIME TIME PRESCRIPTIONS FOR KAREN

Karen was encouraged by her supervisor to discuss her fear with a counselor. Karen's Prime Time Sister and counselor persuaded her to join a group where she could practice overcoming her social phobia.

## Effective Treatment Plans for Phobias

An intervention known as *exposure therapy* can be an effective treatment for phobias. Through this process, which is a form of cognitive-behavioral therapy, you are exposed, in a very gradual way, to objects or situations that frighten you. Armed with training in relaxation and deep breathing, you learn how to replace negative or irrational beliefs with more positive thoughts.

Another technique used is *flooding*, which exposes you in a nongraduated way to what causes your fear, until the fear disappears. For example, in flooding, a therapist might take a patient who is afraid of dogs to a kennel until her fear of dogs dissipates, or have the patient who is afraid of public speaking give a speech in front of strangers until she's no longer afraid.

There is no proven drug treatment for specific phobias (such as fear of water or rodents), but an SSRI such as Paxil (paroxetine) and certain MAOIs and benzodiazepines are being used to treat social phobias; Inderal (propranolol) has been used for stage fright. However, more long-term research needs to be done to determine correct dosage and length of treatment.

## OBSESSIVE-COMPULSIVE DISORDER (OCD)

The hallmark of obsessive-compulsive disorder is recurrent, repetitive thoughts (*obsessions*) or behaviors (*compulsions*) that are irrational and unwanted. Obsessions can range from trivial to terrifying. Common preoccupations are with contamination or "germs," violence toward self or others, safety, sex, or fear of making a mistake. Compulsions often include frequent hand washing, repeatedly cleaning a room, or checking to see if a door is locked or an iron is unplugged. Four million to five million people experience OCD. It is the only anxiety disorder that is equally prevalent in women and men.

---

### DIAGNOSTIC CRITERIA FOR OBSESSIVE-COMPULSIVE DISORDER

*Obsessions*
- *Recurrent, persistent ideas, thoughts, impulses, or images that are experienced, at least initially, as intrusive and senseless*
- *Trying to ignore or suppress such thoughts or impulses or to stop them by substituting other thoughts or using medication*
- *Recognition that the obsessions are the product of his/her own mind and are not imposed by outside forces*

*Compulsions*
- *Repetitive, purposeful, intentional behaviors that are performed in response to an obsession or according to certain rules or in a stereotyped fashion*
- *The compulsions cause marked distress, are time-consuming (take more than an hour a day), or significantly interfere with the person's normal routine, occupational functioning, or usual social activities or relationships with others*

---

*Source:* Harold I. Kaplan, M.D., and Benjamin L. Sadock, M.D., *Pocket Handbook of Clinical Psychiatry,* 1990.

---

African Americans and Caucasians have the same rate of obsessive-compulsive disorder. However, African Americans are underrepresented in studies that focus on OCD. Excessive shame, fear of insanity, a desire for secrecy, and the stigma attached to mental health disorders in our communities can make it more difficult for African Americans to seek treatment.[8]

# CHARLENE'S STORY

Charlene, fifty-three, is a very successful accountant. Thus, her attention to detail and order in her office, car, and clothes was attributed to habits acquired in her profession. Only her partner (who didn't know the full extent of her problem) realized that Charlene was not just meticulous, but often consumed with obsessions and compulsions—especially around clothes. Every morning, Charlene changed her blouse at least three times before she left the house. She was obsessed with the idea that her clothes were dirty even when they had just come from the cleaners. There was always something wrong with the first two blouses—a spot on the sleeve or a smudge on the collar. Her shoes had to be polished at least three times. She had to brush her suit at least three times to ensure that there was no lint on it.

While Charlene's OCD was most apparent in the way she fussed over her clothes, her office chair and the papers on her desk all had to be aligned and in a certain order or she began to feel nervous. Her partner and secretary complained about her fastidiousness, and she felt ashamed and sad about her obsessiveness but believed that she could not change her thoughts or behaviors. Charlene was also too afraid of what people might think to seek the help she needed.

**Rx** **QUICK PRIME TIME PRESCRIPTIONS FOR CHARLENE**

Charlene's fear that she was "going crazy," her drinking, and her depression made her decide to talk to her pastor, who encouraged Charlene to get professional help. The combination of cognitive-behavioral therapy and medication helped her to regain her sense of wellness.

OCD is often associated with depression, other anxiety disorders, and eating disorders, and can lead to substance abuse to help calm the person's fears.

## Effective Treatment Plans for OCD

Cognitive-behavioral therapy can be effective with 50 to 90 percent of those with OCD, but the patient must really commit to keeping to an agreement she makes with the therapist. The therapy works best if family members and friends are encouraging and supportive.

A specific form of cognitive-behavioral therapy uses a technique called *exposure and response prevention*. In this approach, the patient deliberately and voluntarily confronts the feared object or idea, either directly or in imagination, but doesn't engage in the compulsive behavior. For example, if every time the patient touches the front-door knob, she feels she must wash her hands, she would be encouraged to touch the doorknob but wait for hours before washing. The goal is to help dissipate fears of what would happen if the compulsion to wash is not acted on. Before this exposure is encouraged, however, the therapist teaches relaxation techniques and deep breathing so that while the patient waits to wash, she is able to stay calm.

Drugs that affect one of the brain's chemical messengers (neurotransmitters), serotonin, can significantly decrease the symptoms of OCD. Prozac (fluoxetine), Luvox (fluvoxamine), and Paxil (paroxetine) are SSRIs that have been approved for use. Improvement usually takes at least two to three weeks.

## POST-TRAUMATIC STRESS DISORDER (PTSD)

Post-traumatic stress disorder is a debilitating psychological, emotional, and behavioral response to witnessing a traumatic event or being a victim of a trauma, which can include military or street combat, attempted murder or other street attack, rape, child abuse, near-death experience, accident, and natural disasters.

---

### SYMPTOMS OF POST-TRAUMATIC STRESS DISORDER

- *Inability to escape memories and thoughts about traumatic events*
- *Flashbacks and nightmares where the event seems to be recurring; sleep disturbances/insomnia, or difficulty staying asleep*
- *Irritability or unprovoked outbursts of anger*
- *Aggressive or violent feelings and behavior*
- *Intense distress at exposure to situations, events, people, or objects that are reminders of the trauma*
- *Withdrawal, numbness, difficulty in expressing positive feelings, loss of interest in people or things that were once important and enjoyable*

*Source:* John Briere, *Psychological Assessment of Adult Posttraumatic States*, 1997.

---

To be diagnosed as *acute post-traumatic stress disorder*, symptoms of PTSD must appear within thirty days of a traumatic event. If the symptoms persist for more than three months, the diagnosis is *chronic PTSD*; and if the symptoms don't emerge until six months after the trauma, it is called *delayed PTSD*.

Between six million and seven million people experience post-traumatic stress disorder. Women and people of color have higher rates of PTSD than male Caucasians. Women have almost twice the prevalence of PTSD than men. The 1999 report by the Surgeon General also revealed that victims of rape and physical assault and survivors of concentration camps and torture have the highest rates of PTSD.

Because of social and economic disparities, African American women are at higher risk for being victims of traumatic events—rape, physical assault, witnessing violence—than Caucasians. We are also more apt than Caucasians to have experienced childhood traumas—separation from or death of parents, child abuse, substance abuse by parents or siblings—that increase our vulnerability to subsequent traumas and the development of PTSD.

---

## ROSEMARY'S STORY

Rosemary, a forty-six-year-old elementary-school teacher, had decided to finish her lesson plans for the following week and leave them in her desk. She and her husband, sixteen-year-old son, and fourteen-year-old daughter were leaving town for the long Martin Luther King Jr. Day weekend. She wanted to make certain that if her plane was delayed on her return, the substitute teacher would have more than just busywork for the kids. She'd been so occupied that she didn't notice that everyone else had left. When she got to the parking lot, she saw only one other car. The driver pulled up to her and started asking her directions while pointing to a map.

Rosemary felt slightly afraid when he started to get out of the car but didn't back away from him or quickly get into her own car because she didn't want to hurt his feelings. She also didn't want to act as if she believed the myth that all Black men are dangerous. After all, she had a wonderful Black husband and son. However, when he pulled a knife, forced her into his car, and raped her, she repeatedly replayed in her mind the scene of him getting out of the car.

After the rape, Rosemary received tremendous support from her husband, children, family, and friends. She was able to give the police a good description and part of his license plate number. The rapist was apprehended and convicted. Rosemary was encouraged to see a therapist or join a rape survivors support group, but she refused. She didn't want people to think she was upset, which she believed would be acting like a "hysterical" White woman. She just wanted to put the incident behind her. She had done that once before, when she was sixteen and had been a victim of a date rape. She had never told anyone about that rape, and in her own mind, she'd done okay.

Six months after the rapist had been convicted, Rosemary suddenly started trembling and shaking as she walked to her car. She felt as if the rape were occurring again. After a few minutes, she felt better, but over the next few weeks, scenes from the rape began invading her waking and sleeping hours. Rosemary didn't tell anyone about these thoughts, but she became increasingly angry, sad, and withdrawn, especially from her male family members, friends, and colleagues. When she refused to allow her husband or son even to touch her hand, the family confronted her and told her that she had to seek help.

---

**Rx** QUICK PRIME TIME PRESCRIPTION FOR ROSEMARY

A friend urged Rosemary to join the rape survivors support group, and suggested she work with an individual therapist, with whom she focused on her feelings of loss, guilt, and shame over her earlier rape.

Post-traumatic stress is often associated with other emotional difficulties—depression, other anxiety disorders, and substance abuse, especially of alcohol, marijuana, and heroin. These substances are often used to suppress the memory of the trauma.[9]

## Effective Treatment Plans for Post-Traumatic Stress Disorder

Exposure treatment for PTSD involves repeated reliving of the trauma under controlled conditions. One form of exposure therapy is *systematic desensitization*, in which the therapist asks the patient to imagine the trauma or, if possible, takes her back where she experienced it. The therapist encourages the patient, on a graduated basis, to recall the trauma, and as she starts to feel anxious, the therapist instructs her in relaxation and deep breathing exercises. Another form is *imaginable flooding*, where the therapist guides the patient in remembering the details of the traumatic event and simultaneously practicing relaxation exercises.

The antidepressants Elavil (amitriptyline) and Norpramin (desipramine) are used to treat PTSD because it is so often accompanied by depression.

## RISK FACTORS FOR ANXIETY DISORDER

There are competing, complementary theories about the cause of anxiety disorders. Some believe that these disorders are the result of a biochemical imbalance. Others believe that each particular anxiety disorder has multiple causes. The risk factors include genetics, biochemical components, and childhood and adult psychosocial experiences, especially those related to learning, stress, trauma, and psychological factors.

### Family History

A genetic predisposition to certain anxiety disorders is often apparent among family members. In studies of twins, there is an 80 to 90 percent chance that identical twins (both from the same egg and sperm) will both develop general anxiety disorders, while fraternal twins (from two different eggs and sperm) have only a 10 to 15 percent probability that both will develop the disorder. About 20 percent of children and/or siblings of agoraphobic patients have that disorder.

### Biochemical Factors

The *hippocampus* and *amygdala* are parts of the brain in which the memory of events connected with strong emotions—especially fear and anger—is stored. Current research suggests that minor changes in these parts of the brain might be caused by exposure to intense or chronic stressors. Once this region of the brain is impaired, it is more difficult to remember or assess stressful events accurately. Brain scans of post-traumatic stress disorder patients have shown a decrease in the size of the hippocampus. When certain chemical messengers (neurotransmitters) in the brain are affected—when gamma-amino-butyric acid (GABA) is decreased or serotonin is increased, for instance—anxiety disorders may develop.[10]

## Psychological Factors

Various psychological factors are posited as explanations for anxiety disorders, from unresolved childhood emotional conflicts to our perceptions of life experiences.

*Psychodynamic theory* postulates that unresolved, unconscious childhood emotional conflicts—especially with parents—are the base of many adult emotional difficulties. Parents' or guardians' responses to childhood expressions of anger, sexual curiosity, sadness, jealousy, or other emotions have a profound impact on adults' abilities to appropriately express these feelings, especially toward significant people in their lives. The denial or minimization of angry or sexual thoughts or impulses can generate the symptoms associated with anxiety disorders.

*Learning theorists* believe that anxiety disorders develop because of conditioning and positive reinforcement. For instance, Roberta, who had the encounter with the growling dog, unconsciously associated her mother's house with her fear of the dog, so the house had the power to elicit multiple anxiety symptoms in her.

*Cognitive-behaviorists* theorize that negative or irrational thoughts or beliefs play a critical role in the development of anxiety disorders. Parents usually teach these beliefs to us in direct or indirect ways, so that these unconscious thoughts directly impact how we feel and behave. Two irrational beliefs that are often associated with anxiety are "It's awful and terrible when things are not the way I very much want them to be" and "If something is dangerous or dreadful, I should be constantly and excessively upset about it and should dwell on the possibility of its occurring."[11] Negative thoughts can convince you that you are not able to control your response to events that affect your life. They also can increase your sense of helplessness.

## Medical and Neurological Risk Factors

Medical conditions that are particularly problematic for African American women can precipitate anxiety-like symptoms. Thus before undergoing any treatment for anxiety disorders, it's imperative that you get a thorough medical examination to rule out the possibility of any underlying physical problems. These include hyperthyroidism (excessive levels of thyroid hormone), hypoglycemia (low blood sugar; this can be a particular problem with diabetes), premenstrual syndrome (PMS), menopause, iron-deficiency anemia, cardiac arrhythmia (disturbances in the heartbeat), epilepsy, multiple sclerosis, mitral valve prolapse (damage to a valve in the heart), lupus erythematosus, asthma, and a deficiency in folic acid or vitamin $B_{12}$.

## Drugs

Using addictive substances, legal or illegal, can induce an anxiety disorder or mimic its symptoms, as can withdrawal from extended abuse of cigarettes, caffeine, alcohol, heroin, cocaine, amphetamines, or marijuana. Certain medications, such as penicillin and aspirin, can also induce this state in some people.

## Stressful Life Events

The variability of individual responses to even major stressors—such as rape or witnessing a murder—makes it difficult to state that stressful life events cause anxiety disorders. Certain stressors—poverty, racism, sexism, and discrimination, physical illness, being a victim of physical violence, dissolution of romantic or erotic relationships, death of a family member or friend—and combinations of stressors dramatically increase vulnerability to anxiety disorders or exacerbate existing disorders. Multiple stressors tend to make individuals even more vulnerable.

### R̶x PRIME TIME PRESCRIPTIONS FOR ANXIETY AND ANXIETY DISORDERS

*Yize uvalo, ingobo yisibindi.*
*Fear is nothing, the real thing is courage.*

—Ndebele proverb

Recommit to taking care of yourself first, as you did when you began reading *Prime Time*. Remember that you are a unique being, a valuable and valued woman.

It takes courage to confront and overcome the unnecessary fears that hinder our growth and development. Fear and anxiety are part of our survival legacy as human beings and as Black women living in America, but we have also inherited from our ancient and recent forebears the ability, fortitude, and persistence to overcome seemingly insurmountable, frightening, and painful obstacles.

*This very place where I am now the mayor, the [White] people used to go arrest me every day and harass me every day. They turned cars upside down, burned crosses in my yard, threw homemade bombs at us. It wasn't just a song for us, "We Shall Overcome," it was our strength. When I see people heading up organizations and doing all these things, it didn't come about overnight and it didn't come without pain.*

—Unita Blackwell (first Black mayor in Mississippi),
quoted in Diane J. Johnson, ed.,
*Proud Sisters: The Wisdom and Wit of African-American Women*

## Recommendations to Help Reduce or Prevent Anxiety

Many of the prevention steps outlined in the chapters on stress management (Chapter 13) and depression (Chapter 15) can also be used to treat anxiety disorders. The following specific recommendations will help keep you from developing an anxiety disorder.

***Get enough rest.*** Inadequate rest can cause symptoms that mimic anxiety symptoms—irritability, feeling on edge, fatigue, trembling, and difficulty concentrating.

***Eat vitamin- and mineral-rich foods or take supplements.*** Good nutrition is essential to prevent anxiety. The B vitamins are truly good for the nerves. Deficiencies in certain vitamins and minerals can mimic or exacerbate anxiety symptoms:

• *Not enough $B_1$* (thiamin) can cause anxiety, hysteria, nausea, and difficulty concentrating.

• *Not enough $B_3$* (niacin) can increase your sense of apprehension, nervousness, and irritability.

• *Not enough $B_5$* (pantothenic acid) can cause weakness and irritability.

• *Not enough $B_6$* (pyridoxine) can cause depression, which is often associated with anxiety and confusion.

• *Not enough $B_{12}$* (cyanocobalamin) impairs the functioning of the entire nervous system.

According to research from the Natural Medicine Collective, certain other nutrients, such as *biotin* and *magnesium*, help keep your mood stable.[12] Whole-grain cereals, seafood, nuts, potatoes, meat, eggs, and green leafy vegetables are good sources of these vitamins and minerals. If you're a vegetarian or on any kind of a restricted diet, ensure that you're receiving adequate amounts of these nutrients by discussing your diet with your primary-care provider and by taking a daily multivitamin-mineral supplement.

*Stay away from caffeine.* Caffeine in coffee, tea, cola, or chocolate can precipitate anxiety-like symptoms—nervousness, heart pounding, racing pulse, and twitching. If you've got to have something to get going in the morning, limit yourself to just one cup. You can cut back your consumption gradually by substituting decaffeinated coffee at other times so that you avoid the headache of withdrawal.

*Pump up your calming hormones by getting active.* Exercise helps the body release the hormone beta-endorphin, which functions as a natural tranquilizer. Exercise also expels excess adrenaline, which propels the body into action.

*Draw on the support of your Prime Time support system.* Your Prime Time Sister or Prime Time Circle can be invaluable in helping you distinguish between realistic and irrational fears and worries. They also provide support as you confront your fears. For instance, if you're afraid of flying, consider asking your Prime Time Sister to go on a vacation with you that requires taking a plane to your destination. Or perhaps she can role-play your request for a pay raise. Your Prime Time Circle can also be a resource for the names of mental health clinicians, support groups, or books or audiotapes on managing anxiety.

*Take a break from the real world.* Reducing your negative information overload can decrease your level of worry. War, crime, terrorists, natural disaster, and poverty have always existed, but we haven't always been exposed to their reality in such an in-depth and continuous manner. From the time we wake up until we go to sleep, we are bombarded with negative, sometimes terrifying news stories on television, the radio, and the newspaper. Constantly being inundated with this type of information can increase your level of anxiety and leave you more vulnerable to developing or intensifying anxiety disorders.

Remember, you don't have to listen to or watch the news four or five times a day. You also don't have to go to movies or watch television programs that promote the idea that most people are violent or insane. Rationing your exposure to fear or anxiety-producing materials can help you avoid the destructive impact of anxiety disorders.

## DIAGNOSING ANXIETY DISORDER

There are numerous symptoms associated with the various anxiety disorders. The criteria used to determine whether you have a particular anxiety disorder are described in an earlier section of this chapter. However, the Bourne Anxiety Inventory below can function as a screening device to help you assess whether you are feeling any level of anxiety.

## WHAT ARE THE ANXIETY DISORDERS?

Self-Diagnosis Questionnaire

The following questionnaire is designed to help you identify which particular anxiety disorder you may be dealing with. It is based on the official classification of anxiety disorders used by all mental health professionals and known as *DSM-IV* (*Diagnostic and Statistical Manual of Mental Disorders—Fourth Edition*).

1. Do you have spontaneous anxiety attacks that come out of the blue? (Only answer yes if you do *not* have any phobias.) Yes ___ No ___

2. Have you had at least one such attack in the last month? Yes ___ No ___

3. If you had an anxiety attack in the last month, did you worry about having another one? Or did you worry about the implications of your attack for your physical or mental health? Yes ___ No ___

4. In your worst experience with anxiety, did you have more than three of the following symptoms?
___ Shortness of breath or smothering sensation
___ Dizziness or unsteady feeling
___ Heart palpitations or rapid heartbeat
___ Trembling or shaking
___ Sweating
___ Choking
___ Nausea or abdominal distress
___ Feelings of being detached or out of touch with your body
___ Numbness or tingling sensations
___ Flushes or chills
___ Chest pain or discomfort
___ Fear of dying
___ Fear of going crazy or doing something out of control

If your answers to 1, 2, 3, and 4 were yes, stop. You've met the conditions for panic disorder.

If your answer to 1 was yes but your anxiety reaction involved three or fewer of the symptoms listed under 4, you're experiencing what are called *limited symptom attacks*, but do not have full-blown panic disorder.

If you have panic attacks *and* phobias, go on.

5. Does fear of having panic attacks cause you to avoid going into certain situations? Yes ___ No ___

If your answer to 5 was yes, stop. It is likely that you are dealing with agoraphobia. See question 6 to determine the extent of your agoraphobia.

6. Which of the following situations do you avoid because you are afraid of panicking?

___ Going far away from home
___ Shopping in a grocery store
___ Standing in a grocery store line
___ Going to department stores
___ Going to shopping malls
___ Driving on freeways
___ Driving anywhere by yourself
___ Using public transportation (buses, trains, etc.)
___ Going over bridges (whether you're the driver or passenger)
___ Going through tunnels (as driver or passenger)
___ Flying in planes
___ Riding in elevators
___ Being in high places
___ Going to a dentist's or doctor's office
___ Sitting in a barber's or beautician's chair
___ Eating in restaurants
___ Going to work
___ Being too far from a safe person or safe place
___ Being alone
___ Going outside your house
___ Other _____

The number of situations you checked above indicates the extent of your agoraphobia and the degree to which it limits your activity.

If your answer to 5 was no but you do have phobias, go on.

7. Do you avoid certain situations *not* primarily because you are afraid of panicking but because you're afraid of being embarrassed or nega-

tively evaluated by other people? (That is, you worry that your embarrassment could subsequently lead you to panic?) Yes ___ No ___

If your answer to 7 was yes, stop. It's likely that you are dealing with social phobia. See question 8 to determine the extent of your social phobia.

8. Which of the following situations do you avoid because of a fear of embarrassing or humiliating yourself?

___ Sitting in any kind of group (for example, at work, in school classrooms, in social organizations, in self-help groups)

___ Giving a talk or presentation before a small group of people

___ Giving a talk or presentation before a large group of people

___ Parties and social functions

___ Using public rest rooms

___ Eating in front of others

___ Writing or signing your name in the presence of others

___ Dating

___ Any situations where you might say something foolish

___ Other _____

The number of situations you checked indicates the extent to which social phobia limits your activities.

If your answers to questions 5 and 7 were no but you have other phobias, continue.

9. Do you fear and avoid any one (or more than one) of the following?

___ Insects or animals, such as spiders, bees, snakes, rats, bats, or dogs

___ Heights (high floors in buildings, tops of hills or mountains, high-level bridges)

___ Driving

___ Tunnels

___ Bridges

___ Elevators

___ Airplanes (flying)

___ Doctors or dentists

___ Thunder or lightning

___ Water

___ Blood

___ Injections or medical procedures

___ Illness such as heart attacks or cancer

___ Darkness

___ Other _____

10. Do you have high degrees of anxiety usually *only* when you have to face one of these situations? Yes ___ No ___

If you checked one or more items in 9 and answered yes to 10, stop. It's likely that you're dealing with a specific phobia. If not, proceed.

11. Do you feel quite anxious much of the time but do *not* have distinct panic attacks, do *not* have phobias, and do *not* have specific obsessions or compulsions? Yes ___ No ___

12. Have you been prone to excessive worry for at least the last six months? Yes ___ No ___

13. Have your anxiety and worry been associated with at least three of the following six symptoms?

___ Restlessness or feeling keyed up or on edge
___ Being easily fatigued
___ Difficulty concentrating or mind going blank
___ Irritability
___ Muscle tension
___ Sleep disturbances (difficulty falling or staying asleep, or restless and unsatisfying sleep)

If your answers to 11, 12, and 13 were yes, stop. It's likely that you're dealing with generalized anxiety disorder. If you answered yes to 11 but no to 12 or 13, you're dealing with an anxiety condition that is not severe enough to qualify as generalized anxiety disorder.

14. Do you have recurring intrusive thoughts such as hurting or banning a close relative, being contaminated with dirt or a toxic substance, fearing you forgot to lock your door or turn off an appliance, or an unpleasant fantasy of catastrophe? (You recognize that these thoughts are irrational, but you can't keep them from coming into your mind.) Yes ___ No ___

15. Do you perform ritualistic actions such as washing your hands, checking, or counting to relieve anxiety over irrational fears that enter your mind? Yes ___ No ___

If you answered yes to 14 but no to 15, you are probably dealing with obsessive-compulsive disorder, but have obsessions only.

If you answered yes to 14 and 15, you're probably dealing with obsessive-compulsive disorder, with both obsessions and compulsions.

If you answered no to 14 and 15 and most or all of the preceding questions, but still have anxiety or anxiety-related symptoms, you may be dealing with post-traumatic stress disorder or a nonspecific anxiety condition. Use the section in this chapter on post-traumatic stress disorder to determine whether your symptoms fit this category.

If you are feeling more anxious than usual, discuss your physical and emotional experiences with your primary care physician. During your annual physical exam, provide your doctor with information about the physical and emotional aspects of your experience. Be certain to describe—in detail—your anxious feelings and their duration, level of intensity, and impact on your normal activities. As Moms Mabley used to say, "Tell the truth." This is not the time to minimize or deny your symptoms. Let it all hang out! In fact, celebrate the fact that you're taking care of yourself.

For African Americans, being very tight-lipped about our personal and professional business has been necessary to our very survival. There are anecdotal and documented accounts of the negative impact of "loose lips" or talking too freely about anything from attempted slave escapes and uprisings in yesteryear to current business dealings such as securing patents or closing a sale. Thus, our ability to be totally open and candid about our thoughts and feelings to anyone, including our immediate family, has been seriously compromised. However, continuing this legacy of silence and secrecy can be as damaging to our health and well-being as inappropriate forthrightness was in the past.

Once physical health concerns have been ruled out, you can then determine with input from your health-care provider—perhaps in consultation with a mental health specialist—the best course of treatment for you. If your doctor, family, or friends try to discourage you from seeking help, if they say "It's nothing to worry about" or "It's just in your head" or "It's just stress," ignore them. Sometimes even physicians and the people closest to us don't understand the negative and frightening effect that anxiety disorders can have. Get another opinion, talk to some other people, but get the help you need.

## TREATING ANXIETY DISORDERS

Anxiety disorders are treatable. You don't have to live a life that is full of fear and worry.

## Psychotherapy to Treat Anxiety Disorder

*Cognitive-behavioral therapy* is a time-limited treatment that teaches people how to recognize and change irrational or negative thoughts, feelings, fears, or behaviors. Various techniques are used in cognitive-behavioral therapy, such as keeping a diary of negative thoughts or learning relaxation techniques.

Depending upon the severity of your anxiety disorder, you can expect to work with a cognitive-behavioral therapist for one to three hours a week for two to six months. He or she will focus on alleviating current symptoms.

*Psychodynamic therapy* attempts to resolve anxiety symptoms by talking to clients about childhood conflicts that may be connected to current emotional problems. While extensive medical studies have not been conducted on psychodynamic clinical interventions, anecdotal accounts indicate that it can be quite effective. These therapies often are open-ended (no specific time limit) and generally last at least a year.

The therapist will usually start the sessions by taking a very extensive social, emotional, and physical history of you and your biological family (parents, siblings, grandparents, etc.). He or she will focus on family members who have had any emotional difficulties, especially anxiety, depression, or substance abuse. You will also be asked to describe in detail childhood memories, and the therapist will ask you to explore your thoughts and feelings during an anxiety attack and may instruct you in relaxation techniques that can stop an attack before it becomes full-blown. He or she will help you connect these thoughts to current and past conflictual relationships.

## Medications Used to Treat Anxiety Disorders

Of the medications used to alleviate anxiety symptoms, *benzodiazepines*, *buspirone*, and *antidepressants* are the most widely prescribed. The most commonly used benzodiazepines are Xanax (alprazolam), Valium (diazepam), Librium and Libritabs (chlordiazepoxide), and Librax (chlordiazepoxide and didinium). They generally take effect within a few hours, some in even less time. *Always, always tell your doctor and pharmacist what other medicines, vitamins, or herbs you may be taking, including herbal treatments such as ginseng, gingko biloba, Saint-John's-wort, and so on.* Like psychotherapy treatments, medication must be tailored to your specific anxiety disorder.

*Benzodiazepines* are thought to enhance the ability of GABA, one of the brain's chemical messengers, to suppress unnecessary neural activity. The primary side effects of benzodiazepines are drowsiness and loss of coordination, but fatigue and mental slowness can also occur. It can be dangerous to drive when you're just starting on these medications. Combining benzodiazepines with other medications or alcohol can lead to serious, even life-threatening complications. If you are taking any antianxiety drug, you should also check before taking antihistamines, sedatives, muscle relaxants, and some over-the-counter and prescription pain medications. Benzodiazepines have also been associated with abnormalities in babies born to mothers who took these drugs during pregnancy.

Many people become dependent on benzodiazepines (especially Valium and Xanax), so these drugs are generally recommended only as a short-term medication. Taking BZDs should be avoided if you or a close family member has a history of alcohol or illegal substance abuse or if you have chronic pain. If you're currently taking this sort of medication, don't abruptly discontinue it. Stopping this medication suddenly can produce anxiety-type symptoms such as insomnia, shakiness, headaches, and, in some severe cases, hallucinations. So discuss your concerns with your doctor before stopping so that he or she can give you the best plan for cutting back on dosages safely and without side effects.

*BuSpar* (buspirone) is a nonbenzodiazepine medication. It has fewer side effects, it's not habit-forming, and it doesn't cause drowsiness. However, you must take it every day for three to six weeks before it becomes effective. Side effects include headaches, dizziness, nausea, and nervousness. According to recent studies, buspirone is not as effective as the benzodiazepines for treating panic disorders.

*Antidepressants* are often prescribed for anxiety disorders, because depression is frequently a result of these disorders. The most commonly prescribed antidepressants are the tricyclic antidepressants, MAOIs (monoamine oxidase inhibitors), and SSRIs (selective serotonin reuptake inhibitors). For more information on these drugs, refer to Chapter 15.

## Complementary/Alternative Medicine

In addition to the traditional treatments of psychotherapy and medication, there are several natural remedies that can be used to treat anxiety disorders. Many of the interventions described in the stress chapter (Chapter 13) are applicable to treating anxiety disorders. However, there are some natural therapies that are particularly helpful when treating anxiety. A naturopath or herbalist and your primary-care physician should be consulted before using any of these interventions.

*Herbal medicine.* Several herbs function in a way similar to sedatives.

They impact the nervous system, bringing on states of relaxation and tranquillity. Herbs are often made into teas.

The Natural Medicine Collective recommends using one teaspoon of herbs to one cup of boiling water. These herbs can include skullcap, mullein, peppermint, hops, catnip, and chamomile. Allow tea to steep for ten to twenty minutes. Reheat if you prefer hot tea.

*Kava kava*, member of the pepper family, can induce calm feelings and sleep. It's available in an extract and capsule form. There are no U.S. studies of kava kava's effectiveness, but there are several German studies. In one long-term German study, participants showed a 23 percent improvement in their anxiety symptoms. There are some concerns about long-term use of kava kava. Allergic reactions, visual disturbances, and health problems similar to those seen in alcoholics, especially with the liver, have been found in chronic kava kava users.

*Hydrotherapy* (water therapy). Warm baths with the following herbs can be very relaxing: lemon balm, basil, bay, peppermint, rosemary, pennyroyal, chamomile, meadowsweet, yarrow.

*Hypnotherapy.* While the patient is in a hypnotic state, the therapist makes positive and relaxing suggestions to relieve anxiety.

*Acupuncture.* This Chinese healing art can restore emotional wholeness and calm as well as treat chronic pain and other anxiety-producing ailments.

*Tai chi* is an exercise of precise movements that are done in a slow, calming manner. Tai chi can be done by people of any age.

Thankfully, it is possible these days to treat anxiety disorders more successfully than ever before and feel better than you may have felt in years of suffering. You can be helped through the use of these interventions, either with therapy or medications or a combination of both. Today, we have an opportunity to conquer our fears and anxieties and live as Audre Lorde declared: "I am deliberate and afraid of nothing."

# Chapter 15

# DEPRESSION: YOU CAN FEEL BETTER

---

## GAYLE'S STORY

When the intercom buzzed on a busy Monday morning in December 1996, I became very annoyed. I didn't want to talk to anyone. I was trying to finish a major report, but just staying awake was proving a major challenge. I was simply exhausted. For weeks I had been waking up between 2:00 and 3:00 A.M., drenched with perspiration and unable to go back to sleep. During the day I had had to deal with mood swings and hot flashes that certainly felt more like an energy drain than the "power surges" that women's groups like to talk about. Even though I intellectually understood that all these symptoms were temporary and due to the onset of menopause, my nerves were completely rattled. And at that moment on that Monday morning, I just wanted to be left alone!

Still, I snatched up the phone and heard my secretary say in a worried voice: "It's a long-distance call from Chicago." I was immediately concerned. Had something happened to my mother, one of my siblings, nieces, nephews, aunts, cousins, or friends? I knew that if there was a problem, everyone would expect me to solve it. Being the eldest child and female had brought an inordinate amount of love—and an equal amount of responsibility.

The call was devastating. One of my oldest and dearest friends was in critical condition. She had been my teacher, mentor, and role model for almost forty years.

I raced home, packed a few clothes, and flew to Chicago. Even though I was born and raised in Chicago and had made the trip from the airport many times, I made several wrong turns and arrived at the hospital ten minutes after she died. I was devastated. Despite my grief, I started writing my friend's eulogy at the request of her family.

Two days before the funeral, I received another heartbreaking call. Marilyn, my longtime friend and coauthor of *Prime Time*, had been in a serious car accident and suffered a fractured vertebra. Her recovery would require that she remain in an upper-body cast for six months.

I returned home, and over the next two months I divided my time between working and helping to care for Marilyn. It was only while driving from home to work to Marilyn's to home that I would find myself crying. My fatigue was overwhelming. I knew I was sad, but it was only when my internist said, "Dr. Porter, I think you're depressed," that I realized the cost to me—and to so many other Black women—of not stopping to care for myself.

---

Millions of African American women are depressed. And too many of us are turning to alcohol, drugs or, even worse, suicide—including writer Terry Jewel, actress Dorothy Dandridge, songstress Phyllis Hyman, and Chicago journalist Leanita McLain—to ease our pain. Yet we rarely discuss how depression is preventing far too many African American women from experiencing the love, joy, and fulfillment that life should bring.

Almost every one of us knows at least one Black woman who is depressed—a family member, a friend, a colleague, or perhaps yourself. However, it is still a shock to read that research conducted by the Commonwealth Fund Women's Health Survey in 1993 and the National Black Women's Health Project estimates that approximately 50 percent of all African American women report depressive symptoms during their lifetime.[1] This is almost twice the rate of depressive symptoms experienced by all men and almost 42 percent higher than Caucasian women. If research estimated that half of adult Black women had tuberculosis, public health officials would declare an epidemic and mandate widespread treatment! However, a 1994 study revealed that only about 7 percent of African American women with clinical depression receive treatment.[2]

There has been very little research focus on the mental health of Black lesbians, and even less on these women in midlife. However, the information that does exist indicates that the rate of depression and thoughts of suicide among Black lesbians is much greater than those of their Black heterosexual sisters. In fact, their rates of depression have been found to be comparable with those of gay males with AIDS. The primary reasons usually given for their higher rate of depression are their difficulty in finding partners and their actual or fantasied negative experiences related to their family, friends, or coworkers finding out about their sexual preference.[3]

Then why don't Black women ever talk about depression? Why aren't our African American health professionals, ministers, legislators, and other leaders discussing it in private and public forums? Why aren't we demanding that depression be a major national agenda item in the African American and larger community? Maybe it's because there is still stigma, embarrassment, fear, anxiety, and ignorance surrounding mental illness in all our communities. Maybe it's because depression is considered a "weakness" or a "White thing." Maybe it's because the slavery legacy that necessitated ignoring or minimizing emotional and physical pain in order to survive is still operating. Maybe it's because, as African American females, we must always be seen as strong Black women. Maybe, to some extent, all of the above are true.

Whatever the specific origins of our conscious or unconscious decision to mute our pain, we need to listen to poet Audre Lorde, who suggested that our silence has not protected us. Depressed immune systems, elevated blood pressure, impaired mental health, and destructive relationships are deafening testimonials to the cost of our silence. Books written by and about African American women, such as *Willow Weep for Me: A Black Woman's Journey Through Depression*, by Meri Nana-Ama Danquah, describe the toll on the quality and longevity of our lives when we have not chosen or been allowed to respond appropriately to our pain, sadness, or anger.[4]

Therefore, it is imperative that you examine your own thoughts and feelings about depression and increase your knowledge and understanding about this debilitating illness. Your response to depressing thoughts and feelings can have a major impact on your life as well as those of your family and friends.

How do you feel about the various treatments used to help depressed women? For instance, how comfortable are you with the idea of seeing a therapist, a shrink, a "head doctor"—or are you conditioned to believe that psychological or psychiatric care is only for celebrities, bored Caucasian housewives, severely disturbed individuals, or the criminally insane? If unhappiness has drained the joy out of your life, would you seek the guidance of a member of the clergy, agree to take medication such as Prozac prescribed by your doctor, or try a nontraditional/alternative treatment such as acupuncture?

This chapter will help you understand more about depression and its impact on Black women. It will also provide self-tests to help you assess your current state of emotional well-being, offer behavioral strategies that can reduce the chances of your becoming depressed, and help you find and use resources within your community to effectively combat your depression.

## WHAT IS DEPRESSION?

Feeling blue, sad, or down for a day or even a few days isn't depression. Grieving the loss or death of a family member or friend also wouldn't be considered depression. Sadness and grief are normal and temporary reactions to life's difficulties and tragedies. Over time, we tend to feel better and get on with our lives.

Depression, on the other hand, is a *persistent* negative change in how you think and feel about yourself and how you behave—from your eating and sleeping patterns to your use of alcohol, tobacco, or illegal substances.

## COMMON SIGNS OF DEPRESSION

- *A persistent sad, anxious mood*
- *Sleeping too little, especially because of early morning waking or sleeping too much*
- *Reduced appetite and weight loss*
- *Loss of interest or pleasure in activities you once enjoyed*
- *Restlessness*
- *Difficulty concentrating, remembering, and making decisions*
- *Feeling guilty, hopeless, or worthless*
- *Thoughts of suicide*

In general, African American women are most apt to report the following symptoms:

- *Increase in appetite and weight*
- *Fatigue*
- *Irritability and anger*
- *Persistent physical symptoms that don't respond to treatment (such as headaches, chronic pain, constipation or other digestive disorders)*
- *Thoughts of death*

If four of these symptoms have lasted for more than two weeks, make an appointment *today* to see your physician or a mental health professional.

*Source:* American Psychiatric Association, *Diagnostic and Statistical Manual,* 4th ed., 1994

The general public and health professionals often identify sadness or suicidal thoughts and attempts as the symptoms most characteristic of depression, but how depression manifests itself depends on race, class, culture, and age. For instance, midlife African American women are more apt to describe their sadness in nontraditional ways. We are much more likely to say we're angry, frustrated, or stressed rather than sad. **Research also has revealed that depression in middle-class African American women is often associated with poor self-esteem, preoccupation with dependence on others' good opinion, sensitivity to criticism or rejection by others, and a decreased drive in pursuing sources of gratification.**[5] These symptoms are common to other disorders, so recognizing depression in Black women can be very difficult, even for our family, friends, and health-care providers.

Instead of being encouraged to seek therapy or counseling, depressed Black women are more apt to be told by friends and relatives, "You need more exercise," "You should eat a balanced diet," "It's just your nerves," "In time this will go away," "It's just a fact of life for Black women," "Pray," "Ride it out," or "Get a change of scenery."[6] But we've all heard the old saying about killing someone with kindness. It's not that our loved ones don't want to help us; sometimes they are too close to be objective and recognize our pain and suffering. Even more likely, they just don't know the signs of depression.

A person is usually considered *clinically depressed* when he or she exhibits four or more symptoms—such as extreme fatigue, sleeplessness, feeling worthless, and thoughts of death—and these symptoms last for more than two weeks. Clinical depression requires that you *see a mental health professional* to help you to feel better.

Meri Nana-Ama Danquah describes the intractable nature of clinical depression in her poignant, powerful memoir, *Willow Weep for Me*:

> We have all, to some degree, experienced days of depression. Days when nothing is going our way, when even the most trivial events can trigger tears, when all we want to do is crawl into a hole, and ask, "Why me?" For most people these are isolated occurrences. When the day ends, so too does the sadness. But for some, such as myself, the depression doesn't lift at the end of the day, or disappear when others try to cheer us up.
>
> These feelings of helplessness and desperation worsen and grow into a full-blown clinical depression. And when depression reaches clinical proportions, it is truly an illness, not a character flaw or an insignificant bout with the blues that an individual can "snap out of" at will.

There are several types of clinical depression. They vary depending on the number of symptoms you exhibit, how severe these symptoms are, how long they last, and how much they impact your ability to fulfill your personal and professional responsibilities.

Although depression may be the result of many influences, here are the four most prevalent types of clinical depression and some common traits they share:

*Major depression* is characterized by an intense, almost daily combination of the following symptoms: sadness, fatigue, sleep disturbance, hopelessness, and sometimes thoughts of death or suicide. When you experience this form of depression, it is often difficult, if not impossible, to care adequately for yourself or your family, or to be effective in your relationships or jobs. Some people have one episode in their lifetime, but for others, depressive bouts are recurrent.

For severely depressed individuals, such as *Willow Weep for Me* author Meri Nana-Ama Danquah, life can take a major spiral downward when their illness takes over:

> Each wave of the depression cost me something dear. I lost my job because the temp agencies where I was registered could no longer tolerate my lengthy absences. Unable to pay rent, I lost my apartment and ended up having to rent a small room in a boarding house. I lost my friends.

Most of them found it too troublesome to deal with my sudden moodiness and passivity, so they stopped calling and coming around.

*Manic-depression* or *bipolar disorder* is a form of clinical depression in which a person alternates between many of the traditional symptoms of depression—especially guilt, sadness, and irritability—and manic behavior, characterized by uncontrollable or excessive enthusiasm or emotions. During the manic phase, which can last for more than a week, manic-depressives exhibit at least three of the following symptoms:

- *Excessively "up" mood*
- *Inflated self-esteem*
- *Irritability*
- *Increased energy*
- *Racing thoughts*
- *Distractibility*
- *Decreased need for sleep*
- *Increased difficulty making decisions*
- *Increased involvement in risky behaviors, such as unprotected sex, substance abuse, shopping sprees*[7]

*Seasonal affective disorder (SAD)* is a seasonal form of major depression, which usually starts in the fall and intensifies during the winter. This type of depression usually disappears during the spring and summer, but it may be replaced by a mild case of mania, increased activity, or a state of *hyper-euphoria* (feeling extra good). The prevalence of SAD is almost four times greater in women than in men. Generally, SAD initially appears in women in their twenties and thirties. It's hypothesized that certain individuals are sensitive to the hormone melatonin, which is usually secreted at night. Because nights are longer during the winter months, more melatonin is secreted, which has a deleterious effect, including daytime sleepiness, fatigue, difficulty concentrating, and irritability.

Approximately 90 percent of individuals with SAD report major problems at work, and they are very vulnerable to job accidents and compromised relationships. Premenstrual symptoms and overeating—especially carbohydrates and sweets—are also associated with SAD.[8] The diagnostic criteria include:

• A regular seasonal relationship between the onset of an episode of bipolar or recurrent major depression between the beginning of October and end of November

• Full remission of all symptoms, or a change from depression to elevated mood or mania, starting in mid-February to mid-April

• At least three episodes of seasonal mood disturbance in three separate years, with at least two of the years being consecutive

• Seasonal episodes of mood disturbance outnumbering any nonseasonal episodes by more than three to one[9]

*Dysthymia* has symptoms that are similar to—but less severe than—those experienced with major depression, especially fatigue, a limited range of emotions, low self-esteem, and a feeling of hopelessness. With dysthymia, however, the symptoms last much longer, maybe up to two years. People with dysthymia often seem joyless. They do what they have to do, but don't show much enthusiasm.

Women suffering from dysthymia often resemble the ex-slave Sethe, Toni Morrison's protagonist in her best-selling novel-turned-movie, *Beloved:* "A face too still for comfort, irises the same color as her skin which, in that still face, used to make him think of a mask with mercifully punched eyes . . . Even punched out, they needed to be covered, lidded, marked with some sign to warn folks of what the emptiness held."

*Depression not otherwise specified* (**NOS**) is a condition in which an individual does not have symptoms that are severe or long-lasting enough to meet the full criteria for a specific clinical depression and yet is depressed. Women with this condition frequently feel sad, disappointed, angry, fatigued, or sick. They may be overweight or have a tendency to oversleep. But even though depression NOS sufferers exhibit at least two of the typical symptoms of depression, on the surface they appear to be just fine. Their job performance is adequate, and they can usually maintain platonic and romantic relationships. People experiencing depression NOS are often substance abusers, usually alcohol. They're not "falling-down drunks," but they're often the first guest with a drink.

## CAUSES OF DEPRESSION

Why does anyone get depressed? And why are women in general and African American women in particular so vulnerable to depression? There is no simple answer. Numerous factors, from biology to self-esteem, seem to be risk factors for depression. Being female and a minority puts you at risk for depression. Let's review six risk factors that are commonly associated with this illness.

*Genetic background.* A family history of depression—especially bipolar disorder and major depression—tends to increase the risk of becoming depressed. If one of a set of identical twins (from the same egg) is depressed, the other has a 50 percent chance of developing a depression, too; for fraternal twins (from two different eggs), the risk is only 20 percent. Several different genes have been associated with bipolar disorder in certain groups; however, millions of people who have parents or family members who are depressed never become clinically depressed themselves, since social and environmental factors as well as biological ones increase or decrease our vulnerability to depression.

*Biochemical makeup.* An imbalance in the biochemical messengers (neurotransmitters)—especially norepinephrine, serotonin, and dopamine— that allow brain cells to communicate with one another has been found in some depressed individuals. We do not know whether this biochemical disturbance has a genetic origin or occurs as a result of stress, trauma, physical illness, or social stressors including poverty, racism, and sexism.

*Stressful life events.* Difficult or traumatic life events are often linked to depression, especially when these events are unpredictable, interminable, simultaneous, and multiple, according to a 1999 report from the Surgeon General. The death of a significant person is one of the most stressful things we face, but imagine the unbearable pain of facing this kind of tragedy when you are sick or lonely or have recently lost your job. Although both women and men experience the stressful life events we explore in Chapter 13, women are more apt to be impoverished, unemployed, and victims of abuse. Stressful events activate the sympathetic nervous system (the part that gets us moving), but depressed patients often have exaggerated and persistent stress responses.

*Psychological factors.* Having ongoing negative and pessimistic thoughts about yourself, your friends, your family, and the world around you, coupled with low self-esteem, anxiety, excessive dependency, and a sense of powerlessness, is a hallmark of depression. Individuals who believe they have no control or influence over their lives often *exaggerate* the impact of positive and negative things that happen to them and *underestimate* their ability to improve their situations. Whenever Gayle sees these unfortunate souls coming, she thinks of Evilene, the Wicked Witch of the West in *The Wiz*, who shouted: *"Don't bring me no bad news!"*

*Minority status.* The prejudice and discrimination experienced by women and men who are members of racial and ethnic minorities often intensify feelings of powerlessness, helplessness, and low self-esteem. In fact, the legacy of slavery is still expressed overtly through disparities between African Americans and Caucasians on every major indicator—health, education, income, and employment, as well as negative stereotypical characterizations in the media. The internalized aftereffect of slavery—which is apparent in self-destructive behaviors ranging from preoccupation with skin color and hair texture to an epidemic of violent Black-on-Black crime—is equally devastating to us and our community.

*Medications.* Some medications used by women in their middle years have been documented to induce or increase the probability of depression. The most common medications associated with depression are listed in the table below, and are often those used for hypertension and arthritis.

## MEDICATIONS REPORTEDLY ASSOCIATED WITH DEPRESSION

| CARDIOVASCULAR DRUGS | HORMONES | PSYCHOTROPICS |
|---|---|---|
| RESERPINE | ORAL CONTRACEPTIVES | BENZODIAZEPINES (XANAX, VALIUM) |
| PROPANOLOL (INDERAL) | ACTH CORTICOSTEROIDS | |
| CLONIDINE (CATAPRES) | ANABOLIC STEROIDS | NEUROLEPITICS (THORAZINE, HALDOL) |
| DIGOXIN | | |
| MAXZIDE | | |
| **ANTICANCER AGENTS** | **ANTI-INFLAMMATORY/ ANTI-INFECTIVE AGENTS** | **OTHERS** |
| CYCLOSERINE | NONSTEROIDAL ANTI-INFLAMMATORY AGENTS (VIOXX, MOTRIN) | COCAINE WITHDRAWAL |
| | | AMPHETAMINE WITHDRAWAL |
| | | L-DOPA |

| ANTICANCER AGENTS | ANTI-INFLAMMATORY/ ANTI-INFECTIVE AGENTS | OTHERS |
|---|---|---|
| | ETHAMBUTOL (MYAMBUTOL) | CIMETIDINE (TAGAMET) |
| | DISULFIRAM (ANTABUSE) | RANITIDINE (ZANTAC) |
| | SULFONAMIDES | |
| | METOCLOPRAMIDE (REGLAN) | |

*Source:* Depression Guideline Panel, *Depression in Primary Care, vol. 1: Detection and Diagnosis,* 1993.

## WHY MIDLIFE AFRICAN AMERICAN WOMEN ARE PRONE TO DEPRESSION

While the middle years can be a time of spiritual freedom and renewal, it is also a time when depression, for many complex reasons, does present itself more frequently. It's important in your re-visioning of yourself as a miraculous being that you consider all of your life experiences—whether they were positive or negative—as vehicles that helped you learn and grow. Many African American women have been helped to reframe and reassess their lives by reading Iyanla Vanzant's *The Value in the Valley.*

The struggle to balance our lives and needs with the demands of others is ongoing for women in general and for African American women in particular. Numerous studies have indicated that the more that women attempt to juggle multiple roles that require us to sacrifice our own needs, the more apt we are to become depressed.

African American women often get contradictory messages from the people around us. We are expected to be strong, independent caretakers of family and community, but we are often castigated for being *too* strong and *too* independent. Sojourner Truth's scream, "Ain't I a woman?" is a question that many African American women continue to ask.

It's no wonder, then, that a 1997 national survey published by the Centers for Disease Control revealed that more than twice as many African American women as Caucasian women (regardless of where they live) experience feelings of boredom, restlessness, depression, loneliness, abandonment, and distress.[10]

The major physiological changes of menopause are problematic for some women. Many are able to perceive these changes as merely components of another developmental milestone, a new experience from which we can learn about ourselves and our bodies, but others are upset by alterations in their body and childbearing role. These women have trouble adjusting to a new body image and feel a decrease in their self-esteem when they judge themselves against society's standard of womanhood, which includes being young, thin, and fertile.

The medical reasons for the high rate of depression in women are contradictory. Fluctuations in female hormones, especially during menstruation, the postpartum period (shortly after childbirth), and menopause, have been proposed as an explanation by some and rejected by others. However, between 50 and 80 percent of all women experience some mild negative mood or somatic changes after childbirth, such as anxiety, irritability, sadness, and headaches. A 1997 study reported that menopause does not appear to be a risk factor for depression. According to this research, unless you are already clinically depressed or have a history of depression, most of these symptoms are temporary and barely affect your ability to function.[11]

On the other hand, being part of the sandwich generation—caring for parents or elderly relatives while still having some level of responsibility for children, especially young ones—can increase the risk of depression in women.

To further complicate this already difficult situation, HIV/AIDS, drug abuse, and alcoholism among adult children have also forced a growing number of midlife African American women to become the primary caretakers of their grandkids. When these adult children become too sick to care for themselves, they too move into their parents' homes. Thus, it is not surprising that Black women in the sandwich generation are most at risk for becoming depressed.

Midlife is often a time of intensified loss, through separation, divorce, or the death of family members and friends. Separated and divorced women have a higher rate of depression than women who are single or widowed. Many women also describe a decline in their sense of good health, complaining of physical concerns that range from annoying to life-threatening. Most women, whether they welcome becoming older, take it in stride, or panic at the thought, can certainly appreciate this take on aging: "One way I know I'm alive in the morning is that something hurts."

Financially impoverished, less well-educated, unemployed middle-aged women of all ethnic groups who are also in poor health and separated or divorced have the lowest level of self-esteem and are at the highest risk for depression. Interestingly, for midlife and other African American women, employment is the most consistent factor associated with self-esteem.

The necessity of taking care of our children and ourselves is part of the legacy of slavery for African American women. Our mates could be sold at any moment, and thousands of couples were permanently separated before and during the Civil War. Even after the war, racial discrimination made it almost impossible for most African American men to earn enough money to support their families adequately. If these families were to survive and leave the straits of dire poverty, they required *at least* two incomes. Thus, it is not surprising that "the higher self-esteem of black women who are older, with higher incomes and in better health, support the contention that self-esteem or personal worth for these women is determined by their ability to be good providers."[12]

African American women between forty-five and sixty-five years of age who are employed, are well educated, have sufficient family income, are in relatively good health, and are married are most apt to have higher levels of self-esteem and perceive themselves to be in control of their lives. They also indicate that their work is an important contributor to their higher level of self-esteem.

## Rx PRIME TIME PRESCRIPTIONS FOR REDUCING DEPRESSION

Even though we have no control over our sex, race, gene pool, or biochemical makeup, we certainly have input into how we think and feel about ourselves. In fact, we can take charge of most of the influences that increase our risk of being depressed. Taking appropriate action can alleviate the symptoms of clinical depression in at least 80 percent of cases diagnosed.

The causes of depression described earlier in the chapter are *possible* risk factors for all of us, but each one of us has our own family, personal, or professional history, which may leave us vulnerable to depression. That's why we must be willing to acknowledge, own, grieve, and work through our individual and collective experiences. If we can cry with acclaimed journalist Marcia Ann Gillespie, who writes in Diane Johnson's edited volume *Proud Sisters: The Wisdom and Wit of African-American Women,*

**Every time I read *The Bluest Eye*, I weep for that little girl lost in a world of pain and for all the women who carry pieces and parts of that**

little girl buried somewhere in their spirits. For who among us has not at some point in time succumbed to the propaganda, looked in a mirror and felt ourselves to be wanting.

Then we can shout with poet Maya Angelou when she writes in the same volume, "Still I rise."

Life is difficult and it is full of valleys, but it's also full of mountains—love, joy, happiness, and beauty. Our ability to accept this paradox of life is the first step in helping us to respond to difficult, tragic, or painful events in our lives in a more positive and appropriate manner. Here are other steps to take on a daily and long-term basis that will help reduce your vulnerability to depressive experiences.

## Daily

*Find positive things to read.* Start each day with a meditation, an affirmation, or a scriptural reading. Reading books by and about Black women who have survived—better yet, transcended—abusive or stressful situations or who offer suggestions for positive change can be very helpful in changing negative thoughts. (Check out the Resources section at the end of the book.)

*Make affirming self-statements.* Stand in front of the mirror and make three positive statements about yourself.

*Set a manageable personal and professional goal for yourself every day.* This will lift your spirits as you reaffirm your competence.

*Think positive thoughts about the people around you.* Make four positive comments about folks you live, work, socialize, and go to church with—yes, even your arrogant boss or ungrateful child—for every negative comment you make.

*Buy yourself fresh flowers.* Wouldn't it be nice to celebrate your own life once in a while?

## Long-term

*Turn to your Prime Time Sister or Circle for support, advice, and love.* Develop or nurture friendships with positive, active people and see them on a regular basis. Don't bring negative, critical, or cynical people into your inner space.

Talk with a financial advisor if you're having money problems or know these might develop. Money is a major cause of stress and depression for Black women. If you are unhappy with your job or profession, tap your circle of friends, coworkers, and professional associates to identify a career counselor who can help you assess your skills and find other work. Maybe someone in your human resources department at work can help.

Join or start a support group that focuses on your particular type of depression, especially if you have a family history of depression or are vulnerable to depressive episodes. (You can find some support groups in the Resources Section.)

## DIAGNOSING DEPRESSION

If, despite your efforts to prevent a depressive episode, it's time to take charge, your first step will be to schedule a full physical examination to rule out any medical condition or drug combination that can cause or mimic depressive symptoms. If your doctor cannot find a physical reason for your malaise, then you'll need to turn to a mental health professional for help. For more specific advice on finding the right therapist or counselor for you, turn to Chapter 19.

Finding the right therapist and determining the most effective treatment will require knowing the type of depression you have (such as major depression or seasonal affective disorder, described earlier in this chapter) and whether your level of depression is mild, moderate, or severe.

*Mild depression* is diagnosed for individuals who have some of the symptoms of depression and who must exert extra effort to complete tasks.

*Moderate depression* is diagnosed for individuals who have numerous symptoms of depression and who are having difficulty initiating or finishing tasks.

*Severe depression* is diagnosed for individuals who have most of the symptoms of depression and who cannot perform most of their personal or professional activities. *If you're feeling suicidal, immediately call 911, your primary-care physician, or a psychiatrist, or go to an emergency room!*

When my physician suggested that I was suffering from a mild case of depression, I knew it was time to take charge of my life.

My first step was to discuss my symptoms with my Prime Time Circle and my internist. We all agreed that the sadness I was feeling was appropriate given the death of my friend and Marilyn's severe injury. My anxiety over my superwoman role—thinking that I could perform *all* of my intensified personal and professional tasks in a superior manner—was increasing my stress level and exacerbating my menopausal symptoms, including the insomnia.

At their urging, I took a few days of leave, reduced my work hours, started taking estrogen to relieve some of my menopausal symptoms, and increased my time with my Prime Time Circle. I continued to provide support to Marilyn but realized that my anxiety about her injury had made me see her as more helpless than she was. She needed my support, but not to the extent that I had been providing it. I also agreed that a short-term trial on an antianxiety drug would be helpful in restoring my balance.

Within two weeks of implementing the plan, I felt 100 percent better. Had my symptoms not stopped, I would have gone into therapy.

## TREATING DEPRESSION

The most commonly used treatments for depression are psychotherapy, medication, phototherapy (light therapy), and electroconvulsive therapy (ECT). They are often used in combination, especially psychotherapy and medication. Complementary or alternative treatments, such as nutritional therapy and herbal medicines, are increasingly being used in conjunction with, or in place of, more traditional therapies. Although there is a paucity of well-documented information on the clinical treatment of depression in African American women, the limited literature suggests that psychotherapy is the treatment of choice for all women, and that we, like our Caucasian peers, respond well to this treatment.

## Psychotherapy (Talk Therapy)

Psychotherapy is the most widely used clinical treatment for mild to moderate depression. It involves a verbal dialogue between a mental health therapist—who might be a psychologist, social worker, psychiatrist, or counselor—and an individual, a family, or a group of unrelated people who have similar concerns. (For a more in-depth description of these professions, look in Chapter 19.)

The therapist's goal is to help you describe your thoughts, feelings, and behaviors so that appropriate and effective treatment plans can be developed. (As we've discussed earlier, we know that being open and honest about feelings and emotions is difficult and may trigger feelings of shame for many Black women, especially if asked to confide in a stranger. But talk therapy is very effective, and depending on your particular situation, it may be the best treatment for you.) Through psychotherapy you can learn how to recognize and resolve conflicted feelings, change negative or irrational thoughts, and eliminate behaviors that contribute to the development or maintenance of depression. The types of psychotherapy most widely used for treating depression include psychodynamic, interpersonal, cognitive-behavioral, and group therapy.

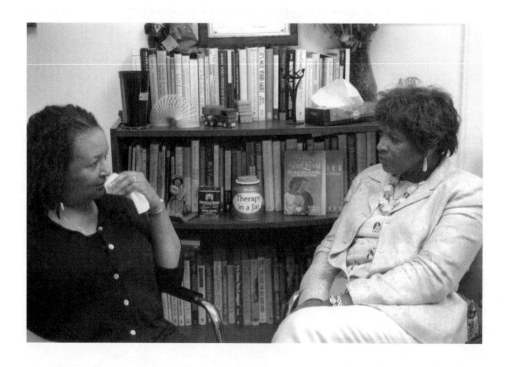

## Psychodynamic Therapy

Psychodynamic therapy, which can last from one to five years or sometimes longer, is based on the premise that unresolved childhood emotional conflicts negatively affect current personal and professional perceptions and relationships. These conflicts are largely unconscious but have a powerful impact on conscious thoughts and behaviors. Understanding and resolving these thoughts, feelings, and patterns of behavior can free up energy for living more openly, optimistically, and productively. Despite the widespread practice of psychodynamic therapy, very few controlled studies have been conducted to assess its effectiveness.

Dr. Sigmund Freud, who developed the initial principles of this theory, hypothesized that the seeds for depression are planted during childhood. He theorized that if a child's early physical needs (such as being fed or changed) or emotional needs (such as being picked up, hugged, kissed, or talked to) were either inadequately met or overindulged, she might become overly dependent on others in adulthood. Freud also maintained that loss—either real or fantasized—of a loved one through death, separation, or divorce leaves one feeling deeply, often unconsciously, angry and unable to express this anger appropriately. This unconscious conflict makes a person vulnerable to depression. If the anger is conscious, however, it can also make one feel guilty and, again, vulnerable to depression.

During your initial visits to the therapist, you will be asked detailed questions about your current and past physical and emotional health and that of your biological relatives. An extensive history of significant developmental experiences will also be gathered during this time, such as the quality of your relationship with your parents, siblings, and other significant people; changes in caretakers; abuse or neglect; and sexual experiences. Current personal and professional relationships are also explored. In traditional psychodynamic psychotherapy, you would lie on a couch and discuss any thoughts, feelings, or dreams you might have about current or past events, but most of this therapy is now done sitting down, face-to-face, one to four times a week. You're encouraged to remember and discuss past and current incidents of loss, guilt, anger, or trauma to help you become aware of any unconscious conflicts and how they are affecting your present thoughts, feelings, and behaviors.

## Interpersonal Therapy

Interpersonal therapy focuses on improving current significant relationships (with your spouse or partner, family member, friend, professional colleagues, supervisor, or boss) that may be causing or exacerbating your depression. Treatment can last from four to six months. Sessions are usually once a week for fifty minutes.

Since the focus of this treatment is improving current relationships, assertiveness training and role-playing are often used. It was actually developed to help women, in particular, cope with midlife transitions—loss, changes in roles and relationships, and reassessment of skills and life choices. Interpersonal therapy is regarded as an effective treatment for women because of the great significance we place on the relationships in our lives.

Various studies have documented that women are more stressed by relationships than men and that our mood is more likely to be affected by problems in our relationships. It's not clear how much of our focus on relationships is part of our female nature and how much is transferred by our society and culture.

## Cognitive-Behavioral Therapy

Cognitive-behavioral therapists contend that depression is caused by distorted or irrational views of oneself, the world, and the future. This type of therapy is usually short-term (ten to twenty weeks, fifty minutes a week), structured, and goal-oriented.

Cognitive-behavioral therapy will help you to identify these negative beliefs and change them for more positive and appropriate thoughts. This therapy incorporates a variety of behavioral techniques, from role-playing to assertiveness training.

Cognitive-behavioral therapy can be particularly effective for women because it challenges and attempts to change some of the irrational cultural beliefs with which women are socialized, such as:

- I must have the love or approval of people who are significant to me.
- I must be competent and successful to be worthwhile.
- My low self-esteem is caused by how others treat me and by events in

my life that I don't control, so I have no power to change how I feel about myself and my life.

Cognitive-behavioral therapists believe that we women are more vulnerable to depression when we assume unnecessary responsibility for negative events (such as "If I were more attractive, my husband wouldn't have had an affair"), minimize or deny our ability to influence what happens to us, or believe that we must please everyone.

The techniques used with cognitive-behavioral therapy that are considered particularly effective treatments for depression in low- and middle-income African American women include:

*Assertiveness training.* This can be an effective intervention for Black women because it teaches us how to express our thoughts and feelings in an open, honest, direct, and spontaneous way. This training helps women assert themselves in a manner that is respectful to others. Although depressive thoughts frequently leave Black women feeling sad and angry, many of us find it easier to express our anger than our sadness. (For more on anger, see Chapter 6.) Assertiveness training provides a mechanism to learn how to express positive and negative feelings.

*Role-playing.* Acting out various situations in which you've felt depressed and practicing an alternative way of thinking and acting is one way to learn new behaviors in a safe environment. It is often combined with assertiveness training.

*Identification of inappropriate behavior.* You can learn to identify inappropriate patterns of behavior by keeping a diary and asking family members or friends to help you identify when your facial or verbal expressions and body movements—foot tapping, nail biting, teeth grinding—indicate that your thoughts, feelings, or behaviors are not consistent with what you are saying.

In cognitive-behavioral therapy, you're expected to take a very active role in and outside of the therapy sessions. Therapists will usually ask you to keep a journal to record your negative thoughts throughout the day. You might be encouraged to wear a rubber band on your wrist and snap it whenever you become aware that you're thinking a pessimistic or negative thought. Snapping the band is a reminder to replace that thought with a more appropriate one. You will also be encouraged to reward yourself for positive thoughts or actions, such as sending yourself a card or buying flowers for your bedroom.

### Group Therapy

Group therapy can focus on a particular issue—bereavement, stress management—or on all aspects of one's life. Most groups meet on a weekly basis for one and a half hours. The group may have a psychodynamic, cognitive-behavioral, or interpersonal focus. This form of therapy allows participants to share thoughts and feelings, give feedback to each other, and learn that they are not alone in the difficulties they experience.

Group therapy is often recommended for people who have relationship problems or difficulty in being assertive. Members are usually expected to sign a contract outlining the expectations to which all group members should adhere. The guidelines governing confidentiality tend to be strictly enforced so that all members can feel safe in sharing even the most personal, painful experiences.

## Medication (Pharmacotherapy)

Medication is often recommended for severe or incapacitating bouts of depression. According to a team of researchers, medication is usually indicated if your symptoms:

- Are persistent and severe
- Prevent you from functioning
- Include suicidal thoughts
- Include hallucinations or delusions
- Have intensified to extreme agitation, anger, anxiety
- Have been alleviated by medication in the past[13]

Each medication affects different chemical pathways of the brain. By increasing or decreasing the brain's chemical messengers (neurotransmitters), depressive symptoms can be eliminated or dramatically reduced. (See box for a list of the most commonly used antidepressant medications.)

While medications for depression are not habit-forming, they may have some side effects, including dry mouth, dizziness, constipation, urinary problems, blurred vision, drowsiness, headaches, heart palpitations, agitation and confusion, weight gain, and decreased sexual drive. They may also interact with thyroid hormone, antihypertensive medication, oral contraceptives, diuretics, aspirin, vitamin C, alcohol, and tobacco. None of the side effects is as dangerous as hallucinations or suicidal attempts, so take the medication if you need to.

## THE MOST COMMONLY USED MEDICATIONS TO TREAT DEPRESSION

*Tricyclics* positively affect the brain's level of norepinephrine and possibly serotonin, giving you a lift and ultimately making you feel better. An imbalance in these biochemical messengers can affect your mood. The drugs most widely prescribed are Elavil (amitriptyline), Pamelor (nortriptyline), Vivactil (protriptyline), Pertofran, and Tofranil (imipramine).

*MAOIs* elevate the levels of chemical messengers by blocking the action of the enzyme monoamine oxidase, which can affect the neurotransmitters. The most prescribed brand names are Marplan (isocarboxazid), Nardil (phenelzine), and Parnate (tranylcypromine). When using MAOIs, foods that contain tyramine must be avoided. The combination of MAOIs and tyramine can cause a dramatic, even life-threatening increase in your blood pressure—a hypertensive crisis. An intense headache, increase in your heart rate, sensitivity to light, nausea, and vomiting are possible. *Call the doctor about the side effects of this mixture.*

All of the MAOIs require that you change your diet. We know it's difficult to change your diet, but if it will increase your emotional well-being, it's worth it. The other positive to changing your diet is that it allows you to eliminate foods that have, to some extent, been obstacles to achieving your optimal nutritional plan. The most problematic foods and beverages when taking MAOIs include: strong or aged cheeses—yes, pizza and grilled cheese sandwiches have to go (but cottage cheese and cream cheese are allowed), smoked, aged, or processed meats and fish; sausages; liver; pickled or salted fish; Asian foods; Korean, Japanese, Chinese, and Thai food that is cooked in soy sauce or MSG (monosodium glutamate); overripe fruits and vegetables; caffeine—coffee, tea, chocolate, cocoa; some dairy products—sour cream and yogurt; alcohol—especially beer, red wines, and sherry.

There are also a number of prescription, over-the-counter, and illegal drugs that should be avoided. Among them are other antidepressants; certain drugs used for hypertension, diabetes, asthma, and weight reduction; Ritalin (methylphenidate); Novocain; stimulants and illegal drugs—amphetamines, cocaine; and nonprescription cold, sinus, and decongestant medications, which contain phenylpropanolamine (e.g., Alka Seltzer Plus, Robitussin C), phenylephrine (e.g., Dristan, Neosynephrine), and pseudoephedrine (e.g., Actifed, Sudafed).

For more specific information about foods, beverages, and drugs to avoid when taking MAOIs, please refer to *What the Blues Is All About—Black Women Overcoming Stress and Depression* and *The Feeling Good Handbook* (see the Resources section).

*SSRIs,* which increase the amount of serotonin in the brain, are increasingly the antidepressants of choice. They have fewer side effects than the other drugs, but they are more expensive. The brand names are Prozac (fluoxetine), Paxil (paroxetine), and Zoloft (sertraline).

*Atypical antidepressants.* This category of drugs affects norepinephrine and dopamine. They are sometimes given when patients don't respond to the usual antidepressants. Wellbutrin (bupropion) is one of the newest antidepressants and has even fewer negative side effects than the SSRIs. However, it is not to be used for anyone diagnosed with a seizure disorder, bulimia, or anorexia nervosa.

*Mood stabilizers.* These medications are used to combat bipolar disorder, commonly referred to as manic-depression. Lithium is the most widely used drug for manic-depressive episodes. It is sometimes used in combination with antidepressants during the depressive phase of the manic-depressive illness. Lithium levels must be monitored on a consistent basis to measure the amount of the drug in the body. An inadequate dose will not be effective; too much can be toxic. Side effects include sensitivity to lowered salt intakes and increased exercise; kidney changes and increased thirst and urination; hypo- and hyperthyroidism; and increased risk during the first trimester of pregnancy of congenital malformations in the fetus. The signs of lithium toxicity are nausea, vomiting, drowsiness, twitching, irregular heartbeat, and blurred vision. Manic-depressive patients who don't respond well to lithium are often prescribed Tegretol (carbamazepine), Depakene (valproic acid) and Depakote (divalproex sodium), and Klonopin (clonazepam).

*Antianxiety medications.* These drugs are sometimes prescribed for depressed patients because anxiety often occurs with depression. These drugs can help with insomnia or panic attacks. Possible side effects can include drowsiness, addiction, and fetal abnormalities. When combined with alcohol, antihistamines, sedatives, muscle relaxants, and some prescription pain medication, serious and even life-threatening complications can result. Brand names include Ativan (lorazepam), Valium (diazepam), and Xanax (alprazolam).

## Self-Help and Support Groups

An increasing number of African American women are joining self-help and support groups that focus on practical ways of dealing with a common problem. These groups can complement more traditional treatments for moderate and severe depression. Support groups are sometimes used as a primary treatment for women with mild depression after their acute episode has subsided. These groups may be led by a professional therapist or facilitator, or the leadership of the group might rotate from member to member. Issues related to confidentiality and logistics are discussed and resolved before the group starts. The National Black Women's Health Project, A Circle of Sisters (a Black women's support group), and various mental health associations can be helpful in locating existing groups or providing materials and personnel to help develop and organize these groups. (Contact information for these national groups is included in the Resources section.)

Support groups often meet in churches, schools, or members' homes. Programs can include group discussions, study groups, visiting speakers, and other activities that inform members and help build their confidence. Along with the personal support gained from meeting together, some groups offer newsletters, a hotline, and a buddy system, which provide additional encouragement and support.

## Phototherapy (Light Therapy)

Phototherapy is used to treat seasonal affective disorder (SAD). Phototherapy suppresses the secretion of melatonin, a hormone to which SAD patients may be sensitive and which is secreted in greater amounts during winter, when hours of daylight are less. Most patients sit under a special broad-spectrum lamp for two to four hours per day during fall and winter.

Specially made light boxes (which cost $300 to $500) or light visors are used. Ask your doctor or pharmacist for recommendations on where to buy a light box. Some caution needs to be exercised with these devices, because some people experience jitteriness and headaches. They have not been approved by the Food and Drug Administration and should always be used under professional supervision.

## Electroconvulsive Therapy (ECT)

ECT, also called shock treatment, is usually reserved for severely depressed patients who have not responded to medications, are at high risk of suicide, have psychotic episodes with agitation, have experienced severe weight loss, or are suffering from a major physical illness that precludes antidepressants. Past misuse as well as negative movie and media depictions of shock treatment have given this therapy an unwarranted bad name. Today, ECT is a safe procedure that uses general anesthesia and special muscle-relaxing medicines to prevent physical harm and pain during the sessions.

Patients wake without pain but might have short-term memory loss, temporary confusion, or headaches. The treatment is usually effective at relieving depression.

## Complementary and Alternative Treatments

Complementary, natural, or alternative medicine and treatments avoid the drugs that Western medicine uses. To treat emotional problems, these alternatives take a more holistic, less invasive approach; usually their treatments can be used as a complement to Western interventions. Some natural, complementary modalities include traditional Chinese medicine (including acupuncture), Ayurvedic medicine, homeopathy, herbal and botanical medicine, psychotherapy, physical medicine (chiropractic and reflexology), aromatherapy, hydrotherapy, and nutrition.

Always discuss your interest in or use of complementary medicines with your primary-care physician because of the potential for negative interaction between different interventions. Health providers who practice complementary medicine can be found through the American Holistic Medical Association (see Resources for contact information), but if you are feeling severely depressed or suicidal, you need to get immediate attention from a traditional health professional.

## Nutritional Therapy

Eating the right foods and taking the proper supplements can help balance the chemicals in the brain. However, before trying to radically change your diet, consult a nutritionist or a naturopath.

Increasing consumption of foods containing the amino acid *tryptophan*, which is used in the synthesis of serotonin, can help reestablish the brain's chemical balance. Tryptophan initially became well known because of its ability to help patients suffering from insomnia. Although turkey is high in tryptophan, it's also a high-protein food. Protein can make it more difficult for tryptophan to reach the brain's sleep center. Until 1989, tryptophan was available as a supplement. However, it was implicated in several deaths from a rare disorder called eosinophilla myalgia syndrome (EMS) and was removed as a supplement by the Food and Drug Administration. Foods containing tryptophan are not a problem. Foods containing this amino acid include bananas, meats, pasta, and pineapple. *Tyrosine*, a precursor of the brain chemicals norepinephrine and dopamine, can be found in eggs, milk, aged cheese, whole-wheat bread, and yogurt. It is available as a supplement.

Deficiency in *folic acid* is often associated with depression. Folic acid can be found in yeast, liver, lima beans, whole-grain products, leafy green vegetables, oranges, oats, peanuts, and beans. Oral contraceptives, aspirin, Tylenol (acetaminophin), and Dilantin (phenytoin) can reduce folic acid in your body. Folic acid is available as a supplement.

Adequate amounts of vitamins C, $B_{12}$, niacin, $B_6$, and riboflavin can help ward off depression. Small amounts of licorice, which naturally contains MAO inhibitors, can also be helpful. Eat too much licorice, though, and you may suffer from headaches and high blood pressure.

## Herbal Medicines

Several herbs are useful in reducing tensions and can complement the treatment of mild to moderate depression. Probably one of the most well known and widely used herbs is Saint-John's-wort (*Hypericum perforatum*). Although the herb has been classified by the *German Commission E Monographs* as an MAO inhibitor, other studies suggest that it might be through serotonin reuptake inhibition. Saint-John's-wort is reported to have fewer side effects than other antidepressants, although it does increase the skin's sensitivity to sunlight and might negatively affect a fetus. Since it appears to function as a mild MAO inhibitor, the same food, beverage, and drug precautions for prescribed MAO inhibitors should be used with Saint-John's-wort. In addition, Saint-John's-wort should not be used with ginger, purslane, borage, thyme, sage, and *fo-ti-lieng*.

### Acupuncture and Acupressure

Acupuncture is an ancient Eastern practice that purports to correct the body's flow of energy or *chi*. Depression indicates an energy imbalance, and the tiny needles used to stimulate energy points work to balance the flow of *chi* by slightly irritating the nerves to release endorphins and enkephalins, facilitating a calming, mood-lifting effect. Acupressure uses hands or feet to put pressure on energy-specific points on the body. To find out more about acupuncture and acupressure, check out the Resources at the end of this book.

### Aromatherapy

Essential oils for treating depression include rosemary, bergamot, basil, Borneo camphor, chamomile, lavender, neroli, and clary sage. They can be added to a vaporizer or boiled in a pot of water.

### Deep Breathing and Yoga

Deep breathing relaxes your mind and body so that you can step back and examine and reformulate your negative or irrational thoughts and feelings. Yoga can help to alleviate depression, especially these positions: plow, shoulder stand, corpse pose, and yoga mudra. To learn more about yoga, turn to the exercise section in Chapter 9.

### Exercise

Exercise can stimulate the production of norepinephrine, which can have a positive effect on mood. Both aerobic (swimming, running, brisk walking) and anaerobic (weight lifting, muscle toning, and stretching) exercises are norepinephrine producers. Choose exercises that fit your style and preferences. For more information on starting an exercise program, review Chapter 9, "Developing Your Prime Time Wellness Plan."

### *Reflexology*

This practice uses finger pressure to stimulate specific points in the feet and hands. To treat depression, a reflexologist presses points that are connected to glands that affect emotional stability—the pituitary, pineal, thymus, thyroid, and parathyroid.

You can begin to take charge of your low mood and depression through any of these holistic techniques and practices, but make sure that if none of them works, you see a health professional to get the support you need. You do not have to feel down, blue, or depressed, but to get through these feelings, you need to acknowledge them and recognize that you *can* ask for help—and you deserve to!

# PART VI

# Coping with Midlife's Passage

# Chapter 16

# MANEUVERING THROUGH MENOPAUSE: A RITE OF PASSAGE

*Girl, I was sitting there about to explode with heat, and the water was dripping off my chin onto my brand-new dress. I was too through—I had been to the hairdresser that morning and I already could feel my hair rising on my head. Sam wondered what was going on, since last night I was freezing to death. Now we're starting to fuss about whether to open or close the windows as I go from one extreme to the other. Then it hit me—I must be going through the change.*

—Gloria

Free at last! Free at last! Thank God Almighty we're free at last! That's exactly how so many of us feel after thirty or forty years enduring the discomfort, tension, and inconvenience of menstrual cycles. Like many of our friends, we couldn't wait to get off the rag. No more super-absorbent, super-big, or heavy-flow pads! No more super-thin sanitary napkins with some kind of super-absorbent crystals in them that never "super-absorbed" anything. No more super-absorbent tampons that were never enough by themselves.

And best of all, no more cramps!

We couldn't wait. And all the while we remembered what we overheard our older aunts, mothers, and grandmothers saying to one another when they sat around the kitchen table: "Honey, I'm really, really starting to enjoy *it* since the change hit me and I don't have to worry about getting pregnant anymore." And they would all agree with a "Honey, hush!"

In truth, menopause is a bridge to the most vital and liberated period in a woman's life. As we have explained earlier, it is a period of rebirth and positive change, a time to rediscover ourselves as spiritual and human beings with a long life ahead.

Midlife and menopause, its rite of passage, is a time of emotional and spiritual transformation. As our bodies and minds prepare for our later years,

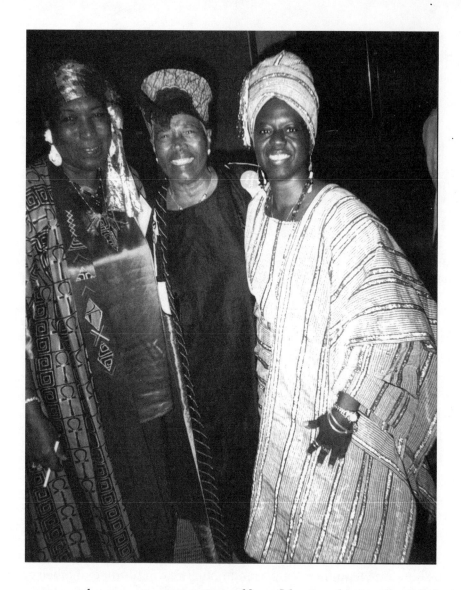

many women become more assertive, self-confident, and in touch with their own needs and wants, and less interested in always pleasing others.

Unfortunately, not all of us celebrate our middle years. Many women buy into negative, stereotypical images and myths of midlife and menopause. Do any of these "menopause myths" sound familiar?

- Menopause will make me sick.
- I will lose my sexual desire during menopause—the light may be on, but the voltage is low.

• I will lose the hair on my head and instead grow hair on my face and chest.

• Menopause will make me fat.

Even though all women go through menopause, your experience will be uniquely your own. When it starts, when it stops, how we perceive it, and how it affects us varies from woman to woman—and it varies a lot. In fact, the menopause experience is so unique, some experts compare it to a thumbprint.

For instance, although menopause may depress libido or sex drive in some women, many more report that sex is more satisfying and gratifying at this time in their lives than ever before. Even though the decrease in estrogen may thin the hair on the head of some women, statements of hair growth in unwanted places are being investigated.

The one myth that does have some teeth may be weight gain. Your metabolism will slow down as you age, especially if you become more sedentary. That's why midlife women must get moving and keep moving—exercise is the key to health and to a healthy menopause. Watching your diet is also critical at this stage. You must eat less and improve the quality of what you eat. You can't afford to indulge yourself anymore with empty calories—you know, foods you love that are high in caloric content and very low in nutritional value, such as potato chips and ice cream.

On the other hand, the myth you should ignore altogether is that menopause will make you sick. Although you may experience some discomfort from hot flashes or lack of sleep, as Gayle did, according to the National Institutes of Health, 80 percent of women experience mild or no menopausal signs at all. Only 20 percent report symptoms severe enough to require medical attention.

Menopause is more than the end of monthly periods—it is a process and a journey during which many things happen. The important point to remember is that even though you don't have a choice about whether or not you go through menopause, *how* you respond to the experience is something you *can* control. To enjoy the journey, though, you must understand the changes taking place and how they affect your body, mind, and spirit. A typical American woman will live one-third of her life after menopause. Think about it—that could mean twenty-five to forty or more years without your period.

Although there has been a tremendous increase in the amount of research on menopause in recent years, we still don't know a lot about it, and the existing studies haven't included an adequate number of African American women. Therefore, many important questions still remain unanswered, such as how much of the changes in our body are due to menopause or just to plain ol' aging.

Thankfully, the National Institute on Aging at the National Institutes of Health has initiated many investigations on menopause, estrogen, and the middle years, with adequate numbers of African American women, and soon we should have some important answers. In the meantime, though, we must go with what we know and be clear about what we don't know.

## MENOPAUSE 101

Menopause comes from the Latin words *meno*, meaning "month," and *pausus*, meaning "cessation," and literally means "the end of menstruation."

Simply put, menopause is the time when your ovaries cease functioning and almost stop producing estrogen. This we know for sure. The average age for menopause in the United States and Canada is sometime between forty-five and fifty-five, usually around fifty-one. By sixty, virtually all women will have experienced menopause. But remember, these are average ages—that means some women experience menopause much earlier, in their forties, and some much later, in their fifties and sixties.

The onset of menopause is influenced by a number of factors. An important indicator is your mother's age when she began menopause. However, studies indicate that women who are less educated, poor, unemployed, or divorced and those who smoke tend to experience menopause somewhat earlier than average—maybe as much as three years earlier. Research also attests that women who undergo early menopause—before age fifty—may be at greater risk for developing heart disease, osteoporosis (bone loss), and other chronic diseases.

Menopause is described in three phases: perimenopause, menopause, and postmenopause.

*Perimenopause* usually means the years immediately *before* your last menstrual period. It usually begins in the mid- to late forties and can last up to five to seven years.

Beginning as early as your mid- to late thirties, your ovaries start producing less estrogen and progesterone, even though you may continue to ovulate. Hormone levels fall even more dramatically when you enter peri-menopause, which may happen as early as age thirty-five. Eventually, when the supply of viable eggs is exhausted, ovulation stops. At this time the levels of estrogen and progesterone produced by the ovaries drop so low that you stop menstruating altogether.

One of the classic signs of perimenopause is *irregular menstrual cycles.* Before you stop menstruating, your periods may be longer or shorter, heavier or lighter, closer together or farther apart. Even though this change is to be expected, *always report unusual bleeding to your doctor,* because irregular bleeding can also be a sign of fibroids, uterine polyps, a thyroid problem, or even cancer. If you are bleeding heavily, be sure to get a blood test to check for anemia, a condition in which the number of red blood cells (which carry oxygen) is below normal.

Since your body is starting to produce less estrogen during peri-menopause, you may also start experiencing hot flashes, night sweats, vagi-nal dryness, mood swings, or depression. (We will explore these symptoms of menopause a little later in this chapter.)

*Menopause* is not official until you have not had a period for at least one year. But menopause includes a number of other physical, mental, and emo-tional changes.

*Postmenopause* represents the period after menopause. The lower levels of estrogen you have at this time can trigger "silent" changes in your body, including bone loss, which could lead to osteoporosis, and rising levels of "bad" (LDL) cholesterol coupled with a decrease in the "good" (HDL) cholesterol in the blood. Over time, this can lead to heart attack and stroke. (We will discuss osteoporosis in depth later in this chapter. You can turn back to Chapter 10 for more information on cholesterol, heart disease, and stroke.)

## WHAT IS SURGICAL MENOPAUSE?

Although most women experience a natural onset of menopause as they age, some women start menopause when both ovaries are surgically removed or are damaged from radiation or chemotherapy treatments for cancer. A sur-gically induced menopause is immediate and often is associated with more severe health problems than when the onset of menopause is natural.

Contrary to what most women think, removing the ovaries is not a standard procedure for a hysterectomy. A *hysterectomy* is the surgical removal of the uterus. A *total hysterectomy* is the removal of the uterus and the cervix (the opening of the uterus). Many women who undergo a hysterectomy still have their ovaries after surgery. And although they don't have monthly periods because they no longer have a uterus, their ovaries continue to function and produce estrogen and progesterone.

*Oophorectomy* is the term for the surgical removal of one or both ovaries. When both ovaries are removed *(bilateral oophorectomy)*, a woman will experience an immediate loss of estrogen and progesterone and the immediate onset of menopause regardless of whether or not she still has her uterus. This is what is known as *surgical menopause*. If a woman keeps one ovary or part of an ovary remains after surgery, that ovary will make up for the loss of the other one by producing additional estrogen and progesterone and prevent a surgical menopause. If your body produces enough estrogen, you will experience a natural menopause around the normal time, or possibly one to two years earlier than average.

Women who experience surgical menopause not only experience more severe symptoms, they are also prone to develop heart disease and osteoporosis at an earlier age than women who have a natural menopause. For these reasons, premenopausal women who have had both ovaries removed are usually strongly advised to take estrogen replacement therapy, both to relieve the immediate symptoms resulting from the loss of estrogen, and also to prevent the long-term health risks associated with surgical menopause.

It is vital for you to understand the issues involved in surgical menopause, because studies show that African American women are twice as likely to have hysterectomies (which may include the removal of one or both ovaries) as Caucasian women. It is not known how many of these hysterectomies are unnecessary, since African American women are always so underrepresented in large-scale studies about menopause. (Statistics also show that hysterectomies are more often performed in the South—so much so that they are called "Mississippi appendectomies.")

The high incidence of hysterectomies may be due to the fact that Black women are more prone to heavy bleeding during our perimenopausal years than White women. Heavy bleeding may lead to anemia, which is why some doctors prescribe hysterectomies. According to the National Black Women's Health Project, another reason for our high number of hysterectomies is that fibroids, which are benign (not cancerous) growths in the uterus, are far more common among Black than White women. Unfortunately, fibroids often lead doctors to recommend that women have unnecessary hysterectomies. However, if you are suffering from large fibroids, bleeding, and constant pain, you may need to have surgery.

Before you have a hysterectomy, make sure you go over all aspects of the surgery with your doctor. You also need to get at least a second opinion. You want to know exactly what the doctor plans to remove and why. If you are premenopausal, discuss whether your ovaries will need to be removed. Your goal, if possible, is to prevent a surgical menopause so that you can have a natural onset of menopause. If you are postmenopausal, you still need to discuss the consequences of having your ovaries removed. At this stage in your life, you may be more inclined to say yes to removal to ensure that you won't have to worry about any possibility of ovarian cancer, which is hard to diagnose.

## HOW CULTURE AFFECTS MENOPAUSE

Most women accept menopause in stride. It's important to think of menopause as a natural process, not an illness, sickness, or abnormal state.

In fact, how you handle menopause may have a lot to do with your cultural background. For example, Asian women report fewer and less severe signs than Western women, perhaps because for many Asian women menopause is a nonevent. In China, for instance, menopause is viewed as a good thing by both women and men, since age is venerated in Chinese culture. One study revealed that 65 percent of Japanese women reported no problems during menopause. The Japanese language does not even have a term for hot flashes. Only 2 percent of Japanese women take hormones.

Another significant reason for the difference in how Asian women handle menopause is dietary. Asian women eat great quantities of soybeans, which are extremely rich in isoflavones, a kind of phytoestrogen. These plant estrogens help balance the drop-off in our body's hormone levels during menopause. Asian women also consume more calcium, and they exercise (walking and biking daily) much more than we do. Their diet and exercise routines both pay healthy dividends, since Asian American women have the longest life expectancy—ninety-seven years!

A study comparing Mayan women with rural Greek women also showed differences in menopausal responses. Mayan women, who also look forward to menopause, eat a diet high in carbohydrates and calcium, but no meat or dairy products. Virtually no Mayan women experience hot flashes. On the other hand, Greek women are much more anxious about menopause and growing older and often report hot flashes. But that's not surprising, since Greek women smoke more than any other women in Europe, and sedentary smokers in any group of women experience more uncomfortable symptoms during menopause than nonsmokers.

Preliminary findings in a study being conducted by the National Institute on Aging (the Study of Women's Health Across the Nation, SWAN), which has a significant representation of African American women, indicates that Black women **have more** problems with hot flashes, night sweats, vaginal dryness, and urine leakage than other women. The study also shows that we **have fewer** headaches, problems with racing heartbeat, and stiffness and soreness in the joints, neck, or shoulders.

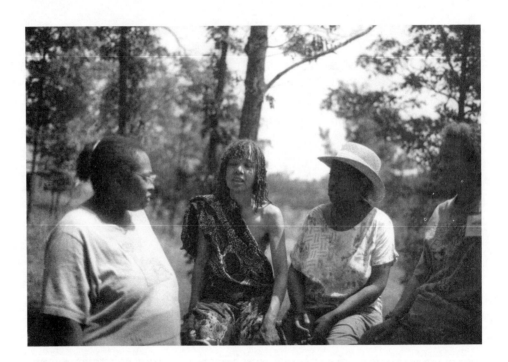

African American women are more likely than White women to pass through menopause without psychological problems. According to Gail Sheehy's survey of women in menopause reported in her book *New Passage: Mapping Your Life Across Time*, we may have an easier time with menopause than White women because:

• African American women tend not to measure our femininity and sensuality only by how we look.

• Young Black women usually have not been made to feel as valued as a symbol of beauty as young White women, and therefore we are more prone to gain in prestige and self-esteem in middle age.

• Our self-worth is not overly attached to our age or how young we look.

• Our self-worth is more tied to our spiritual strength.

• Our sensuality is not related to the European American anorexic body type. (We know well the shamelessly lusty older Black women entertainers—from Della Reese to Patti LaBelle, from Jessye Norman to Etta James.)

The fact that Black women in midlife tend to be heavier than White women may also have a role in how we handle menopause. Estrogen is stored in fat and therefore, as our ovaries start producing less estrogen, our bodies use the estrogen in the body fat. The fact that we carry around more body fat means that we have more stored estrogen to use.

## WHAT ARE THE SYMPTOMS OF MENOPAUSE?

Although we've mentioned hot flashes, night sweats, and a few of the other signs of menopause, we haven't defined what happens when you experience any of these symptoms. Knowing what to expect can help ease you through the discomfort.

## Hot Flashes

Hot flashes are the most common signs of menopause. About 80 percent of menopausal American women experience hot flashes at some time. You may have heard your friends say, "I'm having my own private summer" or "It's not a hot flash—it's a power surge."

Marilyn had very few flashes going through menopause—however, they were a major problem for Gayle, who was often unable to sleep. It's different for every woman. That's why we've included some of frequently asked questions about this annoying symptom.

*What are hot flashes?* Women often describe hot flashes as a sensation of heat throughout their bodies. Some women complain of heavy sweating in the upper part of their body: chest, neck, and face. During a hot flash, your body temperature actually rises, the blood vessels in your skin dilate, the blood flow in your extremities increases, and you may appear flushed. Your heart rate goes up a little, maybe five to ten more beats a minute. Some women say they experience warning signs (such as pressure in the head, anxiety, a tingling sensation, or nausea) when a flash is coming on. Following a flash, body temperature drops and many women experience a chill.

*Why do hot flashes occur?* Changes in estrogen can cause hot flashes. Some pregnant women also complain of flashing. Low estrogen levels affect the *hypothalamus* (your body's climate control center in the brain). A drop in estrogen upsets the ability of the hypothalamus to regulate your internal temperature. Experts speculate that when estrogen levels take a dive, the hypothalamus reads that event as a drop in body temperature and turns up your thermostat. As mentioned earlier, women who have an abrupt loss of ovarian estrogen due to surgery, radiation, or chemotherapy often experience the worst hot flashes.

*How often do hot flashes occur?* Most menopausal women have two or three flashes a day, but some women may "power-surge" as often as once an hour. These usually last from about three to ten minutes. In rare cases, flashes can extend to thirty minutes or even an hour. Most women experience hot flashes for a period of as little as two months to as much as two to four years or more. A handful of women report flashes up to a decade after their last menstrual flow.

*Are there any external triggers that bring on hot flashes?* Triggers for hot flashes include spicy food, hot drinks, alcoholic drinks, white sugar, hot weather, hot tubs and saunas, tobacco and marijuana, stress, and anger, especially when unexpressed.

## Night Sweats

Night sweats are simply hot flashes that occur at night while you sleep, but they can sometimes be so severe that they prevent you from sleeping. If they lead to sleep deprivation, you should seek medical attention.

## Sleep Disturbances

Problems with sleeping are usually caused by big-time hot flashes. Sleep deprivation can be very serious and lead to:

- Ongoing fatigue
- Feeling irritable and anxious
- Forgetfulness
- Poor concentration

**℞ PRIME TIME PRESCRIPTIONS FOR HOT FLASHES, NIGHT SWEATS, AND SLEEP PROBLEMS**

*Add soy protein to your daily diet.* Soy's phytoestrogens (which are hormonelike compounds) can help regulate your body temperature during menopause. A study reported in the *Journal of Obstetrics and Gynecology* revealed that women consuming 60 grams of powdered soy protein daily reported a 45 percent decrease in hot flashes when compared to a control group.

Tuberous (true) yams (not sweet potatoes) and soy-rich diets can ease flashes, but these so-called plant estrogens may be too weak to dramatically improve severe symptoms. Therefore, you must experiment with how much yam or soy works for you. Aim for one serving of soy a day. A good way to start is with a Soy Smoothie for breakfast.

---

### PRIME TIME RECIPE
### SOY SMOOTHIE

*Pour 1 cup of low-fat soy milk in blender with frozen fruit to taste, or 2 tablespoons of roasted soy nuts and mix well.*

---

*Avoid all types of caffeinated drinks and foods,* including coffee, tea, cola drinks, and chocolate. Too much caffeine also causes your body to lose calcium, which will increase your risk for osteoporosis and bone fractures.

*Avoid alcohol, sugary drinks or foods, spicy foods, hot soups, and very large meals.* Consuming any of these may increase the intensity of your flashes.

*Take vitamin E.* Studies show that 400 to 800 IU of vitamin E prevents hot flashes in some women. Try 400 IU per day for one month. If flashes are still a problem, boost your intake to 800 IU per day, though some women report that they experience headaches on 800 IU per day.

*Increase your activity level.* Moving around relieves hot flashes, stress, and depression and helps you sleep better. That's because exercise helps lower the amount of circulating hormones and raises endorphin levels, which drop during a hot flash.

*Reduce physical tension brought on by stress* with deep breathing and massage. (Since stress exacerbates hot flashes, read more Prime Time Prescriptions for reducing stress in Chapter 13.)

*Stay hydrated by drinking eight to ten glasses of water a day.* Always carry mineral water, since drinking water at the start of a flash may stop its progression. Also, keep water by your bed to quench your thirst when you flash in the middle of the night.

*Keep cool.* Make sure you have a fan (hand fan or battery operated) and a small spray bottle filled with water to mist yourself, which will soothe and hydrate your skin. Dress in layers, so clothing can be removed easily when you start to sweat. Sleep in a cool room.

*Meditate.* Take several long, deep breaths and imagine yourself totally naked, sliding through soft, cold snow down the gentle slope of a mountain. Suck on an ice cube. Drink large glasses of ice water.

*Use special herbs in your cooking.* Some herbs, such as ginseng, dong quai, and licorice root, have estrogenic properties, and are often recommended for the discomforts of menopause. Be careful, though. *Do not use ginseng, dong quai, or licorice root if you have high blood pressure!*

*Black cohosh* also has been well studied for its ability to chill out hot flashes. *Cohosh* is an Eastern Abenaki (Native American) word that means "knobby rough roots," and the Native Americans were the first to use black cohosh to treat female ailments. Mild side effects such as upset stomach, headache, dizziness, and weight gain have all been reported. The dose that works best seems to be a supplement capsule of 40 mg of root per day (larger doses may be unsafe) or drinking a tea made with the herb. Herbal and other natural and dietary remedies are increasingly popular for menopausal symptoms.

Herbs are slower-acting than drugs, so you must be patient when starting to use them. Sometimes it can take six weeks or longer for the herbs' healing or soothing powers to kick in. Some herbs are toxic if used in large amounts, so you should consult an herbalist for advice and recommendations. Also be sure that you know the source of the herbs, since 80 percent of dried herbs come from other countries, where pesticides that are banned here may be used. Read labels carefully and ask the supplier for information.

Herbs last longer in the dried form, which is best for making teas. Dry herbs should be almost the same color as when they were fresh, and the herbs should maintain a strong scent. Powdered forms of herbs (often found in capsules) lose efficacy sooner than dried herbs.

*Try herb teas to help you sleep.* Teas made from hops, spearmint, or chamomile can be very soothing. Or try a few drops (up to ½ teaspoon) of tincture of valerian or passionflower in a cup of water or juice forty-five minutes before bedtime. Valerian has an unpleasant odor and taste but may work for you if you're desperate enough. Evening primrose may give relief.

*Consider acupuncture and biofeedback.* Both have helped women find relief from hot flashes. Acupuncture performed by a medical doctor may be covered by your health insurance.

## Vaginal Dryness

Decreased estrogen causes the walls of your vagina to become thinner, drier, and less elastic. The vaginal lining also pales and the vaginal tissues become increasingly fragile. As the vaginal tract becomes drier, sexual intercourse can become uncomfortable, even painful, and consequently your interest in sexual activity may diminish. Because vaginal dryness is often discussed as a symptom of menopause, women mistake this as a sign that their bodies are no longer interested in sex. You can have and enjoy sex as long as you live. If pain from vaginal dryness is a problem, you can find a healing remedy in the different hormonal creams. The dryness also causes itching and irritation and a tendency to develop repeated vaginal infections.

The bladder and urinary tract also can be affected by menopausal changes, and you may lose a little urine while laughing, coughing, or exercising. This condition is referred to as *stress incontinence*. Women suffering from this problem also find themselves running faster to get to the bathroom because they're unable to hold their urine as well as before. (For more information on incontinence, see Chapter 17.)

**Rx** **PRIME TIME PRESCRIPTIONS FOR VAGINAL DRYNESS**
*Schedule a checkup with your doctor.* Do not start any self-treatments before checking with your doctor, so you can be sure any vaginal irritation is not due to an infection.

*Stop douching, if you are!* Douching can irritate the vagina and make matters worse. Douching may even change the acid balance of the vagina, which destroys necessary bacteria that fight infections.

*Have more sex.* Believe it or not, being sexually active helps. Sexual arousal increases the blood flow to the vaginal area and stimulates natural lubrication. It may take longer for the vagina to become lubricated than when you were younger, so be patient and allow time for foreplay—it's more enjoyable that way, anyway. Don't forget sexual fantasy and props—use whatever helps you get aroused. And please don't forget self-stimulation. If you don't use it, you will lose it!

Jellies and creams can help combat dryness and improve sexual intercourse, so spread a small amount of water-soluble jelly on the outside of your vagina. Smart choices: K-Y jelly, Astroglide gel, Maxilube jelly, Replens prefilled applicators, and Lubrin vaginal inserts. Do not use petroleum jelly with condoms, because it can make them more likely to break; also, because it is not water-soluble, it is not good for your mucous membranes. Have your partner help apply the cream or jelly as part of foreplay, and the lubricant will mix with your own natural lubrication.

*Discuss with your doctor the pros and cons of taking estrogen.* Estrogen (whether in the form of a vaginal cream, an estrogen-containing vaginal ring, pills, or patches) increases blood flow to the tissues and restores the natural moisture and acid-base balance of the vagina. (See the section on hormone replacement therapy later in this chapter.)

## Mood Swings

Menopause doesn't necessarily make women moody, but if you do experience temporary mood swings, it's not all in your head. It could be in your hormones. First of all, mood swings can be caused by the symptoms we've already described, especially sleep problems, which can impair your memory and make you irritable and anxious. Studies show that decreasing estrogen levels can trigger biochemical changes in the brain—serotonin levels rise and fall with the increase and decrease in estrogen levels—which may result in bouts of sadness and the blues. Menopause is a time when other stressful life events and circumstances can occur and may provoke sadness, such as elderly parents getting sick, loved ones dying, or difficulties developing in your relationship with your partner. See Chapter 13, on stress, and Chapter 15, on depression, for a variety of Prime Time Prescriptions to battle mood swings.

## Blood Sugar Levels and Diabetes

If you have diabetes, you should pay special attention to menopause because of its effect on blood sugar levels. Estrogen and progesterone blunt the effect of insulin, and so when these hormones drop with menopause, your insulin requirements will go down. In fact, once menopause is complete, your insulin requirements will have dropped about 20 percent. If you have type 2 diabetes and don't use insulin, you may find your doses of medications need to be decreased.

## THE 411 ON HORMONE THERAPY

One of the most important decisions you face during midlife, especially as you traverse menopause, is whether to take *hormone replacement therapy* (HRT). Hormone therapy is defined as treatment with estrogen or a combination of estrogen plus progesterone that replaces the hormones your body is no longer making. Making a decision about HRT may be difficult because you will get conflicting advice about the benefits and risks of estrogen. Some of the controversy is because we simply do not have all the information we need about the side effects of estrogen replacement. We hope that many of the studies currently in progress will help women make more informed choices in the future. However, you may need to make a decision now.

As you investigate the pros and cons of hormone replacement therapy, remember that the final decision of whether to take it or not is yours, although your doctor must manage the dosages. As with many aspects of menopause, there is no single answer that is right for every woman. The decision should be based on *your* individual needs, risks, and anticipated future outcomes. You cannot base your decision on what other women are doing, although you should find out from friends whether their therapy is helping them. Health experts such as former U.S. surgeon general Dr. Joycelyn Elders stress that HRT is not a one-stop cure for all women. Instead, Dr. Elders encourages women to ask themselves this important question: "Although hormone replacement therapy may be a dream come true for women who suffer through the change of life, is HRT right for you?"

Even naturopaths such as Tori Hudson emphasize the importance of making the decision regarding HRT based on the patient's individual needs and risk factors. "Not all women need estrogen, and not all women can just take herbs," says Hudson. "When I'm talking to a patient whose mother had osteoporosis, and she's a smoker and thin—all of which raise her risk of bone loss—my chief concern is not whether a treatment is 'natural' or 'unnatural.' My chief concern is: What do I know will protect her bones and therefore her life? Sometimes estrogen is the best answer." Ultimately, you need to decide whether or not the benefits of estrogen replacement outweigh the risks.

Before you make this decision, you should also get as much medical information as possible. We'll give you the basics in this chapter, but you need to discuss the treatment with your doctor and read up on HRT and alternatives elsewhere. Discuss this issue with your Prime Time Circle, and talk to many different women to learn more about their experiences with HRT.

Be sure you explore and understand all of your options before making any decisions about hormone therapy. Don't make your decision to use HRT or not based solely on another woman's decision. You don't want to mimic someone else's individual reasons for her decision. Also keep in mind that any choice you make can be changed, which is why you must continue to stay abreast of breakthroughs in hormone therapy. New developments are happening all the time, perhaps even as you read this.

Ask lots of questions when you discuss the risks and the benefits of HRT with your doctor. Your family medical history will be helpful in determining whether the benefits of HRT outweigh the risks, as many experts believe. If you had a loved one suffer from osteoporosis and have a low risk of cancer, you may be much more inclined to take HRT. On the other hand, if you have a family history of breast and reproductive cancers, you won't want to take estrogen. Here are some questions you can ask your doctor to start the dialogue.

- Should I take hormones? Why?
- How could hormone therapy improve my risk for heart disease and osteoporosis?
- How old should I be before I consider HRT?
- How long should I stay on the therapy?
- Should I consider HRT if my family has a history of breast cancer?
- Should I take HRT if I have heart disease?
- What follow-up tests or checkups will I need to monitor my reaction to the therapy and how often will I need to take each test?
- Do the benefits of HRT outweigh the risks for me?

Although most people refer to HRT as estrogen therapy, more than likely you will be prescribed an estrogen/progesterone combination pill, such as Prempro. If you haven't had a hysterectomy and still have your uterus, you should be given estrogen and a progesterone-like agent (progestin) to help reduce the risk of uterine problems such as uterine cancer. Estrogen also can be taken in the form of vaginal creams or patches that release estrogen through the skin. The form of estrogen your doctor chooses may depend on your symptoms. For instance, creams are used for vaginal dryness, while pills or patches are used to ease hot flashes or to prevent bone loss.

Doctors may prescribe different schedules for taking HRT. Some women take estrogen for a set number of days, add progestin for a set number of days, and then stop taking one or both for a specific period of time. This pattern, which would be repeated every month, often causes regular monthly bleeding like a menstrual period. On the other hand, some women take HRT every day of the month without any break and there is no monthly bleeding. You and your doctor must decide which program is best for you.

To get you started, we've outlined the benefits of HRT and how doctors are using this treatment to prevent or reduce the risks of developing serious illnesses and diseases associated with the change of life. Later in the chapter we'll explore the risks of HRT and how HRT may affect any ongoing health problems you currently have.

## The Benefits of Hormone Replacement Therapy

HRT is most frequently prescribed to improve short-term discomforts of menopause such as hot flashes, sleep disturbances, and vaginal dryness, but it can help reduce the risk for some women of developing three devastating long-term health problems: *cardiovascular disease (heart attacks and stroke), osteoporosis (bone loss and fractures), and memory problems (such as Alzheimer's disease).* Deciding whether to take hormone therapy to reduce your risk for any of these depends largely on your individual risk factors for them.

The Black Women's Health Project conducted a study that indicated that postmenopausal female hormone supplements are more widely prescribed to Black women in the western United States than to those living in the Northeast.[1] Hormone use among this group in the western United States was associated most strongly with menopause due to the surgical removal of both ovaries. However, even though HRT is recommended for women at greater risk of heart disease, the study found that Black women who were at higher risk for coronary artery disease (due to high blood pressure, cigarette smoking, or family history) do not seem to be adequately represented in the samples of women of color receiving this treatment.

Let's look more closely at how effective HRT is in addressing serious diseases associated with menopause.

### HRT and Cardiovascular Disease

Postmenopausal women are at greater risk of developing heart disease than younger women. More than thirty studies have shown that postmenopausal women on estrogen are at lower risk for coronary disease than those not on estrogen.[2] Researchers believe that estrogen guards against heart disease and stroke by helping to control blood cholesterol levels, which tend to rise as estrogen levels fall during menopause.

On average, estrogen replacement raises the protective or "good" cholesterol (HDL) by 21 percent and lowers the "bad" cholesterol (LDL) by 28 percent. This helps prevent blood vessels from accumulating harmful plaque that narrows and blocks arteries. There is some evidence that estrogen also dilates blood vessels, which inhibits plaque formation and allows the blood to flow evenly. This will decrease your risk of death from blockages in the blood vessels leading to the heart.

The Postmenopausal Estrogen/Progestin Interventions (PEPI) trial conducted during the late 1980s and early 1990s also found that HRT decreased the blood's ability to clot, thereby decreasing the risk of heart disease and stroke.[3] The Nurses' Health Study, the first comprehensive, long-range study of women's health, found that women who took estrogen after menopause had *half as many heart attacks and cardiovascular deaths as women who never used estrogen.* This study, which tracked about 120,000 nurses over several years throughout the 1990s, concluded that "the benefits of estrogen outweigh the risks, substantially."

However, the Heart and Estrogen/Progestin Replacement Study (HERS) found that postmenopausal women with *diagnosed* coronary disease who took HRT had 50 percent more heart attacks than those not on HRT in the first year after starting the treatment. The study also reported a 40 percent drop in heart attacks in HRT patients in the third and fourth years of taking this therapy.[4]

An HRT study reported in the August 2000 issue of the *New England*

*Journal of Medicine* reversed the HERS finding.[5] This study showed no effect from estrogen on women with established heart disease.

Despite the differing research conclusions, most researchers favor HRT for protecting against heart disease for women who are at **risk for cardiovascular problems but who don't show any signs of heart disease**. This is supported by a report in the August 2000 issue of the *New England Journal of Medicine* that showed a 31 percent drop in the incidence of heart disease among postmenopausal women who used estrogen. This study followed eighty-five thousand women (who did not suffer from cardiovascular disease) over fourteen years. (As always, adherence to a healthy lifestyle is a key factor in preventing heart disease.)[6]

If you are not clear about whether you are at risk for heart disease or stroke, review the assessment tools for these diseases in Chapter 10. Your individual risk is the key factor in deciding whether to go with HRT as a way to protect your heart.[7] But for reasons that we discuss later in this chapter, you should only take HRT for a limited time (up to five years), to minimize other complications.

### HRT and Osteoporosis

Over the years you've probably noticed older women who could no longer stand up straight or who have developed a curved spine, often called a "dowager's hump." These are two visible signs of *osteoporosis*, a progressive loss of bone density that weakens bones and makes them more likely to fracture. When women reach age thirty-five or so, their bones begin gradually to lose their strength and density, at the rate of about 1 percent a year. The loss becomes more rapid when we reach fifty to sixty years old.

Unfortunately, bone loss is often detected only after a woman has fractured her hip or some other extremity. Fractures can cause loss of height, deformity, and death, depending on where they occur and how severe they are.

The most common complication of osteoporosis is hip fracture, which is associated with significant disability and death. Approximately 16 percent of patients with a hip fracture die within the first few months after the injury. According to studies on osteoporosis, every year almost as many women die from complications from osteoporotic hip fractures as die of breast cancer.

Although bone loss is part of the aging process and therefore affects both women and men, the majority of osteoporosis patients are postmenopausal women. In fact, most bone loss in women takes place in the first three to eight years after the body's production of estrogen drops.

Estrogen decreases bone loss and plays a major role in keeping bones strong. It helps the body absorb calcium, which is vital for bone strength. More than 95 percent of your body's calcium is stored in your bones. If the body isn't getting enough calcium, it takes the vital mineral from the bones, which become weaker and may collapse and break.

Osteoporosis tends to run in families. But remember, if it runs in your family, that doesn't mean you will definitely get it; similarly, if you have no family history of it, there is no assurance that you won't suffer from weakened bones. Plus, bone loss can be slowed and reversed if you identify your risk factors early and deal with them.

*More Black women suffer from osteoporosis than you think!* Pay attention! This is not only a White woman's illness, or your grandmother's illness—it could affect you.

Genetic background plays a key factor in who is more likely to develop osteoporosis. Women who are light-skinned and very thin with small bones seem to be more prone to osteoporosis, which is why White and Asian women are at greater risk. However, because our bone loss usually occurs later in life, the incidence of osteoporosis in African American women may be greatly underestimated. African American women tend to have higher bone mineral density (stronger bones) than White women throughout life, but when we reach seventy, our risk of developing osteoporosis closely resembles the risk of White women. Dr. Anthony Cannon, an endocrinologist at Rancocas Hospital in Willingboro, New Jersey, warns that by age seventy-five, the incidence of hip fractures in African American women virtually parallels that in White women. And once bone loss begins for us, it progresses at twice the rate seen in White women of the same age.

So as the number of older African American women in the United States increases, there will be more Black women with osteoporosis. Here are some other facts you should know:

• Approximately three hundred thousand African American women currently have osteoporosis.

• Between 80 and 95 percent of fractures in African American women over sixty-four are due to osteoporosis.

• Diseases more prevalent in the African American population, such as sickle cell anemia and systemic lupus erythematosus, are linked to a higher risk of osteoporosis.

• As African American women get older, our risk for hip fracture doubles approximately every seven years.

• African American women are more likely than White women to die following a hip fracture from osteoporosis.

### Risk Factors for Osteoporosis

The leading three risk factors for osteoporosis are:

1. **Too little physical activity**—because exercise, especially weight-bearing activity such as brisk walking or running, strengthens your bone structure.

2. **Low calcium intake**—because calcium plays a crucial role in building peak bone mass and preventing bone loss. Studies indicate that African American women consume 50 percent less than the U.S. RDA of calcium.

3. **Low vitamin D intake**—because vitamin D helps the body utilize calcium and phosphorus (another bone-strengthening mineral) and build bones and teeth. Women over sixty tend to be deficient in vitamin D because as you age, your skin's ability to manufacture vitamin D from exposure to sunlight declines. Also, African American women need twice as much exposure to sunlight as light-skinned people for adequate vitamin D production.

In addition, risk factors that can also lead to fragile bones are:

• **Inadequate amounts of vitamin K** (found in dark green vegetables). Research has also indicated that increasing vitamin K consumption can strengthen bone mineral density.

• **Smoking**. Smoking lowers estrogen levels and increases the risk of heart attack, stroke, and osteoporosis.

• **Excessive consumption of alcoholic beverages.** Excessive drinking suppresses bone formation.

• **Prolonged use of steroids and certain medications** used to treat diseases such as systemic lupus erythematosus, asthma, arthritis, or other inflammatory diseases interferes with how your body handles calcium and reduces the strength of the bones. Ask your doctor about any such side effects from your medications.

• **Thyroid or kidney disease** also interferes with how your body uses calcium, and it can reduce bone strength.

## Rx PRIME TIME PRESCRIPTIONS FOR PREVENTING AND TREATING OSTEOPOROSIS

These prescriptions are preventive and therapeutic. Doctors prescribe HRT and other bone-strengthening medications to prevent osteoporosis when bone density tests (described later in the chapter) indicate a weakening.

*Increase physical activity.* To ward off osteoporosis, your workout should include one hour of weight-bearing aerobic exercise, such as walking, five times a week and thirty minutes of resistance training, such as weight lifting, at least three times a week. Swimming is not as effective in fighting osteoporosis, since it is not a weight-bearing activity.

*Increase calcium intake.* Every day you must ask yourself: "Have I had enough calcium?" And while you're at it, remind your children and grandchildren to eat and drink calcium-rich foods.

Milk and other dairy products such as cheese and yogurt are the best calcium sources. Soy milk and calcium-fortified orange juice and cereal are also quite effective. Nondairy foods that contain calcium (such as turnip greens, mustard greens, and kale), and fish with edible bones such as sardines are good sources of calcium as well. Following are the recommendations made at the National Institutes of Health Consensus Development Conference on Optimal Calcium Intake:

• Women eleven to twenty-four years old: 1,200 to 1,500 mg a day
• Women twenty-five to forty-nine years old (premenopausal): 1,000 mg a day
• Women over fifty years old (postmenopausal): 1,500 mg a day

As a Prime Time woman, you should take calcium tablets—500 mg three times a day. Younger women who are lactose-intolerant (unable to digest lactose, the sugar found in dairy products) also need to get calcium from calcium tablets, or they should find a nondairy source of calcium or drink or eat very small doses of milk or dairy products throughout the day. As many as 75 percent of all African Americans are lactose-intolerant and experience discomfort such as stomach bloating, cramps, or diarrhea when they consume dairy products. If you have this problem, drinking small amounts of milk (such as four half-cups of milk spread throughout a day) may help you avoid any discomfort. You can also drink milk fortified with lactase (the enzyme that helps the body digest milk) or take lactase tablets to help you digest milk products. You may also want to eat more yogurt, since the cultures in yogurt have already broken down the lactose in the milk.

Take calcium supplements in the form of *calcium citrate*, which comes in various forms. Although some doctors recommend calcium carbonate, this is not as easily absorbed as calcium citrate.

Don't take calcium on an empty stomach. If you are taking antacids with a high aluminum content, such as Mylanta or Maalox, do not take calcium citrate. (Citrates bind with the antacid's aluminum and the calcium will not be absorbed.) Instead, take antacids that contain calcium.

If you have a history of kidney stones or kidney disease, speak to your physician before beginning a calcium regimen. Drink eight to ten glasses of water a day when you are taking any type of calcium supplement.

*Increase vitamin D.* Each cup of fortified milk contains 100 IU of vitamin D. Salmon, sardines, egg yolks, and fortified breakfast cereals are other good sources of vitamin D. To make sure you get all the vitamin D your body requires, a daily multivitamin with 400 IU of vitamin D is usually the best solution.

*Increase vitamin K.* We're not sure how much is needed to prevent fragile bones, but it's believed to be much more than the daily recommended allowance of 65 mcg for women. Preliminary research suggests that anywhere from 109 to 420 mcg of vitamin K daily is better for bone health. Green leafy vegetables are the best sources, and collard greens top the list. Attention, Black women! We have finally found something we really love that is *good for us*!

In fact, collard greens are the champion food for us, just as tofu is for Asian women. They need to start eating more collard greens and we need to start eating more tofu. We all need to go out and invite an Asian woman into our kitchen to teach us how to cook the many tofu dishes, especially how to make tofu tasty. And while she's there, we can teach her how to mix up some delicious collard greens—low fat, of course. Gayle and Marilyn plan to learn how to cook collard greens and tofu together from Marilyn's daughter Ami and her friends.

## HAVE YOU HAD YOUR VITAMIN K LATELY?

| Vegetable (½ cup cooked) | Vitamin K (MCG) |
| --- | --- |
| Collard greens | 440 |
| Spinach | 360 |
| Brussels sprouts | 235 |
| Romaine lettuce | 200 |
| Scallions, raw | 150 |
| Broccoli | 113 |
| Cabbage | 75 |

*Source:* Vitamin K Laboratory, Jean Mayeruman Nutrition Research Center on Aging at Tufts University.

Remember, the greener the lettuce, the more vitamin K it will have. Iceberg lettuce, for instance, is very low in vitamin K, whereas romaine lettuce is packed with this critical vitamin.

***Decrease smoking and excessive alcohol intake.*** We know that giving up smoking and drinking can be difficult. For help to stop smoking, turn to the smoking cessation program outlined in Chapter 9. Consider joining a program such as Alcoholics Anonymous or one affiliated with your local hospital or medical center if you are having a problem controlling your drinking.

## WHY YOU NEED A BONE DENSITY TEST

To help assess how your bones are holding up during menopause, get a *bone mineral density study* at the onset of menopause to use as a baseline. Getting one at this stage, along with follow-up tests every few years, will help your doctor monitor your bone density.

This test uses X rays to measure your bone density and predict your risk of fracture. The gold standard in bone-density testing is the *dual-energy X-ray absorptiometry* (DEXA). The test should be done on the most common sites for fractures, such as your spine or hip. Measurements can also be done at peripheral sites such as your wrists, heels, and the bones of your hand. A bone density test is reported as a T-score. Good bone mass is a T-score of +1 or higher. Low bone mass would be a negative score, usually between −1 and −2.5. A T-score at or lower than

-2.5 indicates that you have osteoporosis and you should be treated using HRT or other bone-strengthening medications.

A new test for osteoporosis using ultrasound is quick, portable, and inexpensive and is available in parts of the country where women have no
other access to bone testing. This test assesses your bones by measuring the density of your heel. You put your foot into a small box and the
sound waves painlessly penetrate your foot for a mere ten seconds. The
heel bone scanner is called Sahara. Another similar test is SoundScan.
The entire test costs $40. Check to see if it is covered by your insurance.

*Hormone replacement therapy.* Although there is no cure for osteoporosis, estrogen therapy can help stop further bone loss and lower your risk of
fracture. You should consider starting HRT if your risk for osteoporosis is high
and your bone density test comes out borderline or low. Some studies reported in the *Archives of Internal Medicine* suggest that you may not need to
take the full dose of estrogen to strengthen bones; rather only half the usual
dose may do, which is good news, since low doses minimize the risk of breast
cancer. Also talk to your doctor about the following alternatives to HRT.

*Bisphosphonates* are a family of drugs that prevent bone loss and decrease the risk of fracture if your bone density test shows early osteoporosis.
Fosamax (alendronate) slows the breakdown of bone and is as effective as
hormone replacement therapy in protecting bones. Bisphosphonates will decrease your chance of developing vertebral and hip fractures by 40 to 50 percent. However, it may cause gastric upset, so follow the dosing directions
carefully.

*Raloxifene* (trade name Evista) is an alternative to HRT that mimics some
of estrogen's positive effects without introducing some of the unfavorable
side effects. (See the section on breast cancer in Chapter 11 for more information.) Raloxifene is a *selective estrogen-receptor modulator* (SERM) or "designer estrogen" that increases bone strength and bone density almost as
much as estrogen does. It also decreases the harmful LDL cholesterol, but
unlike estrogen, it doesn't increase the good HDL cholesterol. SERMs don't
cause uterine cancer and may even reduce the risk of breast cancer.

SERMs will not prevent or treat short-term symptoms such as hot flashes,
and in fact may increase hot flashes.

*Soybeans and yams.* Another study reported in the *Archives of Internal
Medicine* in 1998 showed that the phytoestrogens in soybeans and yams

provided the same benefits in treating osteoporosis as high-dose estrogen, without negative side effects.

### HRT, Cognitive Function, and Dementia

Some studies suggest that postmenopausal estrogen therapy might improve intellectual function and prevent dementia as we age. Others report improvement in memory and prevention of Alzheimer's specifically.[8] Large, controlled trials are required to verify these findings.

## Side Effects and Risks of HRT

Some women may have side effects from HRT such as unwanted vaginal bleeding, headaches, nausea, vaginal discharge, fluid retention, swollen breasts, or weight gain. Research also indicates that more serious diseases may be associated with HRT. These include:

*Uterine cancer.* Estrogen replacement after menopause can cause an overgrowth of the uterine lining that could result in cancer. A woman who has had her uterus removed, of course, need not worry about this cancer. *If you still have your uterus, your doctor should prescribe progesterone (progestin) with the estrogen to reduce the risk of uterine cancer.*

*Breast cancer.* Evaluation of many studies suggests that long-term estrogen therapy increases the risk of breast cancer, but the Nurses' Health Study showed a reduced risk of death from breast cancer in women who took estrogen for less than five to ten years. Women who used HRT more than five to ten years were 46 percent more likely to get breast cancer than nonusers and had a 43 percent increase in deaths from breast cancer. *Researchers recommend that women who have a history of breast cancer in their families should not take HRT.*[9]

An article in the June 1999 issue of the *Journal of the American Medical Association* suggested that breast cancer developed while on HRT tends to be less aggressive. The risk of breast cancer may be increased by 2 percent per year, with the most risk after ten to fifteen years of HRT treatment. Keep in mind that a woman between fifty and eighty years old already has about a 10 percent chance of getting breast cancer. Add estrogen and the risk goes up to about 13 percent to 15 percent. That means that out of one hundred women, thirteen to fifteen will likely develop the disease—but only three to five of those cases will be estrogen-related.

Think about this, too: In this same group of one hundred women, HRT may spare thirty of them from an early death from heart disease. Therefore, if your medical history indicates that you are at increased risk of heart disease, the scales tip in favor of estrogen to protect your heart. "Most women who develop breast cancer die of something else, whereas most women who develop heart disease die from heart disease," points out Dr. Nananda F. Col, assistant professor of medicine at New England Medical Center/Tufts University School of Medicine and author of A *Woman Doctor's Guide to Hormone Therapy*.

Although concerns about breast cancer are high, the chances of dying from heart disease are greater for high-risk African American women.

Other problems related to hormone therapy include:

- Migraine headaches
- Risk of deep-vein blood clots and clots in the lung
- Increased risk of gallbladder disease
- Unpleasant side effects—headaches, nausea, bloating, breast tenderness, and weight gain

## OUR FINAL WORDS ON HORMONE REPLACEMENT THERAPY

Throughout the chapter, we have discussed a wide range of HRT studies that explore its pros and cons. At this time, however, most large studies point to positive effects and maybe longer lives with HRT. Here is a summary of what we found:

- If you are at risk for heart disease but don't already have signs of it, you should probably take HRT to prevent its onset—but only if you don't have a personal or family history of breast cancer.
- If you are at risk for osteoporosis, you should probably take HRT to prevent its onset, but only if you don't have a family or personal history of breast cancer.
- Short-term use of hormones (five years or less) to alleviate menopausal symptoms does not increase your risk for breast cancer.
- There is good evidence that long-term hormone use (five to ten years or more) does raise the risk of breast cancer. However, when you stop HRT, your risk drops to the level it would have been before you started.

Whether you take HRT or are considering the treatment to ease your menopausal discomforts or prevent future illness (such as heart disease and osteoporosis), you and your doctor should regularly discuss the benefits and side effects of HRT and consider the findings of any new studies. Above all, regularly reevaluate your treatment with your doctor to determine what makes sense for you at that time.

In December 2000, estrogen was being considered for addition to the listing of the *Report on Carcinogens* (cancer causers), published by the National Institute of Environmental Health Sciences, the National Toxicology Program. Asbestos, secondhand smoke, and alcohol consumption are already listed as human carcinogens.

# Chapter 17

# MIDLIFE'S COMMON CONCERNS

*Of all the things I've lost in my middle years, I miss my mind the most!*
— Naomi Chamberlain

As we age, we all face a slew of annoying changes in our bodies. At one time or another we have difficulty remembering where we put our keys. We start slowing down earlier in the day. We start complaining about our aching feet more than we did in the past. Happily, all of these concerns can be easily addressed with the right Prime Time Prescriptions.

## THE MEMORY CHALLENGE

We all must face it—the increasing loss of our memory. Someone described it as if your brain had become Teflon-coated: Nothing sticks! Our friend Andrea offered this revealing description of her midlife struggles:

*First I lost my waistline,*
*Second, I lost my natural hair color,*
*Third, I lost my memory,*
*And there's a fourth one . . .*
*But I can't remember it.*

We all know that feeling! This is the time in our lives when we have to write everything down—absolutely everything! We seem to make more and more to-do lists. And thank God for Post-its, which we have everywhere—in the workplace, the bedroom, and the car. We can't shop without a grocery list. We can't remember names—though that skill was probably never really well developed in the first place, now it's worse. We're always losing our car keys or our glasses—or both. Sometimes we feel like we're literally losing our minds.

This forgetfulness is not the first sign of Alzheimer's disease. Only 9 percent of Americans over age sixty-five suffer from Alzheimer's, which is a distinct illness, *not* an inevitable part of aging. Short-term memory does seem to worsen with age, the result of changes that take place in the way the brain functions, and these changes have an effect on memory. We admit more often to having a "senior moment," which often feels like a "senior week." According to a Charles A. Dana Foundation survey, 80 percent of people age thirty-five and older reported difficulty with memory or concentration. By age forty-five, 56 percent say they habitually lose things, and 45 percent have difficulty remembering familiar names. But even though a good many of us can count on our memory declining somewhat with age, most memory loss is not severe. And long-term memory remains relatively unaffected.

After age forty-five, it does take longer to recall things. It also takes the brain longer to absorb new information. Older people can still learn new, complicated things, but we may need more time than younger people.

The difference between normal forgetfulness—known as *age-associated memory impairment* (AAMI)—and serious *dementia* or brain damage is that AAMI is neither progressive nor disabling. The memory lapses associated with AAMI are most likely to occur when you are tired, sick, distracted, under stress, or trying to remember many different things at the same time. Sound familiar? In other words, AAMI may cause you to forget where you put your car keys. A more serious memory disorder would cause you to forget what the keys are used for.

When it comes to our memories, we are our harshest critics. Too often, Prime Time women refuse to feel good about the countless facts we recall every day. Instead, we focus on the forgotten few. Under less stressful circumstances, most of us *will* remember things that elude us when we're tired, frustrated, or rushed. In fact, studies repeatedly show that older people who do poorly on timed tests actually do as well or better than their college-age counterparts when permitted to work at their own pace.

Another point of encouragement: If you're worried about memory loss, then probably nothing serious is wrong. People with serious memory impairment tend to be unaware of their lapses, don't worry about them, or attribute them to other causes. However, if the memory lapses interfere with your daily routine or if close friends and relatives believe that your lapses are serious, then have yourself checked, because something more complex may be at fault.

Still concerned about your forgetfulness? Then try to keep this memory trick in mind: When something feels like it's right on the tip of your tongue, relax and stop trying so hard to remember it. More than likely it will soon come to you.

## How Does Our Memory Work?

The *hippocampus*—a small S-shaped structure that resembles a seahorse (*hippocampus* is Greek for "seahorse") appears to play a major role in the process of forging memories. This small section deep within the brain instantly evaluates incoming data from our senses and determines whether any bits of new information should be stored or discarded.

Interestingly, memories don't reside in the hippocampus or in any other specific site in the brain. They are stored throughout the entire brain, particularly in the *cerebral cortex* (the convoluted outer layer of gray matter that constitutes the "thinking" portion of the brain) as well as the *cerebellum* (which controls our movement and balance) at the base of the brain.

Memories exist in the brain in two distinct forms. One is *short-term* or *working memory*, which can hold no more than six to seven items at a time (such as the digits in a phone number.) These data will be forgotten in five to ten seconds unless they are constantly repeated or transferred to long-term memory. *Long-term* or *permanent memory* stores both old and new information, such as the name of your high school or a new acquaintance. The emotions you feel with a particular memory are thought to be stored in a different part of the brain than the memory itself.

## Causes of AAMI (Age-Associated Memory Impairment)

As you age, the nerve cells in your brain (*neurons*) shrink, which slows your mental functions in midlife and older years. Serious memory problems occur when whole clusters of neurons are destroyed by major disorders such as stroke or Alzheimer's disease.

In midlife, the brain also begins producing smaller quantities of *neurotransmitters*, which are chemicals that help brain cells communicate. There is also evidence that blood flow to the brain is reduced by approximately 15 to 20 percent from age thirty to age seventy. Certain areas of the brain, such as the hippocampus, are particularly sensitive to a decrease in oxygen.

Other memory busters include stress, depression, anxiety, information overload, and simply being too tired to pay full attention to our surroundings. Too little sleep, too many sleeping pills, too much alcohol, high blood pressure, or an abnormal thyroid gland also can disrupt the formation of new memories.

### Rx PRIME TIME PRESCRIPTIONS FOR MEMORY LOSS

Although age-associated memory impairment is common and is not a sign of a serious disorder, it is frustrating, annoying, and frightening—but we hope it is less so now that you've read this section. Most important, as with everything we've addressed in the book, you can do something about it.

*Relax and learn to manage your stress.* We are all more likely to remember things when we are calm and relaxed. Review the recommendations throughout the book regarding the relief of stress (specifically, see Chapter 13, "Stress Can Be Managed"). An important, effective stress buster that we repeatedly recommend is deep breathing. Not only does deep breathing calm you down, it also increases the oxygen to the hippocampus, the memory part of the brain that is supersensitive to oxygen levels. Try it right now and you'll see.

*Pay attention to what you're doing.* Make it a conscious habit to observe and note things such as where you have left your coat or umbrella, or where your car is in the parking lot. This also means eliminating distractions. Turn off the television, radio, and petty thoughts—whatever prevents you from paying full attention to what you are doing. When trying to remember if you turned off the coffeemaker or locked the door while rushing out in the morning, pause for a moment, take a deep breath, close your eyes, and relax. Try to recall everything you did before you walked out of the door.

*Rehearse and repeat new information.* Just repeating certain ideas or facts aloud or over and over to yourself will help the information to stick or sink in. For example, when you meet someone for the first time, say his or her name aloud and repeat the name several times to yourself soon afterward.

*Use cues and associations to help jog your memory.* There are many ways to invent visual images, rhymes, or acronyms to recall names, facts, or masses of information that are meaningful only to you. For example, let's say you just met a woman named Harriet Snow. In your mind, imagine Harriet Tubman shoveling snow to free the slaves.

*Group information together.* It's easier to manage small clumps of data than many individual units. For example, when you are trying to remember a series of numbers, group two, three, or four of the digits together. Think about it: Recalling 2-9-5-1-3-6 is much tougher than remembering 29-51-36 or 295-136.

*Get organized.* Taking a few simple steps to structure your life will greatly improve your ability to keep track of details.

• *Write things down.* The mere act of writing notes and making lists reinforces memory. Make lists of things to do and leave notes to yourself around the house. For instance, you can write a note to remind yourself to take your medication.

• *Use a date book, calendar, or electronic organizer that you can keep in your purse.* Even as we age, there's no excuse for constantly forgetting appointments, meetings, and social engagements.

• *Leave important items in the same place all the time.* This includes the small things that we always seem to misplace, such as keys, the mail, and the checkbook, as well as other items that you may use only occasionally, such as the hand vacuum, hammer, or scissors.

• *Use a pocket notepad, wristwatch alarm, voice recorder, or other aids to jog your memory.* Whatever you choose, find something that you can always keep with you so you can use it and refer to it all day long.

*Establish a healthy lifestyle.* Your general physical condition can affect how well your memory is working.

• *Exercise your body to keep your mind fit.* Since the brain is at the mercy of the circulatory system, a heart-healthy lifestyle that increases cardiovascular endurance can improve your mental function. Exercise also helps maintain a normal blood pressure, which increases the level of oxygen and blood flow to the brain. In addition, exercise may boost the body's production of brain-derived nerve growth factor (NGF), which is a molecule that helps keep neurons strong.

• *Eat healthy foods.* A diet rich in fruits, vegetables, and fiber improves brain function.

• *Avoid excessive alcohol, caffeine, and nicotine consumption.* If taken in excess, any one of these three can significantly hasten the destruction of brain cells.

• *Sleep, sleep, sleep.* Lack of sleep is a memory killer. Adequate sleep enhances your alertness, your ability to concentrate, and your overall mental agility.

*Keep mentally healthy.* Depression, grief, anxiety, anger, and stress make it difficult to concentrate, learn, and remember. Counseling, medications or a combination of both can help improve your memory.

*Stay mentally active.* Research shows that mental exercise helps keep your mind alert. Doing crossword puzzles, playing bridge or chess, taking classes, and learning new skills will help you remain mentally agile as you age.

*Utilize your best learning pathway.* Some of us learn and absorb more when information is presented visually. Others tend to remember more of what they hear. If your learning pathway is visual, then making notes and writing every little thing down really helps. If your best pathway is auditory, then talk your way through something you're trying to remember; for example, when trying to remember where the car is parked, say "The car is parked in section three, space twenty-two" several times before you walk into the mall.

*Check your medications.* Some medications that may impair memory include prednisone; heartburn drugs such as Zantac (ranitidine), Tagamet (cimetidine), and Pepcid (famotidine); antianxiety/sedative drugs such as Halcion (triazolam), Xanax (alprazolam), and Valium (diazepam); and even insulin, if the dose you take is too high.

*Check your estrogen level.* Besides lowering the risk of Alzheimer's disease in postmenopausal women, studies suggest that estrogen replacement therapy helps maintain both verbal and visual memory. The reasons are still not clear, but the hormone seems to fuel the development of hippocampal neurons and boost the production of acetylcholine, a chemical that helps brain cells communicate. (See Chapter 16, "Maneuvering Through Menopause," for more information on estrogen-replacement therapy.)

*Ask your doctor about using supplements designed to boost your memory.* Although the research is sketchy, some supplements are recommended as memory enhancers. Here are some you may want to research:

*Vitamin E* is an antioxidant and helps prevent heart disease and boost immune function. It may also slow the progression of Alzheimer's. There is no evidence it helps memory in healthy people.

*B vitamins* help improve how the brain functions.

*Ginkgo biloba* is currently the most popular memory aid and has been used in Asia for thousands of years to improve circulation. Extracted from the leaves of the ginkgo tree (one of the longest-living trees in the world, with a thousand-year life span), ginkgo biloba may help strengthen memory and improve concentration. Ginkgo biloba also increases blood flow to the brain, dilates the arteries, thins the blood, prevents blood clots, and enhances the blood's ability to carry oxygen to the brain.

Dr. Andrea Sullivan, a well-known African American naturopath, recommends taking 40 mg of standardized ginkgo biloba extract three times daily.[1] (Look for a content of 20 to 24 percent ginkgo heterosides or glycosides on the label.) Do not take ginkgo if you are on medication for high blood pressure or heart disease or if you are scheduled for even minor surgery.

*Other brain-boosting chemicals that help improve memory and brainpower* include boron, calcium, magnesium, zinc, lecithin, and selenium. Take them as directed on the supplement bottle. Studies suggest that another supplement, phosphatidylserine, helps the brain release adequate amounts of dopamine and acetylcholine, which are chemicals that carry messages from one cell to the next in the brain. This supplement is available in health-food stores, but check with your doctor before taking any supplement.

## URINARY INCONTINENCE

Of all the annoyances in midlife, this just might be the most embarrassing. While urinary incontinence (an involuntary loss or leakage of urine) may be common among older adults, it is not a normal part of aging. More than eleven million women in the United States suffer from urinary incontinence. The September 1999 issue of the *Tufts University Health and Nutrition Letter* reports that 25 percent of women ages thirty through sixty and 33 percent of older women suffer from incontinence. So don't feel you're the only one wetting herself—there are many of us struggling with this predicament. Bladder control problems can be caused by many medical conditions.

Under a doctor's care, incontinence can be treated and often cured. Even if it is not cured, it can be managed successfully.

Getting over your embarrassment is critical. You cannot suffer in silence, get depressed about it, and become socially isolated because you're having trouble controlling your bladder. Remember, incontinence is a symptom, not a disease, so talk to your health-care provider to find out what is wrong and what you can do.

Two of the most common causes of incontinence are childbirth and lowered estrogen levels in postmenopausal women. Both situations can weaken muscles around the urinary tract that help block urine flow. In addition, the tube from the bladder to the outside (urethra) is shorter in women than in men and provides less resistance to urine flow. The drop in estrogen at menopause thins the lining of the urethra, reducing resistance even more.

Depression, stress, certain medications, infection, lack of exercise, being overweight, caffeine, and alcohol all contribute to incontinence. Untreated lower back pain and sciatica can lead to incontinence because of nerve damage from a disc problem.

## Types of Incontinence

There are many types of incontinence; however, the two most common are stress incontinence and urge incontinence.

*Stress incontinence* occurs with increased pressure on the bladder. For example, small amounts of urine leak out when you cough or sneeze or with physical exertion such as running or lifting. This is the most common type of incontinence and can always be cured. As we explained before, this is especially common in women our age whose muscles around the urinary tract have weakened due to a loss of estrogen.

*Urge incontinence* happens when the body is not able to suppress or delay urination. A stroke or infection sometimes causes the bladder to become overactive and contract repeatedly and inappropriately. Because of this activity, the urine leaks out before you can get to the bathroom.

*To measure your degree of incontinence:* When your bladder is full, hold a brown paper towel (the kind in public restrooms) against your bottom where you urinate. Cough hard three times. If the towel is soaked from end to end, you should see your primary-care doctor and a urologist or gynecologist for a full exam and testing. A wet spot that doesn't go to the edges of the paper towel indicates a moderate to mild level of incontinence. Go to your primary-care doctor for a consultation.

## ℞ PRIME TIME PRESCRIPTIONS FOR URINARY INCONTINENCE

*Talk to your doctor.* Don't get so embarrassed about bladder problems that you simply resort to pads and refuse to talk with your doctor. Your doctor will probably not ask about how your bladder is functioning—so you *must* speak up if you're having problems. To determine the cause of incontinence, you'll need a physical exam and a urine sample to check for infection. Your primary-care physician may refer you to a urologist or a gynecologist for further testing.

According to the National Kidney and Urologic Disease Information Clearinghouse, be sure to tell your doctor:

- What prescriptions and over-the-counter medicines you take
- When the trouble started
- Number of babies you have had
- Date of your menopause
- If you have symptoms of bladder infection, such as burning when you urinate or blood in urine
- How often you are constipated
- Other medical problems you may have: cancer, depression, back pain or sciatica, spinal cord injury, urinary tract infection, smoking, constipation, diabetes, stroke, multiple sclerosis, and so on

*Try exercises that will help strengthen bladder-control muscles.* Kegel exercises strengthen the pelvic muscles and reduce involuntary contractions of the bladder. These exercises work better than drugs, but they must be performed regularly. If you integrate the exercises as part of your daily life, you should notice improvement in about three months.

Before you begin Kegel exercises, you must locate your pelvic floor muscles. One way to identify them is to stop your urine in midstream several times; the muscles you use to do this are your pelvic floor muscles.

To do Kegel exercises, squeeze or contract the muscles for a count of ten, then relax for a count of ten. Repeat ten times for one set. Try to complete four sets each day. Practice holding the contraction while talking, then contract and hold while you gently blow your nose. Then try while you cough.

Practice doing Kegel exercises many times during the day. You can do them in your car, standing in line, or even as you wash the dishes.

*Try urinating on a set schedule instead of waiting for the urge to go.* However, do not cut back on fluids when you try this! Reducing your fluid intake will concentrate the urine, which will irritate the bladder and make matters worse.

*Consider medications or herbs if the suggestions listed above are not successful.* Estrogen replacement alleviates stress incontinence. Bladder relaxants and some antidepressants (such as Tofranil) can also help. A Chinese herbal medicine called Ba-Wei-Wan is the most common Asian therapy.

*If nothing else works and the incontinence is extreme, discuss surgery with your doctor.* Surgery repositions and supports the bladder and urethra. This may be especially helpful for women who have given birth to many children or have really relaxed pelvic muscles.

## ARTHRITIS

We all grew up hearing about someone being in bed with one of those Itis brothers—Arthur being the most well-known one—*Arthur Itis.*

The word *arthritis* comes from the Greek word *arthron*, meaning "joint." The ending *-itis* means "inflammation." So *arthritis* means "inflammation of a joint." Nearly forty million Americans have a form of arthritis. Of those, four million are African Americans. Arthritis is one of the top three self-reported conditions among African Americans, ahead of other common conditions such as asthma, diabetes, and hearing impairment. After age thirty-five, African American women report a higher rate of arthritis than Caucasian women.

In addition, when compared with other groups of people, African Americans develop more physical limitations as a result of arthritis. Arthritis is the reason why many older African Americans must stop working, can no longer keep their own house, and forfeit their independence. By 2020, the estimated number of Americans with arthritis will reach sixty million, of which seven million will be African Americans. A majority of this group will be Black women.

There are many different forms of arthritis. The one most common form of arthritis and the one most often associated with aging is *osteoarthritis*, also known as degenerative joint disease. Virtually everyone over age fifty has osteoarthritis to some degree, but many are without symptoms. It is so common that if you had X rays taken today, you would probably show some signs of it. By age forty, about 90 percent of all people have X-ray evidence of osteoarthritis in the hips and knees.

An estimated sixteen million Americans—mostly women—have been diagnosed with osteoarthritis. This condition is up to four times more common in women than in men, a ratio that increases with age. While osteoarthritis has little or no effect on your longevity (unlike some other forms of arthritis), severe osteoarthritis of the hips, knees, and spinal column may greatly limit your activity and diminish your overall enjoyment of life.

Basically, osteoarthritis is the result of the wear and tear throughout your life on the weight-bearing joints of the body, especially the vertebrae, hips, and knees. Over the years, stress on these joints leads to a breakdown of the shock-absorbing joint cartilage that covers the ends of the bones. Without this protection, a joint loses its shape and the bones no longer align properly. As a result, the ends of the bones thicken, bony growths called *spurs* form, and bits of cartilage float in the joint space. These changes can be painful and reduce your range of motion.

In addition to age and being female, there are several specific risk factors for osteoarthritis:

- Injury or trauma to the joints
- Obesity (which leads to cartilage damage by placing greater stress on the hips and knees)
- Lack of exercise
- Genetic predisposition

## Symptoms of Osteoarthritis

People rarely develop osteoarthritis before age forty or fifty. At first, symptoms are mild—for example, morning stiffness that rarely lasts for more than fifteen minutes. As the disease progresses, the osteoarthritis becomes more painful and activity may be limited.

## Prevention of Osteoarthritis

The only preventive measures for osteoarthritis are:

- Avoidance of repeated joint injury
- Weight reduction (in one study, loss of only an average of eleven pounds by women reduced by half the development of osteoarthritis in their knees)
- Hormone replacement therapy (women taking estrogen had a 38 percent lower likelihood of signs of osteoarthritis on their hip X rays, compared to women never on estrogen)
- Exercise, exercise, exercise

**Rx PRIME TIME PRESCRIPTIONS FOR OSTEOARTHRITIS**

The goals of osteoarthritis treatment are to relieve pain and to maintain as much normal joint function as possible. The key is early detection and early intervention. That means your doctor must perform a complete evaluation to diagnose your type of arthritis. Rheumatoid arthritis, gout, or lupus are other forms of arthritis to consider.

*Take a course to learn more about osteoarthritis.* To develop an effective action plan, you must understand many aspects of this disease. For a nominal fee, local chapters of the National Arthritis Foundation offer an Arthritis Self-Help Course. This course has successfully helped osteoarthritis sufferers reduce the problems associated with the disease by explaining the causes and treatments of arthritis, providing tips that will improve patient-doctor communication, offering suggestions for an eating plan and exercise program, and outlining relaxation and other pain management techniques.

*Get adequate rest and exercise.* The right balance between rest and exercise must be tailored to you and your stage of the disease. While rest is important when joints ache, appropriate exercise is equally essential to maintain joint motion, muscle strength, and fitness. In fact, every study that has ever been done on arthritis patients shows that exercise reduces symptoms and pain. *Do not begin any exercise program without consulting your physician.* In some cases of arthritis, you may need to work with a physical therapist.

*Try relaxation therapy.* The National Institutes of Health recently endorsed relaxation therapy—meditation, deep breathing, biofeedback, hypnosis, and acupuncture—to ease the pain associated with arthritis. These techniques help relax the muscles that support arthritic joints that tighten due to stress and anxiety, and therefore relieve pain.

*Reduce stress on a joint by using a cane, splinting the joint, wearing a sling, or using special shoe inserts to reduce the pain.* A heating pad or hot pack in a towel wrapped around the joint can also provide much-needed pain relief.

*Take a warm bath first thing in the morning to improve your range of motion and flexibility.* Heat relaxes, soothes, and improves blood flow to the area, and may help reduce pain throughout the day. You may want to get out those ol' Epsom salts and see if that also doesn't help. A two-liter carton of Epsom salts is $2, and added to the bathwater, it provides the healing powers of magnesium sulfate, the same mineral that can be found in the waters of the great spas around the world.

*Try over-the-counter drug treatments.* Tylenol (acetaminophen), aspirin, Advil or Motrin (ibuprofen), and Aleve (naproxen) work very quickly to relieve pain in tender joints. Be aware that all of these remedies except Tylenol cause stomach upset and other side effects. However, Tylenol in very high doses can cause side effects, including kidney and liver disease.

*Investigate alternative treatments.* Glucosamine and chondroitin sulfate have been cited as cures for arthritis in two best-selling books, *The Arthritis Cure* and *Maximizing the Arthritis Cure*, both by Dr. Jason Theodosakis. Glucosamine comes from crab shells, and chondroitin sulfate is derived from cow cartilage. Together these two substances may provide the body with the raw materials needed to *make new cartilage*. However, Theodosakis' claim of using this substance to "cure" arthritis has not been generally accepted in the scientific community. Still, experts agree that glucosamine relieves joint pain and increases range of motion in patients with osteoarthritis. Smaller studies with chondroitin sulfate also show some benefit. Trials are currently under way with both drugs. (These substances can cause stomach upset.)

COX-2 inhibitors such as Celebrex (celecoxib) and Vioxx (rofecoxib)—called "superaspirins"—are a promising new class of drugs that treat the symptoms of arthritis without causing stomach bleeding or ulcers, which are the major drawback of aspirin and other anti-inflammatory drugs.

## EYE DISEASE

As we age, our eyes begin to change. Around age forty, most of us begin experiencing a natural visual condition called *presbyopia*, in which the lens of the eye loses its elasticity. Consequently, focusing on objects up close becomes difficult. When this occurs, you'll probably need glasses, or if you wear glasses, you'll need to get your prescription adjusted. It's also around midlife that two of the primary diseases that lead to blindness occur: *glaucoma* and *cataracts*.

## Glaucoma

Glaucoma occurs when increased pressure in the eye damages the optic nerve, resulting in vision loss. The risk of nerve damage from glaucoma is increased with heart disease, diabetes, and nearsightedness. By far, glaucoma is the leading cause of blindness in the United States. For African American women, this harmful disorder can occur even earlier than midlife. Glaucoma is common in West Africa, where many of our ancestors originated, which may explain why this disease is more common in African Americans than Caucasians. Another reason is that African American women typically have more of the risk factors associated with this disease. You are at higher risk of developing glaucoma if this condition runs in your family, you're over forty years old, or you're nearsighted or farsighted.

Glaucoma can be detected in a routine eye exam (which you should be scheduling every one or two years) with tests that check the pressure in your eye. Since glaucoma runs in families, it's critical that you begin getting tested in your early forties. This will let your doctor establish a baseline of what's normal for you before the impact of aging takes place. If you are in your mid-forties or older, get the test as soon as you can. *Don't wait for any symptoms to appear.* Once they appear, you've already developed the disease.

An *ophthalmologist* (a medical doctor who specialize in the function, structure, and diseases of the eye) will use one or more of the following three types of tests to screen for glaucoma, make the diagnosis, and follow patients during treatment:

• A *tonometry test* measures the pressure in the eye. The most accurate way to administer this test is by using an instrument to put pressure on the eye after numbing it with eye drops. Another way is to blow a puff of air at the eye; however, the results of this test are not as accurate.

• *An examination with an ophthalmoscope* (a handheld light) or a *slit lamp* used in a darkened room allows doctors to examine visual changes in the optic nerve that may be caused by glaucoma. Before looking into the eye, the doctor will dilate it with drops. Since glaucoma can occur when the eye pressure is normal, a series of measurements taken and recorded over time (using photographs and drawings of the eye) can help to track damaging changes.

• A *visual field test* will help doctors determine whether your peripheral vision has been diminished due to glaucoma. The tests require you to look at a central spot and indicate when spots of light can be seen on either side. To administer the test, the examiner will use a screen and light pointer or an automatic device that gives off spots of light.

**℞ PRIME TIME PRESCRIPTIONS FOR GLAUCOMA**

Glaucoma cannot be cured, but it can be treated to prevent damage to the optic nerve. Eye drops are the most frequent medical treatment. An ophthalmologist will design your therapy to meet your individual needs, but you have to be vigilant in using the drops and keeping your appointments for eye exams.

## Cataracts

Cataracts are another very common eye problem, especially for men and women over fifty-five or sixty years old. Cataracts are a cloudy formation over the lens of the eye. The lens is located behind the pupil (the dark hole in the center of your eye) and the iris (the colored part of your eye.) The lens focuses light (like the lens of a camera) on the retina, the membrane at the back of the eye that forms the visual images. As you age, the lens can gradually turn opaque, which clouds your vision. As this condition progresses, light can no longer pass through to the retina. Eventually, blindness results because all light entering the eye is blocked from passing through the lens. Blindness is not inevitable, however, and cataracts can be treated.

Cataracts affect 60 percent of Americans over the age of sixty and 70 percent of those over age seventy-five. It is, in fact, the third leading cause of avoidable blindness in the country. In the United States, cataracts are the most common cause of vision impairment, ranking behind only arthritis and heart disease as a leading cause of disability in older adults. Your risk of developing cataracts is increased with smoking, long-term steroid use, prolonged exposure to sunlight, diabetes, and obesity.

You can prevent cataracts by wearing sunglasses that filter out ultraviolet rays from the sun.

The most common symptom of cataracts is a painless blurring of vision. Everything becomes dimmer, as if you constantly need to clean your glasses. Occasionally cataract sufferers experience double vision and feel as if they frequently need to have the prescription for their glasses changed. Some cataract patients see a yellow tinge over objects. Answer these five questions to see if cataracts may be the cause of your visual problems.

---

## CATARACT QUESTIONNAIRE

Despite wearing glasses, do you have difficulty:
Driving at night?
YES          NO
Seeing road signs at dusk?
YES          NO
Seeing in the distance or reading?
YES          NO
Recognizing colors?
YES          NO
Recognizing friends and family at a distance?
YES          NO

If you answered yes to two or more of these questions, you may have cataracts. Make an appointment with an ophthalmologist for a thorough examination now.

---

 **PRIME TIME PRESCRIPTIONS FOR CATARACTS**

The amount of vision loss due to cataracts dictates the treatment.

*Try new eyeglasses or contact lenses.*

*Take medication.* Using antioxidant eye drops to decrease the damage from free radicals may help. L-glutathione is a powerful antioxidant.

*Increase antioxidants in your diet.* The eight-year Nurses' Health Study found that women who take vitamin A supplements lowered their risk of clouded lens by 39 percent. An increase of vitamin C, beta-carotene, and vitamin E can also improve your vision.

**Get cataracts surgically removed.** The clouded lens can be removed and replaced with a clear plastic lens. Cataract removal is considered one of the most effective surgeries available today. Studies are in progress to evaluate the use of drugs so that surgery may not be needed in the future.

## FATIGUE

Be honest—doesn't it seem that another important thing you have lost is your energy? It feels as though the middle years walked through the front door and your energy ran out the back door. Think about how many times a day you say, "Oh, my God, I'm so tired!" or hear one of your friends exclaim, "I've been tired all week, maybe all year!"

---

### MORNING SALUTATION

A middle-aged friend of ours spent the night with a new lover about ten years younger than herself. Upon awaking, our friend went through her usual ritual of calling on the Lord for help to get her arthritic bones moving and to relocate her energy to start her day. Her exclamations woke her younger lover, who expressed concern at her "obvious" distress. In fact, it was a usual day and probably even a good day for our friend. It was at that moment our friend realized the relationship was doomed to end, as she could never explain, and didn't have the energy to try to explain, her daily midlife routine of morning salutation.

---

Haven't you sat on the edge of the bed some mornings and wondered what it would take to really get you going? Have you wished for your bed at two o'clock in the afternoon and realized that you've been struggling to keep your eyes open since lunchtime?

Fatigue is one of the top ten complaints doctors get from women. Who knows what that statistic is for African American women? Dr. Gayle Olinekova in her book *Power Aging: Staying Young at Any Age* calls fatigue "the irrepressible recurring energy deficit." The clever acronym for this is TIRED!

So many Prime Time women are just plain tired. Being tired happens for a number of reasons, and it is a warning sign that we should not ignore.

Most fatigue is caused by too much of something—too much stress, too much work, too much weight, too much junk food. But it's also caused by some "not enoughs"—not enough sleep, not enough exercise, not enough water, not enough joy in your life. Much of the fatigue we experience is due to the inability to pace ourselves, to effectively stagger our workload, or to bring a sense of order to the chaos around us. The magic word is *balance*!

In addition, illnesses such as anemia (low red blood cell count), infection, and thyroid problems can cause you to feel tired. Depression can cause you to wake up very early in the morning feeling lethargic. **See your doctor to be sure nothing is wrong that needs treatment.**

## Rx PRIME TIME PRESCRIPTIONS FOR FATIGUE

*Reduce your stress and learn to relax.* Stress is the number one energy drainer.

*Get more sleep.* The first and most obvious place to look is at your sleep pattern. Increasing the amount of sleep you get is also the easiest way to treat fatigue. However, as we go through menopause, our sleep is usually interrupted when hot flashes wake us up. Reduced levels of estrogen also can affect certain neurotransmitters in the brain and disrupt sleep. Stimulants such as caffeine (even one chocolate bar can keep you awake), stress, and certain medications (including over-the-counter pain medications with caffeine) can inhibit sleep.

Many of us have the misperception that as we age we need less sleep, which leads some of us to go to bed late and wake up early. Even though middle-aged folks tend to sleep more lightly, awaken more frequently, and typically get up more often to go to the bathroom, we still need eight hours of sleep to function at our best, think fast, and enhance our memory. Sleep improves your longevity and helps improve your overall health. Too little sleep impairs your coordination, concentration, and judgment, increases irritability, and weakens your immune system.

**Suggestions for increasing and improving your sleep:**

• *Maintain a regular time for going to bed and waking up.* Turn off those late-night television shows. Go to bed earlier if you must arise early.

- *Relax before going to bed.* Take a warm bath, read a relaxing book, and listen to soothing music. The meditation and relaxation exercises outlined in Chapter 13 also work well.
- *Make your bedroom comfortable for sleeping.* Be sure you're sleeping on the best mattress you can afford. If your mattress is more than ten years old, you may need to shop around for a new one. Also, a neat room can help calm your nerves. Just living around clutter all the time is enough to drive you to distraction.
- *Avoid caffeine, alcohol, and tobacco before bedtime.* Drink warm milk or herb teas such as chamomile. Passionflower herb tea has been used for centuries as a mild tranquilizer and sedative. Valerian root and kava kava teas help relieve anxiety and sedate.
- *Put drops of lavender oil on your pillow to help you relax,* or put drops on a handkerchief and put that in the dryer with your sheets.
- *Don't depend on sleeping pills.* These are addictive and hard to stop once you get started. Take your calcium supplement before bedtime instead.
- *Don't take long naps during the day.* A fifteen- to twenty-minute "power nap" can sharpen attention, enhance decision-making abilities, and improve mood, but sleeping longer than that will make you groggy. Some businesses are encouraging on-the-job naps to improve efficiency and productivity.
- *Exercise regularly.* Regular exercise every day helps you not only fall asleep faster but also sleep more deeply. Exercise is one of the most important elements in having more energy. It increases the delivery of oxygen and nutrients to the cells and carries away more waste products, such as lactic acid and carbon dioxide. This will leave you feeling more energetic.

*Eat meals that are more nutritious.* One common cause of fatigue is undereating. Skipping breakfast will cause you to drag all day long. Always eat a breakfast that has protein in it, to give you energy throughout the morning.

*Stop snacking on cookies and candy.* Sugary snacks will give you a quick boost of energy, but once the surge of insulin dissipates, you'll crash from your sugar high and feel even more tired and hungry than before you snacked. Instead, eat nuts, raw cut-up vegetables or fruit, cottage cheese, yogurt, hard cheese, or tofu for a slower but longer-lasting energy boost.

*Eat less and eat more often.* Digesting big meals two or three times a day is an enormous energy drain. Skipping meals leaves your fuel reserves low. Your body needs fuel in moderate doses spread evenly throughout the day.

*Get adequate amounts of vitamins and minerals.* You need calcium, potassium, iron, magnesium, B vitamins, and chromium. Foods such as honey, whole-grain cereals, and grapes are all energy boosters. Magnesium is a particularly important supplement. British research found that 80 percent of people with chronic fatigue syndrome have low magnesium levels—and their condition improved with magnesium injections. We need 350 to 400 mg of magnesium a day. The best way to obtain it daily is through taking supplemental one-a-day vitamins. Inadequate potassium is an important and common reason for fatigue, especially if you are on diuretics. Watch your daily intake of bananas, oranges, green vegetables, and other foods high in potassium.

*Drink eight to ten eight-ounce glasses of water per day.* Feeling rundown is often the first sign of dehydration. Adequate hydration helps the enzymes in your body as well as other body functions to work more efficiently.

*Watch for burnout.* According to Dr. Thomas Miller, professor of psychiatry at the University of Kentucky College of Medicine, "just dealing with the pressures of everyday life takes a lot of energy. Whenever anyone has a hard time coping—with family problems, relationships, job pressure—there's usually a tremendous burnout factor, physically as well as emotionally."

*Pace yourself.* African American women tend to push ourselves beyond the point where our minds and bodies say no. So think about where you might be overexerting yourself, and cut back. Learn to focus your energy and don't waste time on things you can't change or control. Remember the Serenity Prayer and use it as a guide: "God grant me the serenity to accept the things I cannot change, courage to change the things I can, and the wisdom to know the difference."

*Learn more about the seven specific energy centers in our bodies known as chakras.* Learning how to use these energy centers can energize, refresh, and revive your body and mind. These energy centers connect our nerves, hormones, and emotions, forming a link between our energy anatomy and our physical anatomy. Even though standard Western medicine has not recognized chakras yet, Eastern cultures have long appreciated them and their influence on health and overall energy. To find out more, check out Dr. Christiane Northrup's book *Women's Bodies, Women's Wisdom.*

*Try essential oils.* Aromatherapy has been used to increase energy levels for five thousand years. You can inhale the oils, burn them in candles, dilute and massage them into your skin, or put them in your bathwater. Lavender, peppermint, rosewood, and sandalwood are common essential oils that everyone should have in her home.

*Increase the joy in your life.* Everyone has things she has to do, but how many of us take time to do activities we love to do, each and every day of our life? Try to include pleasure in your daily life and your energy will soar.


## HEARTBURN

Heartburn increases as we get older. As many as 30 percent of all people over the age of sixty have heartburn, which is the primary symptom of gastroesophageal reflux disease (GERD). In people with GERD, acid in the stomach flows backward and upward into the esophagus instead of taking its normal course toward the small intestine. This can happen because:

• The valve between the stomach and esophagus is weak
• Your stomach produces excess acid
• There is too much pressure on your abdomen, from tight clothes, for instance

GERD can cause chest pain that mimics that of a heart attack. At least 180,000 people each year are admitted to the hospital complaining of chest pain from GERD that is so severe, they think they are having a heart attack. It can also cause difficulty swallowing, a feeling of burning after eating and at night, or difficulty keeping food down after meals. Less commonly it causes a sore throat, bothersome coughing, or even hoarseness. If your discomfort is relieved by antacids such as Rolaids or Mylanta, you probably have GERD.

The first step in treating GERD is to modify your diet. Alcohol, coffee, and fatty foods should be avoided, as well as frequent spicy meals. Small frequent meals are best; don't eat close to bedtime. Stop smoking, throw away your girdle, and elevate the head of your bed six to eight inches. (Use some blocks under the bed, not pillows.) Antidepressants, tranquilizers, and calcium channel blockers (for hypertension) increase your susceptibility to GERD.

Next, speak with your doctor and try over-the-counter medications such as Tagamet (cimetidine) or Zantac (ranitidine) for relief. Tagamet interferes with the action of many other drugs, so check with your pharmacist. A prescription drug that works well is Prilosec (omeprazole). If the symptoms continue, you need an endoscopy, a procedure in which a fiber-optic viewing tube is passed down your throat into the stomach to see if anything is wrong. This is performed after putting you to sleep with a strong sedative.

It is important to have your symptoms treated, not only for relief but also because there appears to be an association between GERD over many years and the risk of ulcers of the esophagus and also cancer of the esophagus.

## ACHING FEET

We hope that by middle age you have learned your lesson and have already thrown away and stopped buying those ridiculous, ill-fitting, unhealthy high heels that cause back pain and foot problems. In fact, now's the time to toss any shoes that don't fit well. The American Orthopedic Foot and Ankle Society found that 88 percent of American women wear shoes that are too small. No wonder our feet hurt!

When we reach midlife, the structure of our feet changes after so many years of wear and tear. For example, the bones in the long part of our feet that connect to the toes (metatarsal bones) spread out, and consequently the feet widen. Sometimes that happens to such a degree that you need a larger shoe size. In addition, the pads of fat that cushion the bottom of the feet become thinner, making the soles more vulnerable to pressure.

That's why it is so important to take care of your feet in midlife. You can relate to the fact that when your feet hurt, everything hurts. Foot problems make you feel older and rob you of the vigor and energy you usually have. And let's get real: Hurtin' feet can put a major damper on your dance life. Finally, remember that bad feet can throw your posture out of whack, which contributes to back pain, knee pain, hip pain, and neck pain.

### ℞ PRIME TIME SOLUTIONS FOR ACHING FEET

*Change your shoes.* High heels and tight or pointy-toed shoes cause corns, blisters, and calluses and aggravate bunions. High-heeled shoes constrict the width of the foot by up to one inch. An estimated 75 percent of foot surgery in the United States is needed because of damage caused by constrictive footwear. You must buy shoes for comfort—and the good news is that you can find comfortable and supportive shoes that are also attractive.

*Pamper your feet.* Rub them, warm them, and wiggle them often. Find a good pedicurist to help you take care of them. Regularly remove dead skin on your feet. Cut toenails straight across and no shorter than the edge of the toe or you will develop ingrown toenails.

*Find a podiatrist* (foot doctor) *or orthopedist* (medical doctor trained to treat bone and joint disorders—though some focus on the foot) *if you are suffering from chronic foot problems.*

*If you are diabetic, it is critical that a podiatrist closely monitor the condition of your feet.* (See Chapter 12 to find out more about foot care for diabetics.)

## DERMATOSIS PAPULOSA NIGRA

You've seen them—raised molelike bumps, or flesh moles. More than half of all Black women develop these harmless growths that are flesh-colored or darker. They are called *dermatosis papulosa nigra* (DPN). More than 50 percent of Black women have a family history of DPN.

According to Dr. Harold Minus, director of dermatology at Howard University, there are two types of DPN: the ones on the neck are raised and sit on a stalklike extension, and the ones on the face are usually flat.

**Rx PRIME TIME PRESCRIPTIONS**

It is absolutely essential for you to see your doctor and a dermatologist or skin specialist to be sure that you are not suffering any serious conditions such as skin cancer. Cancer caught early can be cured.

*If you have a light complexion and many moles, it is a good idea to create a map.* A dermatologist examines your skin from head to toe and records the location, appearance, and size of each mole to be able to easily spot changes along the way.

Remember this: A normal mole is round or oval, and flat or slightly raised. It has well-defined edges and is usually less than quarter of an inch across—smaller than a pencil eraser. The color should remain a solid tan, dark brown, or flesh color. The ABCD guidelines help you tell if a mole is abnormal.

## Abnormal Moles

- Asymmetrical shape
- Borders are blurry
- Color is uneven
- Diameter is larger than a pencil eraser

*Consider having the growths removed.* Dr. Minus reports that some spots can be removed easily by simply cutting them off under local anesthesia in a doctor's office if they are on a stalk. Others may be removed by a technique called *electrodesiccation*, where a mild electric current (using a hyfercator) is applied to the growth. The growth will then dry out and fall off in seven to ten days without scarring.

# Chapter 18

# LOVE IS A MANY-SPLENDORED THING: SEXUAL WELLNESS

*Oh what makes my grandpa*
*love my grandma so*
*She's got the same old jelly*
*she had 40 years ago*
— Cleo Gibson, quoted in Terry L. Jewel, ed., *The Black Woman's Gumbo Ya-Ya:*
*Quotations by Black Women*

Our ability as Black women to view our sexuality in a healthy manner, as an important part of our body, mind, and spirit, has been seriously compromised by racism, culture, ageism, homophobia, and religion. In their attempt to justify the rape of Black women during and after slavery, many White male and female slave owners promulgated the notion that Black women were lewd and "sex-starved." As Dr. Gail Wyatt documents in *Stolen Women: Reclaiming Our Sexuality, Taking Back Our Lives*, the stereotyping of Black women did not end with slavery. African American women have usually been depicted in films, in books, and on television as either permissive, promiscuous, and immoral—Welfare Queen, Carmen Jones, "Hoochie Mamas" (extremely short skirt, blond wig, heavy makeup)—asexual "mammies," workaholics, or masculinized, aggressive criminal types.

What is most distressing is that many of these negative sexual stereotypes have been internalized by Black women and men, which has had a deleterious impact on our beliefs and attitudes toward ourselves and our interactions with each other.

Dr. Wyatt's research confirmed that many African American women have abdicated their right and responsibility to integrate assertive sexual thoughts and appropriate behaviors into their life plan. Thus, we see Black women in midlife who go to work wearing thigh-high skirts and too-small sweaters, and who buy and laugh at songs in which they're called "ho" or "bitch." We meet women who have never explored their own bodies, had an orgasm, or expressed to their partners their sexual fantasies or desires. And we've seen patients who engage in risky sexual behaviors—such as not requiring that sexual partners wear condoms or be tested for HIV—despite the fact that our rates of sexually transmitted diseases, including AIDS, are higher than those of other racial or ethnic groups.

---

## NAKIA'S STORY

Nakia, a forty-three-year-old artist, was proud of her reputation as a "free spirit." She considered herself bisexual and had had numerous one-night stands with both women and men. Nakia refused to use contraceptives because she felt they interfered with her "natural rhythm." As a result of her sexual decisions, Nakia had several abortions, a miscarriage, and sexually transmitted diseases—gonorrhea, chlamydia, herpes, and genital warts—before she was thirty. Nakia's repeated bouts of pelvic inflammatory disease caused a major infection in her fallopian tubes that spread to the membrane lining her abdomen and necessitated a hysterectomy. It was after the surgery that Nakia started to question whether her perception of "sexual freedom" wasn't actually a self-destructive trap. She decided to go into individual psychotherapy to look at her long-standing issues about her family and sexual identity. Nakia also joined a Black women's support group focused on discussing midlife.

---

To counter the image of being hypersexed and promiscuous, some African American women adopted or intensified very restrictive sexual practices outside and inside of marriage. Their religions, which often had a puritanical basis, reinforced the idea that sex was only for procreation and that "good" women were sexually naive, dispassionate, and docile. Even when Black women know that the racial and larger cultural stereotypes are grossly distorted or simply untrue, our intraracial cultural and historical legacy, childhood training, and religious beliefs can severely restrict the scope of our sexual activities.

## MILDRED'S STORY

Mildred, a fifty-five-year-old married teacher's aide, had been raised by her grandmother. Throughout her childhood, she heard stories about "loose"—non-church-going or makeup-wearing women—whose behavior "invited" sexual assault. Granny believed that even during slavery, most "good women"—religious, self-effacing, asexual—were able to avoid being raped by the plantation owner. Although Mildred was relatively assertive at work, her dress, demeanor, and actions reflected her grandmother's belief about "good women."

Mildred and her husband, Herb, who had been a widower, had been married for almost five years. Their marriage was a good one overall. However, he was constantly asking her to take a more active role in their sex life. He wanted her to express her desires and fantasies and to initiate sexual contact. Herb had had a very exciting, mutually stimulating sexual relationship with his first wife. He didn't want to compare Mildred to his deceased wife, but he found it difficult to accept her passive, almost uninvolved behavior during lovemaking. Mildred assumed that Herb's attitude about sex stemmed from being a man. "That's all men think about," she would say to herself.

The first time that Mildred heard women discussing sex in a positive way was in a Black women's group she joined. One evening, the topic was sexuality in midlife. The agenda was to take a holistic approach to sexual wellness. The women were encouraged to assess their sexual beliefs, talk frankly about masturbation and oral sex, explore the physiology of orgasms, and share the benefits of trying different sex positions. Mildred listened intently, talked some, and immediately went to buy the books used in the discussion. She was determined to start the exciting journey toward sexual wellness.

---

As women in midlife, we also have had to contend with American culture's obsession with youthful sexuality. Academy Award–winning movies such as *Shakespeare in Love* and *American Beauty* and numerous television programs proclaim the message that thin, young, almost pubescent (and usually White) females are the true "sex goddesses." The media are full of overt and covert messages that imply that middle-aged women (with a few exceptions—Tina Turner, Raquel Welch, and Sophia Loren among them) and sensuous sexuality are mutually exclusive concepts. Often older women are perceived as being less desirable and less sexual and are expected to act as if they are asexual beings.

Toni Cade Bambara provides, in her short story "My Man Bovanne" in *Gorilla My Love*, an accurate and hilarious description of adult children's disapproval of any hint of their mother's sexuality. Ms. Hazel, who is in her sixties, is reprimanded by her children for dancing "too close" to Bovanne, a slightly older blind man, and she responds to them in an assertive manner:

> But right away Joe Lee come up on us and frown [at me for] dancing so close to the man. My own son who knows what kind of warm I am about; and don't grown men call me long distance and in the middle of the night for a little mama comfort? But he frown.
>
> And here come my youngest, Task, with a tap on my elbow like he the third grade monitor and I'm cutting up on the line to assembly.
>
> "Look here Mama," say Task, the gentle one. "We just trying to pull your coat. You were making a spectacle of yourself out there dancing like that."
>
> "Dancing like what?"
>
> "Well uhh, . . . like one of them sex-starved ladies getting on in years and not too discriminating. Know what I mean?"
>
> I don't answer cause I'll cry. Terrible thing when your own children talk to you like that. Pullin me out the party and hustling me into some stranger's kitchen in the back of a bar just like the damn police.
>
> . . . says Joe Lee. "The point is Mama . . . well it's pride. You embarrass yourself and us too dancing like that."
>
> "I wasn't shame." Then nobody say nuthin.

The truth is that enjoying sex can be a lifelong activity. Several studies have confirmed that women who have partners often engage in sexual activity on a weekly basis well into their nineties. In fact, over one-third of women between 80 and 102 years of age reported that they continued to have intercourse.

Many women express increased sexual pleasure, especially after menopause, when they're no longer concerned about pregnancy or experiencing the fatiguing demands of child rearing. According to a study cited in Paula B. Doress-Worters and Diana Laskin Siegal's *The New Ourselves, Growing Older*, 91 percent of people from sixty to over ninety years of age reported that they enjoyed sex for various reasons: "It reduces tension, makes women feel more feminine, helps people sleep, and provides a physical outlet for emotion."

Social and emotional barriers, however, are not the only obstacles to midlife Black women having active and assertive sexual lives. Heterosexual Black women are confronted with the reality that there are more of them and they live longer than men in general and Black men in particular. In midlife, there are approximately three women for every two men. Lesbians, especially those living in small towns or rural areas, often find it extremely difficult to meet other gay midlife women. Older lesbians tend to be more "closeted" (secretive) about their sexual preference than younger ones.

After menopause, vaginal changes often occur because of the reduction in the estrogen our bodies produce. Sexual enjoyment can be temporarily affected (see Chapter 16). Estrogen replacement therapy and vaginal creams can restore the vagina's suppleness and improve its lubricating ability.

Medical problems that are intense or chronic can also reduce our *libido* (sexual desire), as can the medications used to treat them. Thus, it's important to discuss any negative change in your sexual desire or performance with your physician. One of the most common medical problems that interferes with sexual functioning is heart disease. Your fear or your partner's fear of a recurrence of angina or of a full-blown heart attack can cause you to lose interest in sex. Joining a support group or receiving counseling from your physician or a couples therapist can greatly reduce the anxiety associated with lovemaking. Another problem can be arthritis or osteoporosis, both of which can restrict your range of motion. Trying different positions—such as having the lighter partner on top or having both partners lying on their side—can restore or increase your sexual enjoyment.

A myriad of obstacles can interfere with your sexual health, but a myriad of solutions exist to help you regain it. Don't despair or give up. Incorporating the following suggestions into your love life can help you achieve sexual fulfillment.

### ℞ PRIME TIME PRESCRIPTION FOR YOUR SEXUAL WELL-BEING

*I may want love for an hour, then decide to make it two;*
*Take an hour 'fore I get started,*
*Maybe three before I'm through*
*I'm a one-hour mama, so no one-minute papa*
*Ain't the kind of man for me!*

—Ida Cox

Your overall commitment to keeping physically, emotionally, and spiritually well has a profound effect on your level of sexual wellness. Learning to enjoy—in fact, relish—your sexuality requires that you be aware of and responsible for yourself as a sexual being.

Understanding your sexuality is critical to your health. You cannot be sexually healthy and treat your sexual behaviors as if they are disconnected from the rest of your being. In the *Wellness Workbook* by Dr. John Travis and Regina Sara Ryan, sexual awareness, responsibility, and love are necessary components of a holistic wellness approach to sex. They write that healthy sex is:

- Freely chosen
- Conscious of consequences
- Respectful
- Erotic
- Playful
- Expansive
- Unifying

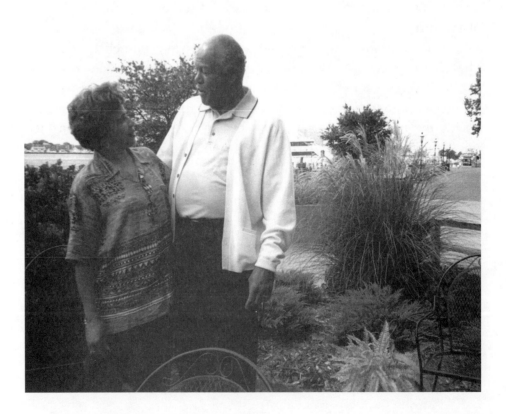

## SEXUAL AWARENESS

Your ability to love and accept yourself unconditionally, which includes accepting your body, is the foundation for living in wellness. (If you're having difficulty accepting this concept, please reread Chapter 3, "The Miracle of You," and Chapter 5, "Self-Esteem: Believing in Yourself.")

Your Prime Time Circle of Sisterfriends can be a terrific resource for gaining or expanding your knowledge about sexual behaviors. Myths and taboos, especially those related to sensuality, sexuality, and menopause, can be topics of discussion. Sisters can explore in depth their feelings about homosexuality, bisexuality, and alternative forms of lovemaking, including oral sex.

Books are another source of information about our sexual development as Black women. Dr. Wyatt's book *Stolen Women* not only discusses historical aspects of our sexual evolution, but provides information about our contemporary practices. She indicates that there are class and racial differences in the sexual practices of Black and White women.

As a group, Black women are less likely to masturbate, less likely to use contraceptives (including condoms), and more apt to have vaginal intercourse as their only form of sexual activity. However, more educated, wealthier, and less religious African American women are more likely to include oral and anal sex in their sexual repertoire.

## SEXUALLY SINGLE

Most Black women will spend some, maybe all, of their middle years alone — either by choice or because of a scarcity of appropriate partners, widowhood, or divorce. Our sexual well-being, however, is not dependent on our relationship status. It is a part of who we are as human beings.

Learning to appreciate and love your sexuality usually requires that you be comfortable being sensuous. Being consciously aware of your senses — touch, smell, sight, hearing, and taste — and how they please *you*, not other people, is a skill that can take practice to acquire. Here are some ideas on how to heighten your sensuality:

- Take a long soothing bath; get a massage; sleep on silk or satin sheets.
- Inhale the scent of your body, oils, perfume, or flowers.

- Look at your body as if it were a piece of art that you love.
- Really listen to the sound of your voice, as if it were music.
- Taste your skin, as if it were your favorite ice cream.
- Use some of the relaxation techniques, such as deep breathing, described in Chapter 13.

Exploring your body through self-touch is another way to become more aware of what gives you sexual pleasure. *Erotic self-touch, masturbation,* and *self-stimulation* are terms used to describe the deliberate touching of your body—alone or with someone. Only you can decide whether this form of sexual pleasure is a choice you would like. We know that many women have been taught that masturbation is wrong or have, for whatever reason, simply never done it. However, we certainly hope that, as you are reassessing other beliefs and attitudes, you will open your mind to the pleasures of self-stimulation.

Using sexual props can also enhance sexual enjoyment. Erotic literature, videos, magazines, music, vibrators, and *dildos* (cylindrical objects that are placed in the vagina) are among the most widely used sexual aids.

## KEEPING YOUR RELATIONSHIP SEXUALLY HEALTHY

There are many strong, loving, and long-lasting Black marriages and partnerships. The authors were recently on a cruise with a large group of single and married African Americans. Seven of the couples had been married for more than forty years. When asked what had helped their marriages endure, they all emphasized the need to reexamine, renegotiate, and reestablish new goals for their relationships after their children became adults.

The couple relationship often suffers while children are being raised. So when the children leave home, the couple comes back into focus and the relationship may need a tune-up, some repairs, or a major overhaul after years of neglect. The changes that often occur during midlife—children leaving, children returning, health issues, "monotony in monogamy"—can exacerbate an already difficult situation.

Refusing to reexamine old sexual attitudes can also affect sexual satisfaction. In her book *Will the Real Women Please Stand Up!,* Ella Patterson discusses some of the myths that interfere with Black women having satisfying heterosexual or lesbian sexual relationships. These include:

- Intercourse is the ultimate sexual satisfaction. Anything else does not count as good sex.
- If a woman takes the lead in sex, it can damage her partner's ego.
- Having to tell your partner what you want isn't necessary. You shouldn't have to touch yourself at all.
- Sex should be man on the top, woman on the bottom to get full satisfaction.
- You have to be available to make love with your partner whenever he or she wants.
- Bad sex is better than none at all.

Another issue discussed in the *Wellness Workbook* by John Travis and Regina Sara Ryan is an overemphasis on performance and orgasm rather than enjoying the sensuous feeling of being with a partner. Remember, as you age, you and your partner need more time to relax and enjoy your sexual interaction.

There are many sexual activities in which couples can engage to enhance and renew their pleasure in each other:

- Everything we recommended earlier for single people can be done with your partner.
- Extend your foreplay time.
- Try new and different positions and behaviors, including oral sex.
- Make love in a different setting.
- Share your sexual fantasies.
- See a sex therapist.

## SEXUAL RESPONSIBILITY

Accepting responsibility for your health must include your sexual health. Being willing to ask assertively for what we want and need, and set appropriate boundaries, is a necessary skill for sexual wellness. (Chapter 6, "Confronting the Two A's: Attitude and Anger," contains information on developing assertiveness skills). Acting in a sexually responsible way requires that you be conscious of the decisions you make, and assertive and informed about sexual behaviors that can protect and harm you. Your failure to know about sexually transmitted diseases and to practice safe sex not only is damaging to your emotional well-being, it can kill you.

Why are Black women reluctant or unwilling to insist that their partners wear condoms? Our professional experiences, focus groups, and Dr. Wyatt's research confirms that even when it comes to sex, we put other people's needs and desires before our own. However, there are some other significant reasons:

- Women in long-term relationships or marriages feel less able than younger women in newer relationships to ask their partner to use condoms. Frequently older women have a compromised sense of themselves as sexual beings, and this decreases their ability to negotiate safer sex practices.
- Some women's financial dependency on their partners precludes them from asserting their desire for protective measures.
- There exists a disparity of power between men and women in sexual decision making.
- Fear of disrupting the relationship by bringing up safer sex practices keeps some women silent despite their apprehensions.
- Our socialization discourages women from questioning the monogamy of their mate. We usually always assume our partner is faithful.
- Demanding use of a condom might inhibit and decrease his enjoyment, and he might then leave the relationship.
- Women who are worried or anxious are least likely to ask their partner to use a condom.

A survey reported that middle-aged Americans showed very low use of condoms—83 percent never used condoms. Middle- and upper-income African American women are *more* likely not to use condoms and less likely to have received sex education about sexually transmitted diseases, and therefore are at higher risk of infection.[1] Only one-third of African American women report consistent condom use—with the older women being least likely to use condoms. Black women who never married (38.3 percent) or who are divorced, widowed, or separated (39.3 percent) are four times as likely as married women (9.9 percent) to always to use condoms.[2]

If you have not consistently practiced safe sex, *now* is the time to begin!

## PRACTICING SAFE SEX

Protecting your sexual health requires that you guard against all sexually transmitted diseases (STDs).

- Role-play asking your partner in an assertive manner to use a condom.
- Limit the number of sexual partners you have—the more partners, the greater the risk of exposure to STDs.
- Use barrier methods of birth control—latex condoms, diaphragms, the sponge—even if you take birth control pills or use an IUD.
- Use a spermicide (agent that kills sperm) that contains nonoxynol-9. Studies have confirmed that it also kills most of the viruses and bacteria spread through sexual contact, as well as sperm. If you have an allergic reaction to it—skin irritation or ulceration—stop using it and call your gynecologist.
- Use only high-quality latex condoms. When used with nonoxynol-9, these condoms offers the greatest protection against infected semen.
- Insist on an HIV test for both you and your partner if you intend to have an ongoing, monogamous relationship. Continue to use latex condoms for at least a year after the test, since the virus can remain undetected for that length of time.

## KNOW YOUR STDs

STDs are caused by bacteria, viruses, or occasionally parasites. Many STDs are easily treated and cured, but others remain chronic. An estimated fifty-six million Americans harbor an STD other than AIDS, and millions more are infected every year. Check out these facts:

- There are more than 650,000 new cases of gonorrhea ("clap") and 70,000 cases of syphilis annually.
- Forty-five million people have chronic genital herpes, and one million new cases occur each year.
- Chlamydia is the fastest-spreading STD in the United States. There are three million new cases each year.
- There are seventy-seven thousand new cases of hepatitis B due to sexual transmission every year, resulting in cirrhosis and cancer of the liver, despite the fact that there is a vaccine to prevent this infection!

• Human papilloma virus (HPV), which causes genital warts and can lead to cervical cancer, infects twenty million men and women, and five and a half million new cases are reported every year.

• There are nine hundred thousand Americans infected by the killer HIV/AIDS virus, with forty-five thousand new cases every year.

**Remember, infection with one STD means that you may have others. So if you have any STD, your doctor must test for all of them.** Here are the STDs you should be aware of:

*Chlamydia.* The most commonly reported STD is not herpes, AIDS, or gonorrhea but chlamydia. The United States has the highest rate of chlamydia in the industrialized world. This fast-spreading STD is caused by a bacterium and is transmitted during unprotected vaginal or anal sex. Untreated, chlamydia can cause pelvic inflammatory disease and infertility in women; in men, painful urination and discharge from the penis. Chlamydia often produces no symptoms and therefore may be difficult to diagnose. In fact, half of all infected men and up to three-quarters of all infected women have no symptoms. It is easy to treat and cure: Just a single dose of the antibiotic azithromycin, or two doxycycline pills a day for a week, will cure it.

*Gonorrhea.* Gonorrhea is caused by a bacterium and is contracted by unprotected oral, vaginal, or anal sex. Infected men have painful urination and a thick puslike discharge from the penis. Some infected women may not have symptoms; others may have vaginal discharge and pelvic pain. Most women are more likely to find out they have it after their male sex partner has been diagnosed. Untreated gonorrhea can cause chronic infection of the genital tract, a form of arthritis, and damage to your heart valves (cardiac patients are especially vulnerable). Penicillin used to be the treatment of choice; however, many strains of gonorrhea are now resistant. Your doctor will probably prescribe ciprofloxacin or azithromycin.

*Syphilis.* This bacterial infection begins with a painless sore at the site of infection, on the mouth or sex organs. This is *primary syphilis*, and it is often mistaken for a harmless cold sore. When this goes away, you think everything is okay. However, after a few weeks or even months, a widespread rash appears—*secondary syphilis*. Then this disappears, and again you are fooled. Eventually, the third stage—*tertiary syphilis*—appears, by which time it is too late to reverse the course of the disease. In this stage, syphilis can damage the heart and brain years after the initial infection. A simple blood test will diagnose this STD, and it can be treated *in the beginning stages* with penicillin.

*Genital herpes.* This STD is caused by one of two viruses, HSV-1 and HSV-2 (most common). You get herpes from oral, genital, or anal sex, and by kissing or touching an infected area when you have a break in your skin. Again, you may be infected and never know it, or you may develop painful bumps and sores at the site of the infection days or weeks after exposure. Don't dismiss this infection, since it cannot be cured. It is also extremely serious for babies if they come into contact with a sore in the birth canal. Although it is not as serious as the other STDs, it can flare up or recur at any time throughout your life. Refrain from having sex when you have a flare-up. Various antiviral drugs can reduce the duration and severity of the disease and delay flare-ups. Acyclovir is used to treat it.

*Genital warts.* The human papilloma virus (HPV) causes a variety of warts in the genital and anal areas. It affects the cervix and can lead to cervical cancer. The warts can be treated directly by lasers, by using chemicals to freeze or burn them, or by surgery. However, there is no cure, and they may reappear at any time. There is an association between HPV and cervical cancer, so every woman with genital warts should have an annual Pap test.

*Trichomoniasis.* This is the most common curable STD, but many women do not experience any symptoms. Sometimes trichomoniasis may cause burning urination, vaginal discharge, abdominal pain, or painful intercourse. Both sex partners should be treated with a single dose of Flagyl (metronizadole).

*HIV/AIDS.* AIDS is the deadliest of all STDs. It is caused by a virus (HIV), and there is no known cure. HIV (human immunodeficiency virus) is spread through infected vaginal fluids, semen, or blood. The most common paths of infection for HIV are:

• Blood transfusions involving infected blood
• Unprotected sex—vaginal, oral, or anal—with an infected partner
• Infected mothers who expose their infants during pregnancy, birth, or breastfeeding
• Sharing a needle with an infected person, intravenous drug use, or skin piercing (tattooing or putting holes in the skin)

Symptoms may not appear for years after the initial infection, but the disease silently progresses. The most common signs of the HIV virus are:

• STDs or other genital infections that are unresponsive to treatment
• Treatment-resistant coughs or fevers

- Chronic fatigue (it feels more intense than just regular midlife tiredness)
- Yeast infections of the mouth or esophagus (thrush)
- Nonmenopausal night sweats
- Swollen lymph nodes
- Skin lesions, hives, rashes
- Diarrhea that does not respond to treatment

Most AIDS patients die from bacterial infection or cancer, which they are unable to resist due to the decline in their immune system.

There are two types of tests for HIV. The ELISA tests for HIV-related antibodies is very sensitive, and 98 percent accurate. The Western Blot test is more specific and more expensive than the ELISA. It is used to confirm a positive ELISA test. You can obtain this test at your doctor's office, hospitals, and local health departments. The Centers for Disease Control National AIDS Hotline (800-342-AIDS) has information on anonymous testing sites in your area, or call your state health department. Many state and county health departments provide these blood tests free of charge. New treatments can delay death and improve the quality of life—specifically the protease inhibitors Retrovir (zidovudine), Hivid (zalcitabine), and Videx (didanosine).

Understanding the information we present on HIV/AIDS is important for everyone, but for African American women at midlife, it is literally a matter of life and death. The risk factors for AIDS and HIV for African Americans are different from those for White populations. Our risk factors include involvement with heterosexual or bisexual men and intravenous (needle) drug users, but for us as midlife African American women, heterosexual contact is by far the most frequent source of HIV transmission.

There has been a shift in the population of HIV-infected African Americans from young, low-income, unmarried homosexual and IV-drug-using men to heterosexual, higher-income, and older women.

- Of infected women fifty and older, two-thirds belong to minority groups.
- The number of new cases among minorities fifty years of age and older is increasing faster than among older Caucasians.
- Between 1985 and 1998 among midlife women, AIDS cases attributed to heterosexual contact increased 106 percent.
- Older people are less likely to practice safe sex. A national AIDS behav-

ior survey found that 10 percent of Americans fifty and older had at least one risk factor for HIV (multiple sex partners, a partner with a known risk factor, or a history of a blood transfusion between 1977 and 1984) but were much less likely to use condoms during sex and get tested for HIV than a comparison group in their twenties.

• Older people are less likely to have had sex education than younger people and don't have accurate information, including the knowledge necessary to protect them from high-risk behavior, such as knowing the effectiveness of condoms or that someone with AIDS can look well and healthy.

• Midlife African American women get AIDS most often through having sex with a bisexual man or a man who uses and shares drug needles. Greater bisexuality is reported among African American husbands and partners than among White men. Yet women in this age group are more likely not to know their partner's risk. Homophobia in the African American community makes it difficult to address these issues openly, and we have a broad-based conspiracy of silence around bisexuality and homosexuality. Religious values make it even more difficult to discuss, especially for older African Americans.

Discussing high-risk behaviors with health-care providers is especially hard for older women, since doctors rarely consider them as sexually active beings. This often leads to life-threatening delays in the diagnosis of HIV, which is why you *must* ask your doctor for the HIV test and discuss your risk factors with your health-care team. You must take charge of your health.

Incorporating the primary principles of sexual wellness into your life—awareness and responsibility—is not easy, but the rewards are certainly worth the effort. You have the power, if you simply use it, to be sexually active, healthy, and fulfilled throughout your middle years and beyond.

## WELLNESS AND SEX

This questionnaire can help you assess your perception of your degree of wellness when it comes to your sexual health. There are no right or wrong answers, but the higher your score, the greater your sense of wellness. Put the number of points that correspond with the answer that best describes your situations in the blank before each statement.

Scoring

3 points: yes

2 points: often

1 point: sometimes, maybe

0 points: no, rarely

_____ 1. I feel comfortable touching and exploring my body.

_____ 2. I think it's okay to masturbate if one chooses to do so.

_____ 3. My sexual education is adequate.

_____ 4. I feel good about the degree of closeness I have with men in my life.

_____ 5. I feel good about the degree of closeness I have with women in my life.

_____ 6. I am content with my level of sexual activity.

_____ 7. I feel good about my body.

_____ 8. I fully experience the many stages of lovemaking rather than focus only on orgasm.

_____ 9. I am informed on issues of birth control.

_____ 10. I am familiar with methods of preventing venereal disease and use them if appropriate.

_____ 11. I communicate any upset feelings with my partner rather than withhold sex as "punishment."

_____ 12. When I'm upset with my partner, I resolve the problem before making love.

_____ 13. I feel comfortable looking at myself nude in a mirror.

_____ 14. I am aware of the difference between needing someone and loving someone.

_____ 15. I am able to love others without dominating or being dominated by them.

_____ 16. I am comfortable consciously abstaining from sexual activity as a way of learning more about myself.

_____ TOTAL POINTS FOR THIS SECTION (MAXIMUM POINTS = 48)

_____ AVERAGE SCORE :(Total points divided by number of statements answered_____ ÷ _____ = _____)

*Source:* Reprinted with permission from *Wellness Workbook*, by John W. Travis, M.D., and Regina Sara Ryan, Ten Speed Press, Berkeley, CA. © 1981, 1988 by John W. Travis, M.D.

# PART VII

# Living in Health and Wellness

# Chapter 19

# BECOME A SMARTER
# HEALTH-CARE CONSUMER

*Each patient carries his own doctor inside him. We are at our best when the doctor who resides within each patient has the chance to go to work.*

—Albert Schweitzer

Dr. Schweitzer said it all. As we have emphasized throughout this book, *your health and wellness depend on you.* In order to receive the quality of service you deserve, however, you must become an informed, outspoken, and active health-care consumer. Your mission is to get the best care you can. That means learning how to navigate this country's rather complicated health-care system (which, unfortunately, includes the almost incomprehensible world of health insurance). It can be tricky, but not to worry—we're here to help guide you along the way.

Remember, everyone in the health-care system is there to serve *you;* they are working with you and *for you!* As part of your new paradigm of making yourself and your health a priority, we want you to view the health-care system as a dynamic partnership between you and your health-care providers. This isn't a partnership among equals, however—you are the boss. What a radical idea! We want you to change your thinking from "The doctor is in charge" to "We are partners and ultimately *I'm* in charge of decisions about my care." Seeing yourself in this new light will make a big difference in your enthusiasm for self-care, in your confidence, and in your healing. Since the idea of an active, assertive patient-as-partner hasn't been universally embraced by the medical community, you must be even more vigilant in getting your needs met.

We believe that your involvement in your own care is even more important these days as the health-care system undergoes major changes. Although the United States spends more on health care than any other industrialized country—over one trillion dollars—forty-three million Americans don't have health insurance, and forty-eight million don't have access to a primary-care provider even if they have an insurance card. Right here in America, there are people who live too far from a medical facility and have no access to transportation to keep routine appointments to monitor their medical conditions. Others live in the midst of a bustling urban center but can't find a doctor nearby who speaks their native tongue.

In addition, certain segments of our population have difficulty finding care with which they are comfortable. For example, lesbian women encounter negative attitudes and discrimination from health-care providers. In fact, surveys show that approximately 70 percent of physicians say they are uncomfortable taking care of lesbians. Therefore, lesbian midlife women have additional reasons to distrust the system. This can result in substandard care from the physicians and failure by lesbian women to disclose their sexual practices, which also compromises their care.

Lesbians in long-term relationships also don't have access to health care through their partners' insurance, as married heterosexual couples do. (Fortunately, more employers and insurers are trying to remedy this discriminatory practice.)

Despite the huge U.S. health-care budget and the greatest medical technology in the world, we lag behind a number of developing countries in the state of our health. For example, our infant mortality rate is higher than Jamaica's, Cuba's, Kuwait's, and that of some other countries. We also have major disparities in death rates (as we discussed in earlier chapters) between minority and nonminority groups and between poor and more affluent populations.

Many of the problems with the health-care system in the United States are due to systemic problems resulting from some rather old-fashioned notions of medicine. Unfortunately, the U.S. health care system is:

- More focused on sickness than wellness
- More focused on treatment than prevention (of the $1 trillion spent on health care, less than 1 percent is spent on prevention)
- More focused on health services than health
- More focused on managing costs than managing care
- More focused on profit than on patients

It's no wonder that many African American women distrust the U.S. medical system. But despite all of this, our health-care system is the best in the world. As health professionals, we authors truly believe this, and we *know* that you can make the system work for you. You don't need to be afraid of the system, but you do need to be assertive and aware if you want top-quality care. We cannot emphasize enough that *you must take charge of your own health and well-being.* The following two essential steps can help you become an empowered health-care consumer:

1. *Find a health-care professional who respects his or her role as your partner in the quest to find the best health-care solutions for you.* Stop thinking that your physician or any other clinician will figure out everything and then tell you what to do. You must ask questions, do your research, and accept the responsibility of working with health-care providers to make medical decisions on your behalf.

Yes, your doctor understands medicine in ways you were never trained to do, but you know more about yourself than anyone else. You have very important information that your doctor needs to know. If your doctor is not receptive to your role as a full partner with decision-making power, then you need to find another physician! Doctors who don't ask or don't tell are dangerous to your health—and they can be lethal if they don't listen. As the former U.S. surgeon general Dr. C. Everett Koop would say, "It's better to put your doctor on the spot than on a pedestal."

2. *Find the best health care possible.* Don't settle for less. Many of us spend more time and energy selecting just the right pair of shoes, just the right outfit, or the right beautician than we do finding the right health professional. Why do so many people spend weeks hunting down the best contractor to remodel their kitchen but take whatever doctor they're referred to without asking a single question? Folks who wouldn't think twice about shelling out $40,000 for a luxury car, buying lottery tickets every week, or going to a casino groan and complain about having to drop a few extra dollars a month to upgrade their health plan for better medical coverage.

# FINDING THE RIGHT DOCTOR FOR YOU

Everyone needs a primary-care physician to provide basic care—from giving physical exams and treating run-of-the-mill illnesses such as the flu to coordinating all of your medical care. In fact, your primary-care physician is your first contact when you need medical attention. A good primary-care doctor will become quite familiar with your physical, social, and emotional situation and serve as your advocate in all health-related problems. He or she will refer you to specialists, monitor tests and evaluations you receive from other doctors, and determine whether there are any other community resources that may benefit your circumstances, such as other insurance alternatives or social service agencies that can assist with particular problems.

At your age, you need a primary-care physician who is trained in *family medicine* or *general internal medicine* (internist). You also need a team of clinicians in different specialties addressing your particular medical concerns. Some gynecologists serve as primary-care physicians, meaning they address all your health-care needs in a comprehensive way and not just your female organs, but you really should have an internist or family physician. (Many gynecologists, however, wish to limit their practice to women's concerns.) After age seventy, you may need to consult a gerontologist, who specializes in treating older patients, or use a gerontologist as your primary-care physician. (See box below for a list of medical specialties.)

## TYPES OF HEALTH-CARE PROFESSIONALS

A critical aspect of self-care and preventive medicine is pulling together a top-notch team of clinicians. This will require a little homework to get a better handle on the wide variety of health-care professionals who can partner with you in your care. Once you've picked your team, it's important to develop a trusting relationship with your physicians, nurses, and other clinicians, and believe that they care about you and will always be working in your best interests. Part of your trust will come from the knowledge that they have a sound medical and health-care background and adequate experience.

Physicians are either *medical doctors* (M.D.'s) or *doctors of osteopathy* (D.O.'s). Medical doctors graduate from medical school, take care of the entire body, and practice standard medicine. Osteopathic physicians graduate from a school of osteopathy, emphasize the importance of the musculoskeletal system (muscles and bones), and practice holistic medicine. D.O.'s frequently manipulate or palpate as part of diagnosis and treatment, but unlike chiropractors or acupuncturists, they can prescribe medicine. Most osteopaths are general practitioners, family practitioners, or emergency medicine specialists.

**1. YOUR PRIMARY-CARE TEAM:** internist or family practitioner, obstetrician-gynecologist, dentist, pharmacist, dental hygienist, nurse-practitioner or physician assistant. Your primary care team can also include practitioners of:

**COMPLEMENTARY/ALTERNATIVE MEDICINE:** naturopath, chiropractor, acupuncturist, massage therapists, reiki masters (the Resources section of this book lists organizations to help find a practitioner)

**2. SPECIALTY CARE TEAM:** ophthalmologist (for annual eye exams); depending on your needs, cardiologist (for high blood pressure and heart issues), endocrinologist (for diabetes), dermatologist, mental health professional, other doctor

## PRIMARY-CARE PHYSICIANS

| | |
|---|---|
| FAMILY PRACTITIONER (M.D. OR D.O.) | Physician trained to treat men, women, and children |
| INTERNIST (M.D.) | Medical doctor trained in internal medicine who treats adults only (pediatricians treat only children) |

### DOCTORS WHO FURTHER SPECIALIZE IN SPECIFIC AREAS OF MEDICINE

| | |
|---|---|
| CARDIOLOGIST | Specializes in heart and vascular diseases |
| DERMATOLOGIST | Treats skin disorders |
| ENDOCRINOLOGIST | Treats endocrine and glandular problems, such as diabetes |
| GASTROENTEROLOGIST | Treats problems with the digestive system |
| GERONTOLOGIST | Provides care for the elderly |
| GYNECOLOGIST | Specializes in the female reproductive system |
| NEUROLOGIST | Treats disorders of the brain and nervous system |
| OBSTETRICIAN | Provides pregnancy care and delivers babies |

| ONCOLOGIST | Treats cancer |
|---|---|
| OPHTHALMOLOGIST | Specializes in caring for the eyes, including treating eye disease (*An optometrist is not a physician; he or she can examine eyes and prescribe glasses but can't treat eye disease.*) |
| ORTHOPEDIST | Performs surgery on bones, joints, and muscles |
| PSYCHIATRIST | Treats mental and emotional problems (*A psychologist treats mental illness, but is not a medical doctor.*) |
| PULMONOLOGIST | Treats lung disorders |
| RHEUMATOLOGIST | Treats arthritis and rheumatism |
| UROLOGIST | Treats urinary system disorders involving the kidneys and bladder |

## DENTAL PROFESSIONALS

| DENTIST | Treats dental problems (teeth, gums, and oral cancer) and provides preventive education, treats diseased gums, and provides instruction on diet, brushing, flossing, and other preventive techniques |
|---|---|
| ORAL SURGEON | Performs surgery on the mouth |
| DENTAL HYGIENIST | Works with dentists and other health professionals to provide education, clinical, and therapeutic services that prevent oral diseases; cleans and applies preventive treatments to teeth and counsel patients on oral health |

## OTHER HEALTH CARE CLINICIANS

| PODIATRIST (DOCTOR OF PODIATRIC MEDICINE, D.P.M.) | Specializes in foot care |
|---|---|

| NURSE PRACTITIONERS (N.P.) | Registered nurses that perform many high-level primary-care tasks, such as physical examinations and treating common medical conditions or illnesses such as colds, infections, chronic diseases (e.g.,diabetes and hypertension) and minor injuries; focus on patient education, health promotion and disease prevention; some specialize in women's health and are very knowledgeable in hormone replacement therapy; in most states, must work under a doctor's supervision, especially to prescribe medication |
|---|---|
| PHYSICIAN ASSISTANT (P.A.) | Trained and licensed to practice medicine under the supervision of a physician and provide a broad scope of medical, diagnostic, therapeutic, and preventive services similar to nurse practitioners: some specialize in women's health and can do Pap smears and even biopsy your cervix; can prescribe medications in more than forty states |
| PHARMACIST | Must be licensed to dispense prescription medications; can provide good advice on dosage and other concerns about medications |

When you reach your Prime Time years, it's critical that you choose a health plan and health facility that allow you to see the same primary-care physician each time you visit. A good primary-care doctor will carefully review your medical history, get to know you as a person, and ask questions about your family, what you do for a living, and your general state of health and well-being. Doctors rely on this vital information to help you improve your health, practice disease prevention and health promotion, treat illness, detect early signs of problems, suggest when specialists are needed, and monitor your care over the years.

Looking for a primary-care doctor or a specialist who will make a good health partner can take some time, so be patient and start now. Begin by tapping your Prime Time Circle, friends, family, coworkers, and any health-care providers you know. Nearby teaching hospitals may have a physician referral service. Also check your local newspapers or magazines—many publish annual rankings of the best area doctors. Go to your public library and check the *Directory of Physicians in the United States*, the *Directory of Medical Specialists*, and the *Compendium of Certified Medical Specialists*. All three publications list physicians by state and provide information on their credentials, including whether they are certified by a professional board in their medical specialty. (Board-certified physicians have undergone additional training in their specialty field and have taken written and oral exams before specialty boards composed of their professional peers.)

If your health plan is provided by your employer, the benefits department may offer some assistance in finding doctors who will take your insurance or health plan. If you're sixty-five or older, your local Medicaid or Medicare office will also tell you which physicians, by specialty, accept a Medicaid or Medicare assignment (that's the jargon used for accepting the fees that Medicaid or Medicare sets for medical care). Look under "Medicaid Information" or "Medicare Information" in the community services section of your telephone book.

## What You Need to Know Before You Decide

Once you've identified some candidates, here's what you need to think about, consider, or check out before you make your decision.

*Decide what are the most important qualities you want in a doctor.* If you can, ask the person who gave you the referral about the doctor's style and personality. Is she willing to answer questions and explain complicated procedures and tests? Would he get annoyed if you asked him to repeat instructions regarding medications? If the doctor has a gruff manner and you need a person who will hold your hand through rough times, than maybe he or she is not the right physician for you. Bedside manner is important.

*Consider whether you feel more comfortable with a male or female doctor.* Several studies have demonstrated that women physicians spend more time with their patients. Research has also found that women physicians may practice more preventive medicine with their female patients than male doctors, such as performing Pap tests (to check for cervical cancer) and scheduling regular visits to monitor any potential problems. Nevertheless, you must make your decision based on your own personal preference.

*Think whether you would feel more relaxed talking to an African American doctor.* A study conducted by researchers at the Johns Hopkins University School of Medicine and reported in the May 1999 issue of the *Journal of the American Medical Association* found that Black patients rated their visits with their White doctors as "significantly less participatory" than did White patients. This means that Black patients were far less satisfied with how their White doctors treated them and communicated with them during office visits than were White patients.

The researchers concluded that "patients who are of the same race or ethnicity as their physician may feel more comfortable talking to their physicians and therefore, have a greater sense of partnership." Likewise, patients who were of a different race or ethnicity than their doctor had lower levels of satisfaction with their physicians. The National Medical Association (NMA) can help you find a black physician.

*Think about the importance of sensitivity to sexual preference if that's an issue for you.* As mentioned, lesbian women have some difficulty obtaining quality care. However, more and more urban areas now have programs and clinicians specializing in lesbian health, so search for them.

There are a number of factors that may account for these problems in partnership and communication. Prejudice and negative attitudes play roles as well. Some doctors may not know that diseases can affect different races in different ways. Also, what doctors expect from the office visit may differ from patients' expectations. In the final analysis, however, what is most important is the quality of your relationship with your doctor. This is why both of us, Marilyn and Gayle, have teams of wonderful, competent African American physicians but also include non–African Americans and both men and women.

*Take into account the pros and cons of going to a physician who is in a solo practice, a group practice, or part of a managed-care organization.* In a solo practice, the physician is the "boss" of the practice, and he or she will be the doctor who sees you every time you visit. When the doctor is on vacation or out of town, you will be referred to another doctor who is on call for your doctor.

The beauty of group practice is that you have several doctors who can work together on your behalf. For instance, if your doctor is away, another doctor from the same group has access to your records and will be on call to handle any medical emergencies. Some group practices consist of internists and specialists who work together to treat patients.

Managed-care practices (like HMO facilities) often offer the benefits of a group practice, but you may not be able to see the same doctor each time you visit. Under managed care, you may also have a number of restrictions that dictate whether you are fully covered to see doctors outside of the practice.

*Make an office visit.* It's essential for you to check out the facilities, get a feel for the office, and see how the doctor deals with you as a patient. Pay particular attention to the office and nursing staff, since you will have to deal with them often! You will need to make an official appointment to actually meet the doctor and talk to the office manager.

# CHECKING OUT THE DOCTOR'S OFFICE

Have a list of questions with you for the staff when you call or visit the doctor's office. The doctor's secretary or office manager should be able to answer most of your questions. Be sure to observe how willing they are to give you clear, detailed responses. Here is what you need to know:

• *At what hospital does the doctor have admitting privileges?* He should be working at the best hospitals in the area or at a hospital that's accessible to you.

• *What are the office hours?* These should match your availability.

• *How much time is allowed for a routine visit?* Flexible time slots are best, but less than fifteen to twenty minutes is not acceptable. You want a doctor who makes it a practice to answer his or her patient's questions— and that takes time.

• *If I called right now for a routine visit, how soon could I be seen?* If the first available appointment is months away, continue looking. Also check how soon you would be seen with an emergency and how it would be handled.

• *What medical insurance do you take?*

• *What are the fees?* If you don't have insurance or your insurance will not cover this doctor's visit, this is a critical question. You will skimp on doctor's visits if you don't have the money to pay.

• *What are the terms of payment? Is there a finance charge if I don't pay all at once?*

• *How long has the doctor been practicing?*

• *What schools did he or she attend?*

• *Is the doctor licensed or board-certified in his or her medical specialty?*

• *Has the doctor written any books or articles?* If so, they may be worth reading.

• *Does the doctor see a lot of midlife women in the practice?* You want a doctor who stays up-to-date on our special health needs.

• *Who covers for the doctor when he or she is not available (on vacation or after hours)? What happens if a patient gets sick in the middle of the night?* Find out who the other physicians are who cover this practice.

• *Who answers patients' routine medical questions when they call—a nurse-practitioner, a physician assistant, or the doctor when he or she gets around to it?* You want timely responses and twenty-four-hour coverage by one of these clinicians, not an administrator who doesn't have any medical training.

Next, you'll need to meet with the doctor. Not many doctors will schedule a free consultation, so you may need to make your assessment and ask questions during your first visit.

*Get a sense of how comfortable you are with the physician.* Assess how comfortable you are asking questions and whether the doctor enthusiastically addresses your concerns. He or she should answer in plain English, using terms you can easily understand.

Think about whether you can establish a trusting, open, and honest relationship with your primary-care physician. Be up front about this and explain that you are looking for a physician who will:

- Treat you as a partner in your wellness journey
- Listen to you
- Explain everything and ensure your understanding
- Encourage your participation in all decisions about tests, referrals, and treatments
- Explain the benefits, risks, and costs of any tests
- Not feel threatened when you seek other opinions
- Give you copies of your test results and consultant reports

Ask if he or she will support all of these points and any others you might have. If you are uncomfortable with his or her response, keep looking!

*Ask the doctor how he or she feels about complementary alternative medicine.* If the doctor isn't receptive to integrating other approaches such as herbal therapy, acupuncture, and massage therapy into traditional care and this is important to you, find another doctor.

*Find out what is expected of you as a patient.* If the doctor doesn't want an assertive, informed patient, walk away.


## FINDING THE RIGHT MENTAL HEALTH PROFESSIONALS FOR YOU

At some point in your life, you may need to partner with a mental health provider. Even if you don't, you will know someone who does. Selecting a mental health professional can be more anxiety-provoking than picking a primary-care doctor. *We rarely get the degree of family, friend, and community support for finding a therapist that we do for finding a provider for our physical health.* Thus we are more apt to ignore or minimize symptoms related to our emotional well-being than those connected to our physical health. You also may be hesitant to work with a therapist out of an ingrained discomfort with talking about your feelings and emotions with people you don't know. That reluctance may be common among the African Americans you know, but don't let fears or shame keep you from getting the mental health care you need.

By now we're hopeful that you're so committed to caring for all aspects of your being that you will fight as hard to get your mental health needs met as you do for your physical health needs.

When seeking a therapist, ask for referrals from friends, family, employee assistance programs, mental health agencies, organizations listed in the Resources section of this book, and university-based departments of psychology, psychiatry, or social work. You'll need to ask your mental health-care provider many of the questions you asked your primary health-care provider to find out his or her expertise, cancellation policy, fees, availability of sliding-scale fees, insurance coverage, length of sessions, referral process (see page 468).

Being a full participant in your treatment is as essential in your mental health care as it is in your physical health care. You must be active and assertive, and you must ask questions. Open communication with your therapist is critical.

Racial biases and sexual stereotyping can influence how African Americans and women are diagnosed and treated. Cultural stereotypes of Black women as Mammy, Sapphire, and Jezebel can influence how we perceive ourselves or how we are perceived by therapists. Before you choose a therapist, you may want to discuss your concerns about being viewed in a stereotypical manner.

For instance, if you or your therapist view Black women as stereotypical mammies, you may have a difficult time discussing your concerns about physical appearance (including obesity) and the impact of being everyone's caretaker. If your therapist sees you as Sapphire (aggressive, constantly angry), this can make it extremely difficult for you to confront and address your aggressive behavior or destructive displays of anger. If you are overly sensitive about the highly sexual Jezebel image, you may have difficulty talking to your therapist about the full range of your sexuality, including any concerns regarding promiscuous or sexually dangerous behavior or repressed sexual feelings.[1]

# MENTAL HEALTH PROFESSIONALS

Most mental health clinicians have at least a master's degree in some form of counseling. However, the criteria for providing mental health services vary greatly from state to state. Thus, it's extremely important that you make certain that your therapist is credentialed by some national accrediting body. Remember, this person is going to work with your mind, spirit, and maybe even your body. You need and deserve the best person you can find.

| | |
|---|---|
| PSYCHIATRIST | A medical doctor (M.D.) who specializes in the problems of mental illness; most use a combination of verbal therapy and medication |
| PSYCHOLOGIST | Diagnoses and treats mental health problems, provides counseling and therapy to patients, groups, and families; generally treats emotional and behavioral problems with some form of psychotherapy (talk therapy); develops, selects, and administers psychological tests; most psychologists who are psychotherapists have a doctorate in philosophy (Ph.D.) or a doctorate in psychology (Psy.D.) |
| SOCIAL WORKER | Helps people and their families adjust to problems in their lives such as serious illness, physical and emotional abuse, poverty; makes referrals to social agencies and resources; has a master's degree in social work (M.S.W.) or obtains a license as a licensed clinical social worker (L.C.S.W.) |
| PASTORAL COUNSELOR | Provides counseling and advice in times of emotional distress; may or may not have formal training in counseling |
| PSYCHIATRIC NURSE | A registered nurse with an advanced degree in counseling |
| PSYCHOTHERAPIST or COUNSELOR | These terms denote no specific degree or training in mental health; thus it's important to ask questions about training and credentials |

## When It's Time to Leave Your Therapist

When you and your therapist agree that the goals you have set have been met, it's extremely important to end therapy in an open and direct manner. However, if you're angry with your therapist or dissatisfied with your rate of improvement, discuss these issues before you stop the sessions. Dropping out of treatment without addressing your concerns is a sign that you may still need help with issues such as assertiveness.

If you feel that the therapist is not really listening to your concerns or is being verbally abusive or dismissive, it's time to leave. But first discuss your frustration with your therapist to determine whether the problem is one of communication rather than one of respect.

Other reasons to leave your therapist and report him or her to a local or national mental health organization:

• If your therapist is routinely (not just occasionally) late, arbitrarily cancels sessions, or talks on the phone during your sessions
• If inappropriate racial, sexual, or stereotyping remarks are made
• If your confidentiality is not maintained
• If there is any indication that the therapist abuses alcohol or any illegal substance

Each of us responds differently to therapy, but it's important to know that no treatment plan works instantly. Even so, you should expect to see some improvement in your symptoms within two to three months, depending upon your particular problems. No intervention can change overnight any problematic patterns of behavior that have been developing for years. If you don't feel better, discuss alternative treatment plans with your therapist. Sometimes it takes a bit of trial and error to find out what works best for you.

### ℞ PRIME TIME PRESCRIPTION TO BECOME A SAVVY PATIENT

Finding the best medical doctor or mental health professional is only part of the challenge of getting the highest-quality care available. **The next part of the challenge requires you to be assertive.** You must not give the doctor all the authority for your care. Don't ever think you are asking a "stupid" question or "bothering the doctor" or "taking up the doctor's time." This is *your* time and *your* body—*not* the doctor's.

As Dr. Koop would say, "Under the present health system, you had better take charge of your health because no one else is going to do it." So here is your prescription for change.

***Be knowledgeable.*** Another aspect of making a commitment to your health is by becoming an active consumer of health information to enable you to understand more about the state of your own health and to better take charge of your activities and be successful. Bookstores, libraries, and the Internet are full of health information, so *do your own research*; don't rely solely on what your physician tells you.

Reading *Prime Time* is a major first step. Watching the health segments on the nightly news, checking out the health shows on cable television, and getting a subscription to a health publication such as *Heart and Soul* (a health magazine for African American women), *Prevention*, *Health*, or *Health Quest* (for African Americans) are great ways to stay current on what's happening in health care and medical science. Join the National Black Women's Health Project and read the organization's publication. Your Prime Time Circle is a wonderful vehicle to research certain topics and discuss them—like a book club. Discuss and share what you're learning with your Prime Time Sister. The Resources section lists books to read and organizations dedicated to specific health issues.

Hang out on the World Wide Web. Surfing Web sites makes the information you need just a few clicks away. But be careful—bad health information can be worse than no information. Always know the source of any advice or information you receive. If it's not coming from a well-known, reputable organization, try to find out the credentials of the researcher or group. We provide a list of reputable sites in the Resources section.

***Be open and honest with your health-care providers.*** If you are afraid to take a certain test, tell your doctor or nurse. If you don't want to take a certain medication, talk about it with your doctor or therapist. Tell them what alternative therapies you are trying, such as herbs, acupuncture, or therapeutic massage and reiki. Be honest about your sexual activity and whether you're practicing safe sex, smoking, using drugs (legal and illegal), and how much alcohol you're drinking in a week. Hiding this information can be detrimental to your care and even life-threatening. Remember, clinicians see and hear all kinds of stories from their patients—there is nothing you can tell us health workers that will surprise us or make us think less of you. We are there for you.

*Keep your own records of past visits, tests, medications, and treatments.*
As we discussed earlier in this book, start a health journal, and use the calendar in Chapter 8 to record dates of examinations, follow-up instructions, and test results. Obtain and keep copies of results of tests and procedures—e.g., PAP smears, mammograms, and others. Note any changes in your general health (such as your blood pressure readings that you take at home) and well-being so that you can remember to discuss them with your doctor. Keep a record of your monthly breast self-exams, exercise schedule, pulse rate, blood pressure, and severe mood swings. If you are having symptoms, keep a diary of how you feel, specifically, When? For how long? What precipitates the symptom? What relieves it?

*Prepare for office visits.* Even with the most caring doctors, visits are getting shorter and shorter. Therefore, you must go in prepared to get what you want and need from the visit. Three to five days before your visit, sit down and write out the questions you want answered. Don't try to memorize the questions; just write them down. Put the most important questions first, in case you don't get through the entire list.

Plan to update the doctor on things that have happened since your last visit. Take your journal, calendar, and test results with you to make sure your discussion is accurate. Point out any changes in your lifestyle, even if it's something you're not proud of, such as smoking or drinking too much. Don't be ashamed or shy. Never withhold information. Mention any changes you have noticed in your appetite, sleep, stress, or energy level, as well as changes in your life such as a divorce or death of a loved one. (To refresh your memory on what to expect in a typical office visit, especially for examinations, turn back to Chapter 8, "The Ultimate Checkup," and take a look at the chapters in Part V, "Staying Sane in a World that Can Seem Insane.")

*Don't leave the doctor's office until all your questions are answered.*
"What" and "why" should become your mantra. For example:

- What else can I do to improve my health?
- What do these symptoms usually mean?
- What else could they mean?
- What can we do to find out?
- What treatment do you recommend?
- Why are you recommending that treatment?
- What other options do I have?
- What are the benefits/risks of this test/procedure/medication?

*Make sure you understand all instructions.* Don't hesitate to say, "I want to make sure I understand. Could you explain that in more detail?" It may help to repeat in your own words what you think the doctor means, and then ask, "Is this correct?" If your doctor has an accent and you are having difficulty understanding what is being said, ask the doctor to write out the instructions. Remember, both you and the doctor have a responsibility to make certain the information is understood.

*Take notes in your journal during your visit so you will remember the answers to your questions.* When you are anxious or fearful, you may not re-

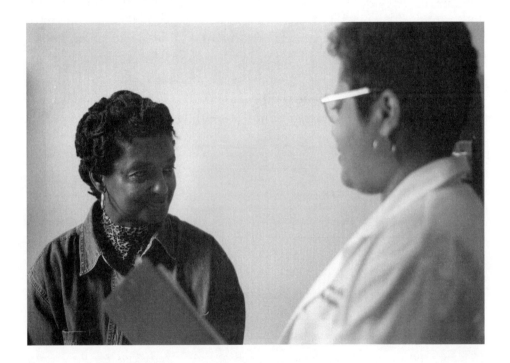

member what is being said. If taking notes is difficult, consider using a tape recorder, or take your Prime Time Sister or a relative with you when you're feeling anxious or afraid. She can provide support but also listen with a set of ears that knows, you very well.

*Always ask for brochures, cassette tapes, videotapes, or written information* from the doctor or staff regarding your condition, treatment, or medication.

*Talk to other members of your health-care team.* Spend some time with the nurse-practitioner or physician assistant, pharmacist, and whoever else plays an active role in your health care. They may have more time to explain something about your situation than the doctor can give you.

*Always get a second and possibly third opinion if your primary-care physician or specialist is having difficulty making a diagnosis, or recommends surgery or specific interventions or tests that are not routine, e.g., an angiogram of your heart.* You want to hear how another doctor would diagnose your condition and which treatment he or she would recommend and his or her take on your expected outcome. Sometimes your current doctor will help you find someone who can give you a second opinion. Even if he or she doesn't help or you feel uncomfortable about seeking another opinion, *DO IT!*

Getting another opinion does not mean you do not trust your doctor or that you are dissatisfied with your care. In fact, you might mention this point with your doctor when discussing why you want a second opinion. You have an obligation to yourself to seek different opinions so that you can make the most informed decision about your care. Use the same procedures as outlined earlier in this chapter for finding the appropriate doctor.

*Know your rights to demand quality care.* In fact, the American Hospital Association has spelled them out in its Patient Bill of Rights.

---

## PATIENT BILL OF RIGHTS*

You have the right:

- *To be spoken to in words that you understand*
- *To be told what's wrong with you*
- *To read your medical record*
- *To know the benefits and risks of any treatment and its alternatives*
- *To know what a treatment or test will cost*
- *To make all treatment decisions*
- *To refuse any medical procedure*

*Marilyn and Gayle would add that you have the right to seek other medical opinions.

*Source:* Developed by the American Hospital Association.

---

*Trust your instincts.* If you feel that your doctor doesn't care or isn't working in your best interests, or if you're not getting the right vibe, it's time to find another doctor or practice. You also need to consider finding another clinician if your doctor:

- Doesn't explain medical terms and concepts you don't understand
- Always seems rushed and ready to leave
- Discourages your questions
- Gets an attitude if you want to participate in decisions or want another opinion
- Acts like he or she knows everything and isn't interested in finding out more about a particular condition

We know how hard it is to change doctors, but sometimes it's necessary. Ask your Prime Time Sister and your Prime Time Circle for support.

## UNDERSTANDING THE REAL DEAL WITH MEDICATIONS

These days, there never seems to be quite enough room to fit all of our prescriptions and over-the-counter medications into our medicine cabinets. In addition, as we age, medicines can affect us differently. That's why learning as much as possible about the medications we take is so important in our Prime Time years.

Ask lots of questions whenever your doctor prescribes a medication. Not only should you drill your doctor, but buttonhole your pharmacist. Make sure you know the name of the drug recommended by your doctor, why it was prescribed, and how it can help you get better or control your condition. Get the dosage in writing, including how often and how long you should take it and whether it should be taken with food or on an empty stomach. Ask whether certain foods or alcohol should be avoided while you take this prescription. Ask about potential side effects and what to do if they occur.

Finally, find out whether a generic version of the medication can be substituted for a brand name that the doctor has recommended. (Generic drugs are medicines that are not sold under a brand name; they are less expensive than brand-name drugs but in most cases are interchangeable.)

Whenever you start taking a new drug, be sure to remind the pharmacist to review the medications you're already on—including over-the-counter medications. The pharmacist is an important member of your health-care team, too, so feel free to consult him or her whenever you have a question. Here are some additional pointers regarding medications:

***Keep a record of all your medications and always show it to your doctor and your pharmacist.*** A suggested format is as follows:

## MEDICATION CHART

| Date Started | Medication | Dosage (amount) | Schedule | Used for | Side Effects |
|---|---|---|---|---|---|
| Example: 1/26/01 | Name of | 1 tablet medicine = 400 mg | 3 times/day (after meals) | Arthritis | Nausea |
|  |  |  |  |  |  |
|  |  |  |  |  |  |
|  |  |  |  |  |  |
|  |  |  |  |  |  |
|  |  |  |  |  |  |
|  |  |  |  |  |  |

Note: List both prescription and non-prescription (over-the-counter) medicines.

The Food and Drug Administration's Office of Women's Health and the National Association of Chain Drug Stores also have a format to list your medicines and keep in your pocketbook. Call 888-8PUEBLO to receive up to 250 free copies of the pamphlet *My Medicines.*

*Always read the label and printed instructions that come with your medications.* This applies to prescription and over-the-counter medications. Always follow label directions. Up to half of all patients on medication don't follow the directions. This is a major concern, since using the wrong dosage can be lethal. Also, it is extremely important to complete the course of medication, unless you're having negative side effects. Stopping the medication too soon can prevent you from being fully healed.

*Check to see if the medication contains any ingredients that you are allergic to or interacts with other meds you are taking.* Also ask your doctor and pharmacist whether the medication could have an adverse effect on you because of another condition or illness. *Discard all medications that are not used up by the expiration date.*

*Don't share your medicines with others or take someone else's medicine.* Just because you are taking medications for similar conditions, the type and dosage of medication you are on may be vastly different.

## WHAT ABOUT YOUR INSURANCE COVERAGE?

No matter what type of health insurance coverage you have, you won't be able to take full advantage of any plan unless you read your manual. No, this is not exciting reading, but knowing your options can save your life. Also be sure to review your plan with your benefits department from time to time to check for any additional coverage. Note that some employers only offer a short period of time each year (usually in October or November) when you can change plans, so if you are not satisfied with your current coverage, find out when this window of opportunity opens.

Health-care coverage is divided into two basic plans: *fee-for-service* and *managed care.* While both plans pay for basic medical expenses such as doctor's visits and hospitalizations, there are important distinctions that will affect your coverage, your costs, and your care. Also, be sure to check to see what exactly is covered in your plan. If your health insurance comes from your employer, find out if you have a separate plan for mental health, dental, and vision care coverage.

### Fee-for-Service

Under these systems, providers receive a fee for each medical service they render, as opposed to receiving a salary or a flat payment for every patient they have under their care (as in managed care). Fee-for-service plans offer a wide discretion to choose the doctors and specialists you want. You pay for the service provided by the doctor and then submit the receipt to your insurance company for reimbursement for some, but usually not all, of the cost. Most companies will pay 80 percent of what your doctor charges; you will be expected to pay the remaining 20 percent (which is called the copayment).

Most fee-for-service policies have an *annual deductible*, which is the amount you must pay out before the reimbursements kick in. The higher the deductible, the lower your monthly premiums will be.

Fee-for-service policies vary in their coverage of hospital care, and this is very important when you select a plan. Some plans will cover the total cost of hospitalization, while others will require a separate hospital deductible, which could be several hundred dollars.

## Managed-Care Plans

Managed care is a prepaid health-care delivery system where different services are offered for a fixed amount of money. The purpose of managed care is to control the costs of health care. Although keeping health costs from zooming sky high is a good thing, doing so by limiting access to specialists, tests, medicines, and treatments is not the best way to practice medicine. Managed care sets the primary doctor up as a gatekeeper between the patient and medical services. Unfortunately, some insurers dole out incentive bonuses or payments to encourage doctors to withhold services deemed unnecessary, to shorten stays in the hospital for treatment or recovery, and to deny expensive tests or consultations with specialists. Stay away from any practices using these types of incentives.

Under managed care, doctors are expected to see more patients, which decreases the amount of time spent with each individual patient. There is limited or no choice for a second opinion with a provider outside the plan. (However, many plans provide a second opinion within the plan.) And if you seek treatments (even for routine illnesses) that your plan considers unnecessary, you may be denied care or have to pay for the care in addition to your premiums. Therefore, it is up to you to manage with care!

## Four Types of Managed-Care Plans

• *Health maintenance organizations* (HMOs) are the most widely known type of managed-care plans. They combine insurance coverage and delivery of health care for a fixed, prepaid premium. The doctors are employees of the plan.

• *Point-of-service* (POS) plans combine the HMO prepaid concept and the flexibility of fee-for-service. A number of HMOs offer POS options, allowing members to seek care outside the HMO network for a higher premium. Consumers are given strong financial incentives to choose among doctors who are members of the HMO, but are allowed to select nonmember doctors if they are willing to pay higher fees for care.

• *Preferred provider organizations* (PPOs) are networks of physicians, hospitals, and other health-care providers who contract with an insurance entity to provide care on a fee-for-service basis at discount rates. You have more freedom of choice in picking a doctor or location with a PPO. Although you can choose clinicians who are outside the network, you will probably pay a higher out-of-pocket cost. These plans are good choices for empowered health-care consumers.

• *Independent practice associations* (IPAs) are groups of doctors who provide managed care in their private offices and usually contract with an HMO to provide services.

## What Does All This Insurance Stuff Mean for You?

It sounds complex and cumbersome, but being a knowledgeable health-care consumer requires that you examine each of these individual policies closely and spend time shopping for the one that is right for you. Remember, there is no health plan that is best; there is only the one that is best for you. Some questions to ask before choosing a plan:

• *How does the referral system work?* Seek out plans that guarantee access to specialists and emergency care. Avoid HMOs that, by contract, forbid their physicians from informing you of treatments and alternatives unavailable at the HMO.
• *What access do I have to specialists and who controls the visits?* The best plans allow your doctors, not an administrator, to determine whether you require the aid of a specialist. You should also be able to obtain second opinions outside the plan. If you have a medical problem, find out if certain consultations that you may need to manage your disease (such as a nutritionist if you have diabetes) are covered by the plan. Also find out if medical specialties such as podiatry (foot care), ophthalmology (eye doctor), and mental health are covered.
• *Does your plan work with patients to develop individual programs for health promotion and disease prevention?* This includes identifying any risk factors you may have for serious disease and routinely scheduling preventive screening tests, such as mammograms, Pap smears, cholesterol tests, diabetic

screening, and so on. Find out whether any or all of these are covered by the plan.

- *What are the fees?* Is there a copay or deductible?

- *Does the HMO offer prescription benefits?* What is the policy regarding using generic medicines, and can I use brand-name medicines when they are needed? Is there a drug formulary or approved list of medications that dictates that I can use only the drugs listed? (In some plans, doctors must get permission to prescribe drugs not on the formulary.)

- *What is the procedure for changing HMOs?* How soon and how often can you change your plan if you don't like it?

- *How does the HMO ensure quality and minimize mistakes?* Find out how it ensures that proper treatment is given and follow-up is done. Ask who gives medical advice over the phone. A clinician, nurse, physician assistant, or nurse-practitioner are the best choices. If you won't be able to talk to a health-care provider, then how qualified is the individual who will be giving you advice? **Don't choose a plan where you can't talk with a clinician.**

- *Be sure to ask about the HMO's administrative policies.* What is the time limit for visits? Are clinicians limited to only ten minutes a visit? How close to my home is the hospital that I must use? If it is far away, ask if the plan provides transportation or if you can switch to a closer hospital. Does it serve patients of different races and ethnic groups? Has its staff been trained to do so? What's the racial makeup of its staff? Find out if the HMO has recently conducted a customer satisfaction survey, and ask for the results!

- *How do I appeal decisions made about my care?* This is very important, since you may need care that isn't readily covered by the plan. You want to know to whom you should make the appeal, how appeal decisions are made, and how quickly decisions are made. Some appeals are heard by an independent committee outside of the plan; other HMOs use a committee of plan members, who probably have a vested interest in the outcome. It's important to understand this before you sign up.

You have the right and the responsibility to obtain the best care possible. If you find yourself in an HMO that isn't meeting your needs, complain until someone hears you. HMOs are increasingly competing with one another based on patient-doctor satisfaction levels. Some groups give a report-card grade to doctors based on the results of patient satisfaction surveys. Use every appeal mechanism available. One dissatisfied patient who tells twenty other people can result in change for the better. Talk to a lawyer to understand other options. Use your support network.

• *How well does your HMO serve the community and address social aspects of health care?* Does it conduct surveys to find out what the community needs? Does it partner with community efforts? Does the plan have cultural competency programs to better serve everyone? Does it have racial/ethnic/gender/economic diversity on the staff? Does it give back to the community with free mammograms, blood pressure screenings, and educational health forums?

## Making an HMO Work for You

When you choose an HMO, be persistent about getting whatever you need. That goes for getting an appointment or for demanding certain tests. The key is to take time to learn your way around your HMO and establish relationships in the system, so that when you call, the staff knows who you are. As with all things, building relationships helps you get what you want.

---

### WHERE TO GO IF YOU *DON'T* HAVE HEALTH INSURANCE

If you are part of the growing number of uninsured in this country, there are community health centers throughout the country that will provide comprehensive, ongoing, quality care regardless of your ability to pay. Call your state health department—specifically ask for the primary-care office for help in finding a physician or health-care center that is taking care of uninsured women. If they're unable to help you contact mental health providers, call your local mental health association. If you think you're eligible for Medicare or Medicaid, call your state offices for these programs.

---

### PRIME TIME FINAL WORD

Your goal is comprehensive, ongoing, efficient, effective, high-quality health care at a price that you can afford, in a place of your choosing, with you as an active partner in a well-trained medical team.

---

# Chapter 20

# REACHING THE NORTH STAR

*There will come a day
it is not far off now
when you wake in the morning and know
you were meant to be happy
and that you want it
more than you want
things, or memories
any concrete place called home
all the strings of the past that fasten you,
more than you want
justice or pride:
your old clay image of yourself
or the faint chance
that all that has gone wrong
may still change.*

*It is you who hold
the power to change.
And whatever it is that holds you
whatever it is you think you cannot live without
the time has come to open your hands and
let it go.*

*Run*
*Flee*
*Disappear*
*Break loose*
*Take wing*

*Fly by night*
*Move like a meteor*
*Be gone.*
*If you fear it will never be possible*
*think of Harriet*
*who traveled alone*
*the first time*
*who finally freed three hundred people*
*but first*
*had to free*
*herself.*

—Becky Birtha, "Poem for Flight," in Patricia Bell-Scott, ed.,
*Flat-Footed Truths: Telling Black Women's Lives*


There's a Harriet in all of us and the middle years give us the opportunity to finally free her.

We hope that you will use this book, your Prime Time Sister, and your Prime Time Circle of Sisterfriends as North Stars to guide you on your journey toward wellness—a journey that will empower you to take charge of your emotional, physical, and spiritual health. Some of you started this journey years ago, so for you this book is an affirmation, and maybe a reminder, of why you chose your wellness path. However, for many of you, this book may serve as the catalyst that jump-starts your wellness journey. The beauty is that you can start *right now*!

We know that not every day, week, month, year will go smoothly, and **freedom, especially from lifelong habits, does not come easily.** There will be times, just as there were with Harriet's charges, when you will want to turn back. And there will be times when you are encouraged overtly or covertly by your partner or spouse, children, extended family, friends, and coworkers to turn back. Your power, especially if it's newly expressed, will evoke fear, anger, sadness, suspicion, and envy in some of those closest to you. But once you're free, your own power and greater happiness and satisfaction—and health—might encourage some of them to start on their own path.

The following steps will help you to stay focused on your journey no matter what internal or external obstacles you face. Remember, obstacles are those frightening things that surface when you take your eyes off your goal. You can get over, under, or through them.

1. Actively give and receive support from your Prime Time Sister and Circle.

2. Reread those chapters of *Prime Time* that you found particularly helpful—and we hope that includes Chapter 3, "The Miracle of You."

3. Focus on your achievements and give yourself praise.

4. Remember that few journeys, especially difficult ones, are as short as we think they're going to be.

Your chance for success will be improved if you practice daily. D. J. Taylor's Prime Time Ten Commandments of Change:

## PRIME TIME TEN
## COMMANDMENTS OF CHANGE

1. Find time to exercise, or illness will find time for you.

2. Put your oxygen mask on first.

3. Give from your abundance.

4. Make dates with yourself.

5. Destress three times daily: ten minutes in the morning, ten minutes at noon, ten minutes at night.

6. Be still.

7. Do eight twice: eight glasses of water *and* eight fruits and vegetables.

8. Change how you think today for a better tomorrow.

9. Transform midlife challenges into midlife corrections.

10. Act now!

We have enjoyed taking this journey with you. We hope that it has helped you and will continue to help you focus on the beauty, joy, and amazing grace of life. We also hope that you truly believe that you have a divine right and responsibility to take charge of your spiritual, emotional, and physical health. That's why we encourage you to remember Ecclesiastes 3:1: "To *everything there is a season, and a time to every purpose under the heavens.*"

   *Now is your time!*

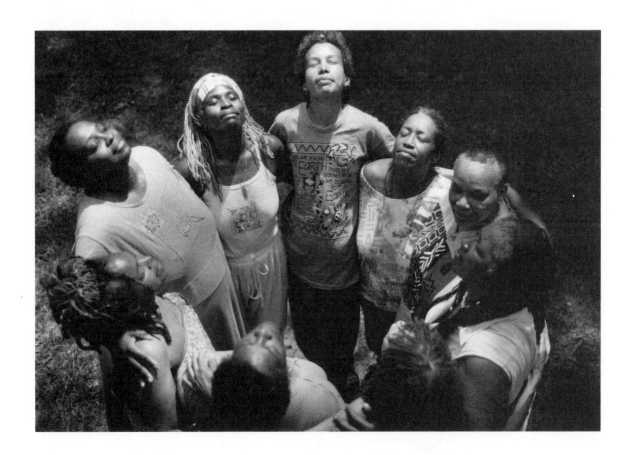

# Notes

## Chapter 4: Now Your Journey Begins

1. Dr. Orville Gilbert Brim, "The MacArthur Midlife Study Finds Tales of Midlife Crisis Greatly Exaggerated," *Philanthropy News Digest* 5(7), February 17, 1999.

## Chapter 7: The Power of Prevention

1. P. A. Sytkowski, R. B. D'Agustino, A. Belanger, and W. B. Kannel, "Trends in Cardiovascular Disease Incidence and Mortality: The Framingham Heart Study, 1950–1989," *American Journal of Epidemiology* 143(4), February 15, 1996.

## Chapter 8: The Ultimate Checkup

1. Joan Kenley, *A Woman's Right to Know—Health and Hormones After 35* (California: A Nancy Hicks Maynard Book, 1995); Morris Notolovitz and Diana Tonnessen, *Menopause and Midlife Health* (New York: St. Martin's, 1993).

## Chapter 10: Controlling Cardiovascular Disease

1. National Heart, Lung, and Blood Institute, *Heart Disease and Women* (Bethesda, MD: National Institutes of Health, 1996); Editorial, "Studies of Acute Coronary Syndromes," *New England Journal of Medicine* 341(4), July 1999.

2. Kevin A. Shulman et al., "The Effect of Race and Sex on Physicians' Recommendations for Cardiac Catheterization," *New England Journal of Medicine* 340(8), February 1999.

3. Marilyn Wimbleby, Thomas Robinson, Jan Sundquist et al., "Ethnic Variation in

Cardiovascular Disease," *Journal of the American Medical Association*, 281(11), March 17, 1999; B. L. Rosamond et al., "Trends in the Incidence of Myocardial Infarction," *New England Journal of Medicine*, 339(13), September 24, 1998; Judith Hochman, Jacqueline Tanis, and Trevor Thompson, "Sex, Clinical Presentation and Outcome in Patients with Acute Coronary Syndromes," *New England Journal of Medicine*, 341(4), July 22, 1999.

4. Frank Hu, Meir Stampfer, and JoAnn Manson, "Nurses Health Study," *New England Journal of Medicine* 337(21) November 1997.

5. K. M. Rexrode, V. J. Carey, and C. H. Hennekens, "Abdominal Adiposity and Coronary Heart Disease in Women," *Journal of the American Medical Association*, 280(21), December 1998.

6. T. L. Branford and E. Ofili, "The Paradox of Coronary Heart Disease in African American Women," *Journal of the National Medical Association*, 92(7), July 2000.

7. JoAnn Manson et al., "A Prospective Study of Aspirin Use and Primary Prevention of Cardiovascular Disease in Women," *Journal of the American Medical Association*, 266(4), July 24, 1991.

8. Carlos Iribarum, "Association of Hostility and Coronary Artery Calcification," *Journal of the American Medical Association* 283(19), May 17, 2000; Stephen Sidney, and Diane Bild, "Taking Anger to Heart," *Johns Hopkins Medical Letter, Health After 50*, July 1999.

9. Daniel Ford, Lucy Mead, and Patricia Chang, "Johns Hopkins—Depression and Heart Disease," *Archives of Internal Medicine* 158(13), July 1998.

10. Alexander H. Glassman and Peter A. Shapiro, "Depression and Coronary Artery Disease," American *Journal of Psychiatry* 155(1), January 1998; Mary Whorley and Warren Brower, "Association Between Depressive Symptoms and Mortality in Older Women," *Archives of Internal Medicine*, 158(19), October 26, 1998.

11. Dean Ornish, *Program for Reversing Heart Disease* (New York: Ballantine Books, 1990); Dean Ornish et al., "Intensive Lifestyle Changes for Reversal of Coronary Heart Disease," *Journal of the American Medical Association*, 280(23), December 1998.

12. Paul M. Ridker, Charles Hennekens, and Julie Buring, "Homocysteine and Risk of Cardiovascular Disease Among Postmenopausal Women," *Journal of the American Medical Association*, 281(19), May 10, 1999.

13. Paul M. Ridker, JoAnn Manson, and Julie Buring, "C-Reactive Protein and Other Markers of Inflammation on the Prediction of Cardiovascular Disease in Women," *New England Journal of Medicine*, 342(12), March 23, 2000.

14. E. Saunders and A. Brest Jr., "Cardiovascular Disease in Blacks," *Cardiovascular Clinics* (Philadelphia: F. A. Davis, 1991); W. Dallas Hall, Elijah Saunders, and Neil B. Schulman, *Hypertension in Blacks* (Chicago: Year Book Medical Publishers, 1990).

15. Vernon Barnes, Robert Schneider, and Charles Alexander, "Stress, Stress Reduction and Hypertension in African Americans: An Updated Review," *Journal of the National Medical Association*, 89(7), July 1997.

16. "Hypertension and Stroke," Johns Hopkins White Papers, 1999.

17. "Prevention of a First Stroke: A Consensus Statement," *Journal of the American Medical Association*, 281(12), March 24–31, 1997.

## Chapter 11: Combating Cancer

1. "Cancer Facts," National Cancer Institute, National Institutes of Health, January 1998.

2. John Ayanian and Paul Cleary, "Perceived Risks of Heart Disease and Cancer Among Cigarette Smokers," *Journal of the American Medical Association*, 281(11), March 17, 1999.

3. J. W. Eley, H. A. Hill, V. W. Chen et al., "National Cancer Institute Black/White Cancer Survival Study," *Journal of the American Medical Association* 272(12), September 28, 1994.

4. James T. Dignam, "Differences in Breast Cancer Prognosis Among African Americans and Caucasian Women," *CA: A Cancer Journal for Clinicians*, 50(1), January/February 2000.

5. Wendy Dermark-Wahnefried et al., "Awareness of Cancer-Related Programs and Services Among Rural African Americans," *Journal of the National Medical Association*, 90(4), April 1998.

6. Donald R. Lannin, Holly Matthews, Jim Mitchell et al., "Culture, Race and Breast Cancer Stage," *Journal of the American Medical Association*, 279(22), June 10, 1998.

7. American Institute for Cancer Research, newsletter, October 1999.

8. B. Fisher, J. P. Costantino, D. L. Wickerham et al., "Tamoxifen for the Prevention of Breast Cancer," *Journal of the National Cancer Institute* 90, February 1998; Collaborative Group, "Tamoxifen for Early Breast Cancer: An Overview of the Randomized Trials," *Lancet* 351, June 1998; Steven Cummings et al., "The Effect of Raloxifene on Risk of Breast Cancer in Postmenopausal Women," *Journal of the American Medical Association*, 281(23), June 16, 1999.

9. D. A. Lieberman, D. G. Weiss, J. H. Bond et al., "Use of Colonoscopy to Screen Asymptomatic Adults for Colorectal Cancer," *New England Journal of Medicine*, 343(3), July 2000.

10. J. A. Baron et al., "Calcium Supplements for the Prevention of Colorectal Adenanas," *The New England Journal of Medicine*, 340(2), January 14, 1999.

## Chapter 12: Dealing with Diabetes

1. Fred Brancati, Linda Kao, Haron Folsan et al., "Incident Type 2 Diabetes Mellitus in African Americans and White Adults," *Journal of the American Medical Association*, 283(17), May 3, 2000.

2. Centers for Disease Control, U.S. Department of Health and Human Services, "Diabetes—A Serious Public Health Problem," 1999.

3. Todd W. Griess, Javier Nieto, Eyal Shaker et al., "Hypertension and Antihypertensive Therapy as Risk Factors for Type 2 Diabetes Mellitus," *New England Journal of Medicine*, 342(13), March 30, 2000.

4. Michael Beyer and Ingrid Muhlhauser, "Diabetes Care and Patient-Oriented Outcomes," *Journal of the American Medical Association*, 281(18), May 12, 1999.

5. John West, "Closing the Gap," newsletter of the National Diabetes Education Program, March 1999.

6. K. Z. Walker et al., "Effects of Regular Walking on Cardiovascular Risk Factors and Body Composition in Normoglycemic Women and Women with Type 2 Diabetes," *Case* 22, April 1999.

7. Marvella Ford, Barbara Tilley, Patricia McDonald et al., "Social Support Among

African-American Adults with Diabetes—A Review, Parts 1 and 2," *Journal of the National Medical Association* 90(6–7), June 1998.

## Chapter 13: Stress Can Be Managed

1. Meyer Friedman and Ray Rosenman, *The Columbia University College of Physicians and Surgeons Complete Home Medical Guide* (New York: Crown Publishers, 1989).

2. Frank Treiber, quoted in *Newsweek* (special issue on stress), June 14, 1999.

3. Dr. Jay Gidd, quoted in *Newsweek* (special issue on stress), June 14, 1999.

4. Jacqueline S. Mattis, Carl C. Bell, Robert J. Jagers, and Esther Jenkins, "A Critical Approach to Stress-Related Disorders in African Americans," *Journal of the National Medical Association*, 91(2), February 1999.

5. Donald F. Tapley, Thomas Q. Morris, Lewis P. Rowland, et al., *The Columbia University College of Physicians and Surgeons Complete Home Medical Guide* (New York: Crown Publishers, 1989).

6. Vickie M. Mays, Lerita M. Coleman, and James S. Jackson, "Perceived Race-Based Discrimination, Employment Status, and Job Stress in a National Sample of Black Women, Implications for Health Outcomes," *Journal of Occupational Health Psychology* 1(3), July 1999.

7. Mary Beth Snapp, "Occupational Stress, Social Support, and Depression Among Black and White Professional-Managerial Women," *Women and Health* 18(1), January 1992.

8. T. H. Holmes and R. H. Rahe, "The Social Readjustment Rating Scale," *Journal of Psychosomatic Research* 11 (2), August 1967.

## Chapter 14: Overcoming Worry, Fear, and Anxiety

1. Rodney Clark, Norman B. Anderson, Vernessa R. Clark, and David R. Williams, "Racism as a Stressor for African Americans," *American Psychologist* 5(10), October 1999.

2. Angela M. Neal and Samuel Turner, "Anxiety Disorders Research with African-Americans. Current Status," *Psychological Bulletin* 109(3), May 1991.

3. Sheryle Gallant, Gwendolyn Puryear Keita, and Renee Royak-Schlaer, eds., *Health Care for Women—Psychological, Social, and Behavioral Influences* (Washington, D.C.: American Psychological Association, 1997).

4. Angela M. Neal, Leslie Nagle Rich, and William D. Smucker, "The Presence of Panic Disorder Among African-American Hypertensives: A Pilot Study," *The Journal of Black Psychology* 20(1), February 1994.

5. Lisa C. Smith, Steven Friedman, and Jeffrey Nevid, "Clinical and Sociocultural Differences in African American and European American Patients with Panic Disorder and Agoraphobia," *Journal of Nervous and Mental Disease* 187(9), September 1999.

6. Ibid.

7. Neal and Turner, "Anxiety Disorders Research."

8. Ibid.

9. John Briere, *Psychological Assessment of Adult Posttraumatic States* (Washington, D.C.: American Psychological Association, 1997).

10. Simeon Margolis and Karen L. Swartz, *Depression and Anxiety—The Johns Hopkins White Papers* (New York: Medletter Associates, 1999).

11. Lynn Clark, *SOS—Help for Emotions: Managing Anxiety, Anger, and Depression* (Bowling Green, KY: Parents Press, 1998).

12. The Natural Medicine Collective with Diana L. Ajjan, *Stress, Anxiety, and Depression* (New York: Dell, 1995).

## Chapter 15: Depression: You Can Feel Better

1. The Commonwealth Fund, *Selected Facts on U.S. Women's Health: A Chart Book* (New York: Commission on Women's Health, College of Physicians and Surgeons, Columbia University, 1997); Linda Villarosa, ed., *Body and Soul: The Black Women's Guide to Physical Health and Emotional Well-Being* (New York: Harper Perennial, 1994).

2. Angela Mitchell with Kennise Herring, *What the Blues Is: Black Women Overcoming Stress and Depression* (New York: Perigee, 1998).

3. Ellen McGraph, Gwendolyn Puryear Keita, Bonnie R. Strickland, and Nancy Felipe Russo, *Women and Depression: Risk Factors and Treatment Issues* (Washington, D.C.: American Psychological Association, 1990); National Institute of Mental Health, *National Lesbian Health Care Survey* (Washington, D.C.: U.S. Department of Health and Human Services, 1987); Susan D. Cochan and Vickie M. Mays, "Depressive Distress Among Homosexually Active African-American Men and Women," *American Journal of Psychiatry* 151(4), April 1994.

4. Meri Nana-Ama Danquah, *Willow Weep for Me—A Black Woman's Journey Through Depression* (New York: W. W. Norton, 1998).

5. C. H. Carrington, "Depression in Black Women: A Theoretical Appraisal," in L. Rogers-Rose, ed., *The Black Woman* (Beverly Hills, CA: Sage Publications, 1980).

6. Jones Warren, "Experience of Depression."

7. American Psychiatric Association, *Diagnostic and Statistical Manual of Mental Disorders*, 4th ed. (Washington, D.C.: American Psychiatric Association, 1994).

8. McGraph, Keita, Strickland, and Russo, *Women and Depression*.

9. American Psychiatric Association, *Diagnostic and Statistical Manual*.

10. B. S. Jonas and R. Wilson, "Negative Mood and Urban Versus Rural Residence: Using Proximity to Metropolitan Statistical Areas as an Alternative Measure of Residence," advance data from *Vital and Health Statistics*, no. 281, National Center for Health Statistics, Hyattsville, MD, 1997.

11. Sheryle Gallant, Gwendolyn Puryear Keita, and Renee Royak-Schlaer, eds., *Health Care for Women—Psychological, Social, and Behavioral Influences* (Washington, D.C.: American Psychological Association, 1997).

12. Vickie M. Mays, Lerita M. Coleman, and James S. Jackson, "Perceived Race-Based Discrimination, Employment Status, and Job Stress in a National Sample of Black Women: Implications for Health Outcomes," *Journal of Occupational Health Psychology* 1(3), July 1996.

13. Mitchell and Herring, *What the Blues Is*.

## Chapter 16: Maneuvering Through Menopause

1. The National Black Women's Health Project, personal communication; Rosenberg et al., "Correlates of Postmenopausal Female Hormone Use Among Black Women in the United States," *Obstetrics and Gynecology* 91(3), March 1998.

2. Michael Francine Grodstein, Meir Stampfer, JoAnn Manson et al., "Postmenopausal Estrogen and Progestin Use and the Risk of Cardiovascular Disease," *New England Journal of Medicine* 335(7), August 15, 1998.

3. "Unity Group for PEPI Trial, Effects of Estrogen with Estrogen/Progestin Regiments on Heart Disease Risk Factors in Postmenopausal Women," *Journal of the American Medical Association* 273 (3), January 1994.

4. Stephen Hulley, Deborah Grady, Trudy Bush, et al. for the HERS Research Group, "Randomized Trial of Estrogen Plus Progestin for Secondary Prevention of Coronary Heart Disease in Postmenopausal Women," *Journal of the American Medical Association* 280 (7), August 19, 1998.

5. David M. Herrington, David Reboussin, Bridget Brosnihan et al., "Effects of Estrogen Replacement on the Progression of Coronary Artery Atherosclerosis," *New England Journal of Medicine* 343(8), August 24, 2000.

6. Frank Hu, Meir Stampfer, JoAnn Manson et al., "Trends in the Incidence of Coronary Heart Disease and Changes in Diet and Lifestyle in Women," *New England Journal of Medicine*, 343(8), August 24, 2000.

7. Michael Mendelsohn and Richard Karas, "The Protective Effects of Estrogen on the Cardiovascular System," *New England Journal of Medicine*, 340(23), June 10, 1999.

8. Kristine Yaffe, George Sawaya, Ivan Lieberbury et al., "Estrogen Therapy in Post-menopausal Women—Effects on Cognitive Function and Dementia," *Journal of the American Medical Association* 279(9), March 4, 1998; Sally Shaywitz et al., "Effect of Estrogen on Brain Activation Patterns in Postmenopausal Women During Memory Talks," *Journal of the American Medical Association* 281(13), April 7, 1999; Ruth Mulnard et al., "Estrogen Replacement Therapy for Treatment of Mild to Moderate Alzheimer Disease," *Journal of the American Medical Association* 283(8), February 23, 2000.

9. Susan Gapstur, Marcia Morrow, Thames Sellas et al., "Hormone Replacement Therapy and Risk of Breast Cancer with a Favorable Histology," *Journal of the American Medical Association* 281(22), June 9, 1999; Catherine Schauer et al., "Menopausal Estrogen and Estrogen-Progestin Replacement Therapy and Breast Cancer Risk," *Journal of the American Medical Association* 283(4), January 26, 2000; Collaborative Group on Hormonal Factors in Breast Cancer, "Breast Cancer and Hormone Replacement Therapy: Collaborative Reanalysis of Data from 51 Epidemeological Studies of 52,705 Women with Breast Cancer and 108,411 Women without Breast Cancer," *Lancet* 350 October 11, 1997; R. K. Ross, A. Paganin-Hill, P. C. Wan, et al., "Effect of Hormone Replacement Therapy on Breast Cancer Risk: Estrogen Versus Estrogen Plus Progestin," *Journal of the National Cancer Institute* 92(4), February 16, 2000; C. Schairer, J. Lubin, R. Troisi, et al., "Menopausal Estrogen and Estrogen-Progestin Replacement Therapy and Breast Cancer Risk," *Journal of the American Medical Association* 283(4), January 26, 2000.

## Chapter 17: Midlife's Common Concerns

1. Andrea A. Sullivan, *A Path to Healing—A Guide to Wellness for Body, Mind and Soul* (New York: Doubleday, 1998).

## Chapter 18: Love Is a Many-Splendored Thing

1. Marge Berer, *Women and HIV/AIDS: An International Resource Book* (London: Harper Collins, 1993).

2. Denise O. Shervington, "The Acceptability of the Female Condom Among Low-Income African-American Women," *Journal of the National Medical Association* 85(5), May 1993.

## Chapter 19: Become a Smarter Health-Care Consumer

1. Angela Mitchell with Kennise Herring, *What the Blues Is: Black Women Overcoming Stress and Depression* (New York: Perigee, 1998); Cassandra Worthington, "An Examination of Factors Influencing the Diagnosis and Treatment of Black Patients in the Mental Health System," *Archives of Psychiatric Nursing* 6(3), June 1992.

# Resources

## MEDICAL ASSOCIATIONS

### National Medical Associations and Organizations

American Academy of Nurse Practitioners
P.O. Box 12846
Austin, TX 78711
512-442-4262
E-mail: admin@aanp.org

American Academy of Physician Assistants
950 N. Washington St.
Alexandria, VA 22314-1552
703-836-2272
www.aapa.org.

American Medical Association
515 N. State St.
Chicago, IL 60610
www.ama-assn.org/consumer.htm

American Osteopathic Association
212 E. Ontario St.
Chicago, IL 60611

Association of American Medical Colleges
2450 N Street NW
Washington, DC 20037-1126

National Association for Health and Fitness
201 S. Capitol Ave., Suite 560
Indianapolis, IN 46225
317-237-5650
www.physicalfitness.org

National Black Nurses Association
1511 K Street NW, Suite 415
Washington, DC 20005
202-393-6870

National Medical Association
1012 10th St. NW
Washington, DC 20001
www.nmanet.org
African American physicians.

National Pharmaceutical Association
The Courtyard's Office Complex
107 Kilmayne Dr., Suite C
Cary, NC 27511
800-944-6742
E-mail: bamc@interpath.com

## Specific National Medical Associations and Organizations

Alliance for Aging Research
2021 K St. NW, Suite 305
Washington, DC 20006
202-293-2856

American Academy of Orthopedic Surgeons
6300 N. River Rd.
Rosemont, IL 60018-4262
800-346-AAOS
847-823-7186
www.aaos.org

American College of Cardiology
9111 Old Georgetown Rd.
Bethesda, MD 20814-1699
800-253-4636

301-897-5400
www.acc.org

American College of Obstetricians and Gynecologists
P.O. Box 96920
Washington, DC 20090-6920
202-484-3321
Publishes *Managing Menopause*, an excellent periodical full of sound medical information on signs and symptoms and what to do about them, and the issue of whether or not to take hormones.
   Send correspondence to:
   Editor, *Managing Menopause*
   P.O. Box 96920
   Washington, DC 20090-6920
Another good pamphlet: *Hormone Replacement Therapy, Preventing Osteoporosis, and the Menopause Years.*

American Dental Association
211 E. Chicago Ave.
Chicago, IL 60611
312-440-2500
E-mail: publicinfor@ada.org

American Heart Association
7272 Greenville Ave.
Dallas, TX 75231
888-MY HEART (888-694-3278)
800-242-8721
www.americanheart.org

American Lung Association
800-586-4872

American Physical Therapy Association
1111 N. Fairfax St.
Alexandria, VA 22314-1488
800-999-2782

American Stroke Association
800-553-6321
www.strokeassociation.org
A division of the AHA.

Arthritis Foundation
1330 W. Peachtree St.
Atlanta, GA 30309
800-283-7800

404-872-7100
www.arthritis.org

Melpomene Institute
1010 University Ave.
St. Paul, MN 55104
www.melpomene.org
Women's health research.

National Association for Continence
P.O. Box 8310
Spartanburg, SC 29305-8310
1-800-BLADDER
www.nafc.org

National Dental Association
3517 16th St. NW
Washington, DC 20010
African American dentists.

National Osteoporosis Foundation
1232 22nd St. NW
Washington, DC 20037-1292
800-223-9994
www.nof.org

The North American Menopause Society
P.O. Box 94527
Cleveland, OH 44101
216-844-8748
900-370-NAMS
www.menopause.org

Simon Foundation for Continence
P.O. Box 835
Wilmette, IL 60091
800-237-4666

## National Mental Health Associations and Organizations

American Association of Pastoral Counselors
9504-A Lee Hwy.
Fairfax, VA 22031-2303
703-385-6967
E-mail: info@aapc.org

American Psychiatric Association
1400 K St. NW
Washington, DC 20005
888-357-7924

American Psychological Association
750 1st St. NE
Washington, DC 20002
800-374-2721
202-336-5500

Association of Black Psychologists
P.O. Box 55999
Washington, DC 20040
202-722-0808

Black Psychiatrists of America
2201 Oxford Ave., Suite 201
Lubbock, TX 79410
806-725-6559

Educare Systems, Inc.
1155 Connecticut Ave. NW, Suite 400
Washington, DC 20036

National Association of Black Social Workers
8436 W. McNichols Ave.
Detroit, MI 48221
313-862-6700

National Association of Social Workers
750 1st St. NE, Suite 700
Washington, DC 20002-4241
800-742-4089
202-408-8600

National Mental Health Association
1021 Prince St., 3rd Floor
Alexandria, VA 22314-2971
800-969-6642
703-684-7722

## Specific Mental Health Organizations

American Association for Marriage and
   Family Therapy
1133 15th St. NW, Suite 300
Washington, DC 20005-2710
202-452-0109

American Foundation for Suicide Prevention
120 Wall St., 22nd Floor
New York, NY 10005
888-333-AFSP
Fax: 212-363-6237
www.afsp.org

American Group Psychotherapy Association
25 E. 21st St., 6th Floor
New York, NY 10010
212-477-2677
Fax: 212-979-6627

American Mental Health Foundation
2 E. 86th St.
New York, NY 10028
212-737-9027

Anxiety Disorders Association of America
11900 Parklawn Dr., Suite 100
Rockville, MD 20852-2624
301-231-9350
Fax: 301-231-7392
www.adaa.org

National Depressive and
   Manic-Depressive Association
730 N. Franklin Street, Suite 501
Chicago, IL 60610-3526
800-82-NDMDA
312-642-0049

National Foundation for Depressive Illness, Inc.
P.O. Box 2257
New York, NY 10116
800-248-4344
212-268-4260
Fax: 212-268-4434

## Gay and Lesbian Organizations

Astraea Lesbian Action Foundation
116 E. 16th St., 7th Floor
New York, NY 10003
212-529-8021

Black Lesbian Support Group
c/o Whitman Walker Clinic
1407 S. St. NW
Washington, DC 20009
202-939-1580

Gay and Lesbian Medical Association
459 Fulton St., Suite 107
San Francisco, CA 94102
415-255-4547
www.glma.org

Hartford Gay and Lesbian Health Collective
P.O. Box 2094
Hartford, CT 06145
860-278-4163
Fax: 860-278-5995
www.hglhc.org

National Black Lesbian and Gay Leadership Forum
1247 S. LaBrea Ave.
Los Angeles, CA, 90019-1627
323-964-7820

United Lesbians of African Heritage
1626 N. Wilcox Ave., #190
Los Angeles, CA 90028
323-960-5051

## Gay and Lesbian Health Centers

Chase-Brexton Health Services, Inc.
1001 Cathedral St.
Baltimore, MD 21201
410-837-2050
Fax: 410-837-2071
www.chasebrexton.org

Fenway Community Health
7 Haviland St.
Boston, MA 02115
617-267-0900
Fax: 617-267-3667
www.fenwayhealth.org

First Family Medical Group
1444 West Bethany Home Rd.
Phoenix, AZ 85013
602-242-4843
Fax: 602-433-7712

Howard Brown Health Center
4025 N. Sheridan Rd.
Chicago, IL 60613
773-388-1600
Fax: 773-388-8689
www.howardbrown.org

Jeffrey Goodman Clinic
Los Angeles Gay and Lesbian Center
1625 N. Schrader Blvd.
Los Angeles, CA 90028
323-993-7400
323-993-7640
Fax: 323-993-7699
Anti-violence hot line: 323-993-7673
www.gay-lesbian-center.org

Michael Callen/Audre Lorde
Community Health Center
356 W. 18th St.
New York, NY 10011
Patient care: 212-271-7200
Administration: 212-271-7250
Fax: 212-271-8111
www.callen-lorde.org

Montrose Clinic
215 Westheimer Blvd.
Houston, TX 77006
713-830-3000
Fax: 713-528-4923
www.montrose-clinic.org

Nelson-Tebedo Clinic
(Foundation for Human Understanding)
4012 Cedar Springs Rd.
Dallas, TX 75219
214-528-2336
Fax: 214-528-8436
www.resourcecenterdallas.org

Whitman-Walker Clinic, Inc.
1407 S Street NW
Washington, DC 20009
202-797-3500
www.wwc.org

## HEALTH SUPPORT/ADVOCACY GROUPS

Alcoholics Anonymous World Service
475 Riverside Drive
New York, NY 10115
212-870-3400
Fax: 212-870-3003
www.aa.org

American Association of Retired Persons
Women's Initiative
601 E St. NW
Washington, DC 20049
202-434-2400

Health Watch Information and Promotion Service, Inc.
3020 Glenwood Rd.
Brooklyn, NY 11210
718-434-5411
Mainly for African Americans.

National Black Women's Health Project
600 Pennsylvania Ave. SE, Suite 310
Washington, DC 20003
202-543-9311
www.nbwhp.org

Nicotine Anonymous
415-750-0328

Weight Control Information Network
6101 Executive Blvd., Suite 300
Rockville, MD 20852
800-WIN-8098
Fax 301-984-7196
www.niddk.nih.gov/health/nutrit/win.htm

## MENTAL HEALTH SUPPORT/ADVOCACY GROUPS

Al-Anon Family Group Headquarters
1600 Corporate Landing Parkway
Virginia Beach, VA 23454-5617
800-344-2666
World Directory Meeting Line: 888-425-2666
Fax: 757-563-1655

A Circle of Sisters
45 Park Ave., Suite 7L
Mt. Vernon, NY 10550
212-459-4806
www.acircleofsisters.com
African American women.

Emotions Anonymous
P.O. Box 4245
St. Paul, MN 55104-0245
651-647-9712

Lithium Information Center
Madison Institute for Medicine
7617 Mineral Point Rd., Suite 300
Madison, WI 53717
608-827-2470
The Lithium Information Center collects, organizes, and disseminates information about
the biomedical uses of lithium and other treatments for manic-depression.

National Alliance for the Mentally Ill
Colonial Place Three
2107 Wilson Blvd., Suite 300
Arlington, VA 22201-3042
703-524-7600

National Mental Health Consumer's Self-Help Clearinghouse
1211 Chestnut St., Suite 1207
Philadelphia, PA 19107
800-553-4539
215-751-1810
Fax: 215-636-6312
www.mhselfhelp.org

## GOVERNMENT AGENCIES FOR HEALTH CARE

Bureau of Primary Health Care Health Resources
    and Services Administration
4350 East-West Hwy., 8th Floor
Bethesda, MD 20814
301-594-4100
Fax: 301-594-5008
www.bphc.hrsa.gov

Health Care Financing Administration
500 Security Blvd.
Baltimore, MD 21244
410-786-3000
www.hcfa.gov

National Committee for Quality Assurance
2000 L St. NW, Suite 500
Washington, DC 20036
202-955-3500
Fax: 202-955-3599

National Heart, Lung, and Blood Institute
P.O. Box 30105
Bethesda, MD 20824-0105
800-575-WELL
301-592-8573
www.nhlbi.nih.gov

National Institute on Aging
P.O. Box 8057
Gaithersburg, MD 20898-8057
800-222-2225
www.nih.gov/nia

National Institute of Arthritis and Musculoskeletal and Skin Diseases
Information Clearinghouse

National Institutes of Health
One AMS Circle
Bethesda, MD 20892-3675
301-495-4484
www.nih.gov/niams

National Kidney and Urologic Diseases Information Clearinghouse
3 Information Way
Bethesda, MD 20892-3580
1-800-891-5388
www.niddk.nih.gov/health/urolog/uibcw/index.htm
Call for a free copy of *Let's Talk About Bladder Control.*

Osteoporosis and Related Bone Diseases—National Resource Center
1232 22nd St. NW
Washington, DC 20037
202-223-0344
1-800-624-BONE
www.osteo.org

## GOVERNMENT MENTAL HEALTH AGENCIES

NIMH Public Inquiries, National Institute of Mental Health
NIH Neuroscience Center
6001 Executive Blvd., Room 8184, MSC 9663
Bethesda, MD 20892-9663
301-443-4513
Fax: 301-443-4279
Mental Health Fax-4-U: 301-443-4536
E-mail: nimhinfo@nih.gov
www.nimh.nih.gov

Substance Abuse and Mental Health Services Administration
Center for Mental Health Services
Department of Health and Human Services
5600 Fishers Lane, Room 1799
Rockville, MD 20857
800-789-2647

## PROFESSIONAL ASSOCIATIONS AND GOVERNMENT AGENCIES FOR INFORMATION ON CARDIOVASCULAR DISEASES

Alliance for Aging Research
2021 K St. NW, Suite 305
Washington, DC 20006
202-293-2856
Call for a free copy of *Controlling High Blood Pressure: A Woman's Guide.*

American College of Cardiology
9111 Old Georgetown Rd.
Bethesda, MD 20814-1699
800-253-4636
301-897-5400
www.acc.org

American Heart Association
7272 Greenville Ave.
Dallas, TX 75231
888-MY HEART
800-242-8721
www.americanheart.org

American Stroke Association
800-553-6321
www.strokeassociation.org
A division of the AHA.

National Heart, Lung, and Blood Institute
P.O. Box 30105
Bethesda, MD 20824-0105
800-575-WELL
301-592-8573
www.nhlbi.nih.gov

National Institute of Neurological Disorders and Stroke
NIH Neurological Institute
P.O. Box 5801
Bethesda, MD 20824
800-352-9424
www.ninds.nih.gov

National Rehabilitation Information Center
1010 Wayne Ave., Suite 800
Silver Spring, MD 20910
800-346-2742
301-562-2400
TTY: 301-495-5626
Fax: 301-562-2401
www.naric.com

National Stroke Association
9707 E. Easter Lane
Englewood, CO 80112
800-STROKES
303-649-9299

Fax: 303-649-1328
www.stroke.org

## SUPPORT/ADVOCACY GROUPS FOR CARDIOVASCULAR DISEASE

Mended Hearts
7272 Greenville Ave.
Dallas, TX 75231-4596
800-AHAUSA1 (ask for Mended Hearts)
214-706-1442
www.mendedhearts.org/
A support group for heart disease patients and their families with more than 250 chapters in the United States.

## FOR MORE INFORMATION ABOUT CANCER

American Cancer Society
1599 Clifton Rd. NE
Atlanta, GA 30329
404-320-3333
800-ACS-2345 (Cancer Response System)
www.cancer.org

American Lung Association
1740 Broadway
New York, NY 10019
212-315-8700
800-LUNG-USA
www.lungusa.org
Publishes *Quit Smoking Action Plan*, which has information on how to prepare to quit, how medications help, and how to stay smoke-free.

Centers for Disease Control and Prevention
National Center for Chronic Disease Prevention and Health Promotion
Office on Smoking and Health
Public Information Branch
Publications Catalog, Mail Stop K-50
4770 Buford Highway NE
Atlanta, GA 30341-3724
800-CDC-1311
770-488-5705
Fax: 800-CDC-1311
www.cdc.gov/tobacco
Publishes and distributes materials on smoking and health, including the surgeon general's annual reports.

National Cancer Institute
Cancer Information Service
Office of Cancer Communications
9000 Rockville Pike
Bethesda, MD 20809
800-4CANCER
www.cancernet.nci.nih.gov


## SUPPORT/ADVOCACY GROUPS

African American Breast Cancer Alliance (AABCA)
P.O. Box 8981
Minneapolis, MN 55408
612-825-3675

National Alliance of Breast Cancer Organizations
9 East 37th St.
New York, NY 10016
888-806-2226
www.nabco.org

Reach to Recovery
1599 Clifton Rd, NE
Atlanta, GA 30329-4251
800-ACS-2345
www.cancer.org

Rise Sister Rise
2005 Belmont Road NW
Washington, DC 20009
202-463-8040
Fax: 202-463-8015
African American breast cancer support group.

Sisters Network
8787 Woodway Drive, Suite 4206
Houston, TX 77063
713-781-0255
Fax: 713-780-8998
E-mail: sisnet4@aol.com
www.sistersnetworkinc.org
Sisters Network has thirty-five chapters across the United States.

Y-Me
212 W. Van Buren St.
Chicago, IL 60607-3908

800-221-2141
312-986-8338
National organization for breast cancer information and support.

## AFRICAN AMERICAN ACADEMIC INSTITUTIONS (RESEARCH AND TREATMENT)

Drew-Meharry-Morehouse Consortium Cancer Center
1005 D. B. Todd Blvd.
Nashville, TN 37208
615-327-6927

Howard University Cancer Research Center
2041 Georgia Ave. NW
Washington, DC 20060
202-806-7697

Texas A&M University
Department of Health and Kinesiology
College Station, TX 77843-4243
979-845-3109

## BREAST CANCER INFORMATION CLEARINGHOUSE WEB SITES

www.cancernews.com
www.cansearch.org
www.oncolink.upenn.edu

## FOR MORE INFORMATION ON DIABETES

American Diabetes Association
Customer Service
1701 N. Beauregard St.
Alexandria, VA 22311
800-DIABETES
www.diabetes.org

Bureau of Primary Health Care
Health Resources and Services Administration
4350 East-West Highway, 8th Floor
Bethesda, MD 20814
301-594-4100
www.bphc.hrsa.gov
Call for information on the LEAP (lower extremity amputation prevention) Filament.

National Diabetes Education Program
800-438-5383
indep.nih.gov

National Diabetes Information Clearinghouse
1 Diabetes Way
Bethesda, MD 20892-3600
301-654-3327
Email: ndic@info.niddk.nih.gov

Diabetes Public Health Resource
www.cdc.gov/diabetes
877-CDC-DIAB

## RESOURCES FOR INFORMATION ON MENOPAUSE

American Menopause Foundation
350 Fifth Ave.
New York, NY 10118-0110
212-714-2398
Operates a national network of support groups that deal with alternative treatments.

## COMPLEMENTARY ALTERNATIVE MEDICINE GROUPS

Acupuncture and Oriental Medicine Alliance (AOMA)
14637 Starr Rd. SE
Olalla, WA 98359
253-851-6896
Fax: 253-851-6886
www.acuall.org

American Association of Naturopathic Physicians
8201 Greensboro Dr., Suite 300
McLean, VA 22102
703-610-9037
http://aanp.net

American Black Chiropractors Association
1918 E. Grand Blvd.
St. Louis, MO 63107
314-531-0615

American Chiropractic Association
1701 Clarendon Blvd.

Arlington, VA 22209
800-986-4636

American Holistic Medical Association
6728 McLean Village Dr.
McLean, VA 22101-8729
703-556-9245
www.holisticmedicine.org
They will send you a publication, *How to Choose a Holistic Health Practitioner.*

American Massage Therapy Association
820 Davis St., Suite 100
Evanston, IL 60201-4444
847-864-0123
www.amtamassage.org

The Herb Research Foundation
1007 Pearl St., Suite 200
Boulder, CO 80302
303-449-2265

Integral Yoga Institute
227 W. 13th Street
New York, NY 10011
212-929-0586

National Center for Homeopathy
801 N. Fairfax St., Suite 306
Alexandria, VA 22314
877-624-0613
703-548-7790

National Commission for the Certification of Acupuncturists
1424 16th Street NW
Washington, DC 20046
202-232-1404

## HELPFUL HEALTH WEB SITES

There are many health-related Web sites—some estimate 15,000 and rising. You must scan them carefully and weigh the site's validity and its author's credentials. We have provided credible sites below. Remember, always verify information from the sites with your health professionals.

**www.cbshealthwatch.com** (Run by Dr. George Lundberg, former editor of the *Journal of the American Medical Association*, this is an excellent site that covers a broad range of health concerns.)

**www.intelihealth.com** (The Web site of Johns Hopkins University and Aetna U.S. Healthcare, it addresses questions about common ailments.)

**www.healthquestmag.com** (*Healthquest* is a Black health and wellness magazine.)

**www.MD.com**

**www.nih.gov/health** (The National Institutes of Health offers a list of resources of federal agencies.)

**www.4healthylife.com** (This site features information on both traditional and alternative care.)

**www.health.gov/healthypeople** (Department of Health and Human Services website for Healthy People 2010)

**www.4woman.gov** (The National Women's Health Information Center is the federal government's most comprehensive women's health resource. To get brochures and fact sheets, call 1-800-994-WOMAN.)

# Bibliography

## General Health

Arnot, Dr. Bob. *The Breast Cancer Prevention Cookbook*. Boston: Little, Brown, 2001.

Barnard, Neal, M.D. *Foods Can Save Your Life*. Dallas, Tex.: The Magni Group, 1996.

Bauman, Alisa, and the Editors of *Prevention*. *Fight Fat: Secrets to Successful Weight Loss*. Emmaus, Pa.: Rodale Press, 1998.

Castleman, Michael. *The Healing Herbs*. New York: Bantam Books, 1995.

Cooper, Robert K., and Leslie Cooper. *Low-Fat Living*. Emmaus, Pa.: Rodale Press, 1996.

Crute, Sheree, ed. *Health and Healing for African-Americans—Straight Talk and Tips from More Than 150 Black Doctors on Our Top Health Concerns*. Emmaus, Pa.: Rodale Press, 1997.

Dixon, Barbara M., L.D.N., R.D. *Good Health for African Americans*. New York: Crown Publishing Group, 1994.

Dunnavant, Sylvia. *Celebrating Life: African American Women Speak Out About Breast Cancer*. Dallas, Tex.: USFI, 1995.

Gaines, Fabiola Demps, and Roniece Weaver. *The New Soul Food Cookbook for People with Diabetes*. Alexandria, Va.: American Diabetes Association, 1999.

Goor, Ron, and Nancy Goor. *Eater's Choice: A Food Lover's Guide to Lower Cholesterol*, 5th edition. Boston: Houghton Mifflin, 1999.

Jonas, Wayne B., M.D., and Jeffrey S. Levin, Ph.D., M.P.H. *Essentials of Complementary and Alternative Medicine*. Philadelphia: Lippincott, Williams & Wilkins, 1999.

Keane, Maureen, and Daniella Chace. *What to Eat If You Have Cancer.* Chicago: Contemporary Books, 1996.

Krichheimer, Sid, and Gale Maleskey. *Energy Forever.* Emmaus, Pa.: Rodale Press, 1997.

Lane, Nancy E., M.D. *The Osteoporosis Book: A Guide for Patients and Their Families.* New York: Oxford University Press, 1999.

Link, John, M.D. *The Breast Cancer Survival Manual.* New York: Henry Holt and Company, 1998.

Mae, Eydie. *How I Conquered Cancer Naturally.* New York: Avery Publishing Group, 1992.

Margolis, Simeon, and Jonathan Samet. *Johns Hopkins White Papers: Cancer.* Baltimore, Md.: Medletta Associates, 2000.

Nixon, Daniel. *The Cancer Recovery Eating Plan.* New York: Times Books, 1996.

Ornish, Dean, M.D. *Reversing Heart Disease.* New York: Ballantine Books, 1990.

———. *Love and Survival: The Scientific Basis for the Healing Power of Intimacy.* New York: HarperCollins Publishers, 1998.

———. *Eat More, Weigh Less,* rev. edition. New York: Quill, 2000.

Pauling, Linus. *How to Live Longer and Feel Better.* New York: Avon Books, 1990.

Quillin, Patrick, Ph.D. *Beating Cancer with Nutrition.* Tulsa, Okla.: Nutrition Times Press, Inc., 1998.

Reese, Sara Lomax, Kirk Johnson, and Therman Evans, M.D. *Staying Strong—Reclaiming the Wisdom of African-American Healing.* New York: Avon Books, 1999.

Steinberg, Alan J. *The Insider's Guide to HMOs: How to Navigate the Managed-Care System and Get the Health Care You Deserve.* New York: Plume, 1997.

Steinman, David, ed. *Life Extenders and Memory Boosters Incorporating the Research of Hans Kugler et al.,* 2nd edition. Reno, Nev.: Health Quest Publication, 1994.

Sullivan, Andrea. *A Path to Healing: A Guide to Wellness for Body, Mind and Soul.* New York: Doubleday, 1998.

Tull, E. S., and J. M. Roseman. *Diabetes in America,* 2nd edition. Bethesda, Md.: National Institutes of Health, 1995.

U.S. Preventive Services Task Force. *Guide to Clinical Preventive Services.* Washington, D.C.: U.S. Department of Health and Human Services, 1995.

Weil, Andrew, M.D. *Health and Healing.* Boston/New York: Houghton Mifflin, 1998.

———. *Spontaneous Healing: How to Discover and Embrace Your Body's Natural Ability to Maintain and Heal Itself.* New York: Ballantine Books, 2000.

## Women's Health/Black Women's Health

Adams, Diane L., M.D., ed. *Health Issues for Women of Color—A Cultural Diversity Perspective.* Thousand Oaks, Calif.: Sage Publications, 1995.

Alcena, Valiere, M.D. *The African-American Health Book.* New York: Citadel Press, 1996.

Aldridge, Delores P., and La Francis Rodgers-Rose, eds. *River of Tears: The Politics of Black Women's Health.* Newark, N.J.: Traces Publishing, 1993.

Allen, Karen Moses, Ph.D., R.N., and Janice Mitchell Phillips, Ph.D., R.N. *Women's Health Across the Lifespan—A Comprehensive Perspective.* Philadelphia: Lippincott-Raven Publishers, 1997.

Berer, Marge. *Women and HIV/AIDS.* London: Pandora Press, 1995.

Crawford, Andrea McQuade. *The Herbal Menopause Book.* Santa Cruz, Calif.: Crossing Press, 1996.

Doress-Worters, Paula B., and Diana Laskin Siegal, in cooperation with Boston Women's Health Book Collective. *The New Ourselves, Growing Older—Women Aging with Knowledge and Power.* New York: Simon & Schuster, 1994.

Epps, Rosalyn Payne, M.D., Susan Cobb Stewart, M.D., and The American Medical Women's Association. *The Women's Complete Health Book.* New York: Delacorte Press/Bantam Doubleday, 1995.

Gallant, Sheryle J., Gwendolyn Puryear Keita, and Renee Royak-Schaler, eds. *Health Care for Women—Psychological, Social, and Behavioral Influences.* Washington, D.C.: American Psychological Association, 1997.

Gladstar, Rosemary. *Herbal Healing for Women.* New York: Fireside, 1993.

Henkel, Gretchen. *Making the Estrogen Decision.* Los Angeles: Lowell House, 1992.

——. *The Menopause Sourcebook: Everything You Need to Know,* rev. edition. Los Angeles: Lowell House, 1998.

Kenley, Joan, Ph.D., with John C. Arpels, M.D. *A Woman's Right to Know: Health and Hormones After 35.* San Francisco: A Nancy Hicks Maynard Book, 1995.

Lucks, Naomi, and Melene Smith. *A Woman's Midlife Companion.* Rocklin, Calif.: Prima Publishing, 1997.

Northrup, Christiane, M.D. *Women's Bodies, Women's Wisdom.* New York: Bantam Books, 1998.

Notelovitz, Morris, and Diana Tonnessen. *Menopause and Midlife Health.* New York: St. Martin's Press, 1994.

Olinekora, Dr. Gayle. *Power Aging: Staying Young at Any Age.* New York: Thunder's Mouth Press, 1998.

Reichman, Judith. *I'm Too Young to Get Old: Health Care for Women After Forty.* New York: Times Books, 1997.

Sachs, Judith. *What Women Should Know About Menopause.* New York: Dell Medical Library, 1991.

Santa Fe Health Education Project. *Menopause: A Self-Care Manual.* Santa Fe, N. Mex.: Santa Fe Health Education Project.

Sheehy, Gail. *The Silent Passage: Menopause.* New York: Pocket Books, 1998.

Snyderman, Dr. Nancy, and Margaret Blackstone. *Nancy Snyderman's Guide to Good Health for Women: What Every Forty-Plus Woman Should Know About Her Changing Body.* San Diego, Calif.: Harcourt Brace & Co., 1996.

Solarz, Andrea L., ed., and Institute of Medicine. *Lesbian Health—Current Assessment and Directions for the Future.* Washington, D.C.: National Academy Press, 1999.

Thornton, Yvonne S., M.D., M.P.H. *Woman to Woman: A Leading Gynecologist*

*Tells You All You Need to Know About Your Body and Your Health.* New York: Penguin, 1998.

Villarosa, Linda, ed. *Body and Soul: The Black Women's Guide to Physical Health and Emotional Well-Being.* New York: HarperPerennial, 1994.

Weed, Susan S. *Menopausal Years: The Wise Woman Way, Alternative Approaches for Women 30–90,* rev. edition. New York: Ash Tree Publishing, 2001.

White, Evelyn, ed. *The Black Women's Health Book: Speaking for Ourselves,* rev. edition. Seattle, Wash.: Seal Press, 1994.

## Mental Health

Bourne, Edmund J., Ph.D. *The Anxiety & Phobia Workbook.* Oakland, Calif.: New Harbinger Publications, 1995.

Boyd, Julia A. *In the Company of My Sisters—Black Women and Self-Esteem.* New York: Dutton Books, 1993.

Branden, Nathaniel, Ph.D. *The Power of Self-Esteem.* Deerfield Beach, Fla.: Health Communications, 1992.

———. *The Six Pillars of Self-Esteem.* New York: Bantam Books, 1994.

Burns, David D., M.D. *Ten Days to Self-Esteem.* New York: William Morrow and Company, 1993.

Clark, Lynn. *SOS—Help for Managing Anxiety, Anger, and Depression.* Bowling Green, Ky.: Parents Press, 1998.

Danquah, Meri Nana-Ama. *Willow Weep for Me—A Black Woman's Journey Through Depression.* New York: W. W. Norton, 1998.

Gallant, Sheryle, Gwendolyn Puryear Keita, and Renee Royak-Schlaer, eds. *Health Care for Women—Psychological, Social, and Behavioral Influences.* Washington, D.C.: American Psychological Association, 1997.

Gandy, Debrena Jackson. *Sacred Pampering Principles—An African-American Woman's Guide to Self-Care and Inner Renewal.* New York: William Morrow and Company, 1997.

hooks, bell. *Sisters of the Yam—Black Women and Self-Recovery.* Boston: South End Press, 1993.

Jackson, Leslie C., and Beverly Greene, eds. *Psychotherapy with African American Women: Innovations in Psychodynamic Perspectives and Practice.* New York: Guilford Press, 2000.

McGraph, Ellen, Gwendolyn Puryear Keita, Bonnie R. Strickland, and Nancy Felipe Russo. *Women and Depression: Risk Factors and Treatment Issues.* Washington, D.C.: American Psychological Association, 1990.

Mitchell, Angela, with Kennise. *What the Blues Is: Black Women Overcoming Stress and Depression.* New York: Herring Perigee, 1998.

Natural Medicine Collective with Diana L. Ajjan. *The Natural Way of Healing Stress, Anxiety, and Depression.* New York: Dell, 1995.

Sanford, Linda Tschirhart, and Mary Ellen Donovan. *Women and Self-Esteem.* New York: Viking, 1985.

Travis, John, M.D., and Regina Sara Ryan. *Wellness Workbook*, 2nd edition. Berkeley, Calif.: Ten Speed Press, 1988

Vanzant, Iyanla. *The Value in the Valley—A Black Woman's Guide Through Life's Dilemmas.* New York: Simon & Schuster, 1995.

## Spirituality

Afua, Queen. *Sacred Woman—A Guide to Healing the Feminine Body, Mind, and Spirit.* New York: One World Books/The Ballantine Publishing Group, 2000.

Avery, Byllye. *An Altar of Words: Wisdom, Comfort, and Inspiration for African American Women.* New York: Broadway Books, 1998.

Bryant, Rev. Cecelia Williams. *Kiamsha—A Spiritual Discipline for African-American Women.* Baltimore, Md.: Akosua Visions, 1991.

Copage, Eric V. *Black Pearls: Daily Meditations, Affirmations, and Inspirations for African-Americans.* New York: Quill/William Morrow and Company, 1993.

Gleason, Judith. *Oya: In Praise of an African Goddess.* San Francisco: Harper SanFrancisco, 1992.

Higginbotham, Evelyn Brooks. *Righteous Discontent: The Women's Movement in the Black Baptist Church, 1880–1920.* Cambridge, Mass.: Harvard University Press, 1993.

hooks, bell. *Sisters of the Yam: Black Women and Self-Recovery.* Boston: South End Press, 1993.

Jakes, T. D. *The Lady, Her Lover, and Her Lord Bishop.* New York: G. P. Putnam's Sons, 1998.

Peck, M. Scott. *The Road Less Traveled.* New York: Simon & Schuster, 1978.

Shervington, Denese, M.D., and Billie Jean Pace, M.D. *Soul Quest: A Healing Journey for Women of the African Diaspora.* New York: Crown, 1996.

Taylor, Susan L. *In the Spirit: The Inspirational Writings of Susan L. Taylor.* New York: HarperCollins, 1994.

Van Sertima, Ivan, ed. *Black Women in Antiquity.* New Brunswick, N.J.: Transaction Publishers, 1984.

Vanzant, Iyanla. *Acts of Faith—Daily Meditations for People of Color.* New York: Fireside/Simon & Schuster, 1993.

———. *The Value in the Valley: A Black Woman's Guide Through Life's Dilemmas.* New York: Simon & Schuster, 1995.

———. *Faith in the Valley: Lessons for Women on the Journey to Peace.* New York: Simon & Schuster, 1996.

———. *One Day My Soul Just Opened Up: 40 Days and 40 Nights Toward Spiritual Strength and Personal Growth.* New York: Simon & Schuster, 1998.

Weems, Renita. *Just a Sister Away: A Womanist Vision of Women's Relationships in the Bible.* San Diego, Calif.: LuraMedia, 1988.

———. *I Asked for Intimacy: The Stories of Blessings, Betrayals and Birthings.* San Diego, Calif.: LuraMedia, 1993.

*Women of Color Study Bible—Created by and for Contemporary Women of African Descent.* Atlanta, Ga.: Nia Publishing, and Iowa Falls, Iowa: World Publishing, 1999.

Zukav, Gary. *The Seat of the Soul.* New York: Simon & Schuster, 1989.

# Index

cholesterol level, 114, 206–10
depression, 20–21, 212
diabetes, 203
family history, 108, 203
hypertension, 115, 204, 215
inactivity, 109, 204
obesity, 111, 113, 204
predictors of, 213–14
secondhand smoke, 245
smoking, 109, 189, 203–4, 247
stress, 204, 210–12, 293
and sexual function, 445
signs and symptoms, 200
tests and procedures, 151, 204–6, 213
vitamin/mineral supplements, 181, 222
*See also* Heart attack; Stroke
Heart and Estrogen/Progestin Replacement Study (HERS), 406
Heart rate, during exercise, 165
Heart rhythm, abnormal, 228, 232, 347
Hemmorrhoids, 141
Hepatitis B, 156, 451
Herbal remedies
for anxiety, 355, 356–57
and blood pressure, 224
for depression, 374–75, 383–84
for menopause symptoms, 400–401
in nicotine treatment, 193
for stress, 310
Herbs, in diet, 183, 221
Herpes, 267, 453
High blood pressure. *See* Hypertension
High-definition imaging (HDI) ultrasound, 145, 256
High-density lipoprotein (HDL) cholesterol, 113, 114, 147–48, 154, 179, 180, 209, 212, 393, 406
Hip fractures, 111, 407, 409
Hippocampus, 345, 419
HIV/AIDS, 105, 119, 369, 452, 453–55
HIV test, 152, 155, 442, 451
Holistic wellness philosophy, 51–55
Homocysteine, 181, 213
Honesty, and self-esteem, 77
hooks, bell, 11, 71, 76, 82, 87, 297, 317
Hormone replacement therapy (HRT)
benefits of, 405–14, 413, 414, 415–16, 422, 428
and cancer, 250, 264, 266, 268, 414
decisionmaking on, 403–4
estrogen/progesterone combination, 405
side effects/risks, 414–15
after surgical menopause, 394
Hot flashes, 397–98, 399–401, 434
Hudson, Tori, 403
Hughes, Langston, 296
Human papilloma virus (HPV), 267, 452, 453
Hurston, Zora Neale, 10, 46, 61
Hydrogenated fat, 179
Hydrotherapy, 357
Hypertension
and cardiovascular disease, 115
control of, 138–39

defined, 215–16
and diabetes, 276
diagnosis of, 138, 139
and diet, 175, 177, 219–21
and exercise, 111, 119–20, 209
and heart disease, 115, 204, 215
incidence of, 20, 115, 138, 215
medications for, 223–25, 276
and panic disorder, 334
relaxation techniques for, 312
risk factors for, 216–17
cholesterol level, 114
medications, 224, 276, 380–81
obesity, 113, 223
smoking, 109
and stress, 286–87
and stroke, 115, 227, 231, 233
and uterine cancer, 268
vitamin/mineral supplements for, 221–23
and weight loss, 113
*See also* Blood pressure
Hyperthyroidism, 141, 153, 346
Hypoglycemia, 332, 346
Hypothyroidism, 140, 152–53
Hysterectomy, 149, 393–95

Immune system, 239, 260, 261, 287
Immunizations, schedule of, 155–56
Inactivity
and colon cancer, 264
and diabetes, 276
and heart disease, 109, 204
and obesity, 109
and osteoporosis, 409
*See also* Exercise
Incontinence, 401, 423–26
Independent practice associations (IPAs), 481
Indoles, 258
Infection, 213–14, 278
Inflammatory bowel disease, 265
Influenza, 105, 155
Information overload, negative, 349
Insomnia, 309–10, 325
Insulin, 274, 277
Integrity, and self-esteem, 77
Interceptive exposure, 335
Interpersonal therapy, 376
Iodine, 183, 185
Iron, 185
Irritable bowel syndrome, 334
Isis, 23

Jackson, Jesse L. Sr. and Jr., 303
Jobs. *See* Work
Johnson, Diane, 61, 348, 370
Johnson, Edwin, 249
Johnson, Wista, 61

Karasek, Robert A., 299
Kava kava, 357
Keen, Sam, 41
Kegel exercises, 425–26

# About the Authors

DR. MARILYN H. GASTON's professional career has been dedicated to improving the health of children and their families, especially underprivileged and minority families. As a primary care pediatrician with a subspecialty in ambulatory pediatrics, she has devoted her career to providing medical education, to involvement in clinical research, and to the administration of local and federal programs directed to services to the underserved.

A former Assistant Surgeon General of the United States, Dr. Gaston is the Associate Administrator for the Bureau of Primary Health Care (BPHC) within the Health Resources and Services Administration. She is the first African American woman to direct a Public Health Service Bureau. BPHC has total resources of close to two billion dollars and is responsible for improving access to quality, preventive, primary health care to millions of underserved minority, underprivileged, disadvantaged people in the United States and its territories, and improving the health status of ten million people.

Prior to her appointment as Bureau Director, she was the Director of the Division of Medicine, which provides funding for training grants in Family Medicine, Internal medicine and Pediatrics, etc. Early in her career, Dr. Gaston helped to establish a community health center serving a large African American, low-income population.

Dr. Gaston is internationally recognized for her leadership in combating sickle cell disease. Through her work at the National Institutes of Health, changes in management of children with this illness have resulted significantly in decreasing illness and mortality in young children. Dr. Gaston is a much sought after speaker on topics close to her heart: improving health care access and eliminating health disparities for vulnerable people, African American women's health, sickle cell disease, and the needs of youth (health and otherwise).

Her awards are numerous and include all awards in the Public Health Service, the institution of Marilyn Hughes Gaston Day in Cincinnati and Lincoln Heights, Ohio, and the Living Legend Award presented by the National Medical Association. Dr. Gaston is a member of the prestigious Institute of Medicine of the National Academy of Sciences. She received an Honorary Doctor of Science degree from the University of Pennsylvania, College of Pediatric Medicine and the Daniel Drake Medal, the highest award bestowed by the University of Cincinnati, College of Medicine. In May 1999, Dr. Gaston received the Scroll of Merit from the National Medical Association, their highest honor. Most recently, the University of Cincinnati, College of Medicine, named a scholarship in Dr. Gaston's honor. Two recipients each year will be selected from underprivileged and minority applicants to receive full, four-year medical school scholarships. The first "Gaston scholars" began medical school in September 1999. In May 2000, Dr. Gaston was awarded the prestigious American Medical Association's Dr. Nathan Davis Award in the category of Career Public Service.

Dr. Gayle K. Porter is a licensed clinical psychologist. She is currently a Principal Research Analyst and a Senior Mental Health Advisor for the Technical Assistance Partnership (TAP) of The American Institutes for Research. The TAP is funded by the Comprehensive Community Mental Health Services for Children and Their Families of the Substance Abuse Mental Health Services Administration (SAMHSA). Technical assistance is provided to forty-five grant communities that offer mental health services to children with emotional disturbances and their families.

Until May 2000, Dr. Porter was the director of the School Based Program of Johns Hopkins' University/Hospital. She was on the faculties of Johns Hopkins' Child and Adolescent Psychiatry Department and Howard University. Before joining the staff at Johns Hopkins, Dr. Porter directed two outpatient mental health clinics for children and families for the Washington, D.C., Commission on Mental Health Services. Prior to completing her graduate education, Dr. Porter was a reading and human sexuality teacher in a junior high school and a school counselor. Dr. Porter has given numerous presentations on various topics related to children and women's mental health, especially poor children and minorities.

Dr. Porter has received numerous prestigious professional and community awards including the St. Benedict Award for Community Service, in Chicago, IL, the Ebenezer AME Church Award for Services Rendered to the Single Parents' ministry in Fort Washington, MD, a Mayor's Citation, Certificate and Award of Merit in Baltimore, MD, and a Certificate of Appreciation from the Department of Health and Human, Substance Abuse and Mental Health Services Administration in Rockville, MD. She has also been honored with the Dr. Addison Pope Award from the Black Mental Health Alliance for Education and Consultation, the Maryland House of Delegates House Resolution, the Distinct Imprint Award from the National Association of University Women in Washington, D.C., and Lifelong Commitment to Black Women's Health from the International Black Women's Congress.